Aging

VOLUME 39

Guidelines for Drug Trials
in Memory Disorders

Aging Series

Aging
VOLUME 39

Guidelines for Drug Trials
in Memory Disorders

Editors

Nicola Canal, M.D.
Department of Neurology
University of Milan
Istituto Scientifico H. San Raffaele
Milan, Italy

**Vladimir C. Hachinski,
M.D., D.Sc.Med.**
Department of Clinical Neurological
Sciences
University Hospital
London, Ontario, Canada

Guy McKhann, M.D.
Johns Hopkins School of Medicine
Department of Neurology
Baltimore, Maryland

Massimo Franceschi, M.D.
Department of Neurology
University of Milan
Istituto Scientifico H. San Raffaele
Milan, Italy

Raven Press   New York

Raven Press, Ltd., 1185 Avenue of the Americas, New York, New York 10036

Made in the United States of America

Library of Congress Cataloging-in-Publication Data

Guidelines for drug trials in memory disorders / editors, Nicola Canal
    ... [et al.].
        p.   cm. — (Aging ; v. 39)
    Includes bibliographical references and index.
    ISBN: 0-7817-0108-2
    1. Memory disorders—Chemotherapy—Testing—Methodology.
    2. Nootropic agents—Testing—Methodology.
    3. Neuropsychopharmacology—Methodology.   I. Canal, Nicola.
    II. Series.
        [DNLM: 1. Memory Disorders—drug therapy—congresses.   2. Clinical
    Trials—methods—congresses.   W1 AG342E v.39 1993 / WM 173.7 G946
    1993]
    RC394.M46G85   1993
    616.8′4—dc20
    DNLM/DLC
    for Library of Congress   93-24715
                                                                         CIP

9 8 7 6 5 4 3 2 1

Foreword

Impairment of memory is probably the earliest and the most constant neuro-psychological disturbance that characterizes the dementia syndromes, and the disturbance that most significantly affects the quality of life of patients. Therefore, it is a symptom of primary importance in investigating in depth the pathogenetic mechanisms of the dementia and in trying new pharmacologic treatments.

Memory disturbances are the clinical element on which various pathogen-eses converge—especially degenerative, but also vascular, traumatic, and even metabolic types. The considerable gap in our knowledge about the anatomic circuits and the neuromediator mechanisms that regulate memory means that we must be pragmatic in organizing therapeutic trials aimed at correcting memory disorders. The essential element in conducting trials of this type, which admittedly can be carried out in patients with various types of dementing diseases, is to use rigorous and uniform methods.

The abundant literature of the last decade shows that the incongruities and inconsistencies of the results of the numerous published trials result mostly from the nonuniformity and inappropriate design of the trials them-selves. This book represents the proceedings of a workshop held in Decem-ber 1991 in Cannes, France, in which the various problems that arise in evaluating treatments of memory disturbances were examined critically. The purpose of the workshop was to establish general criteria necessary for con-ducting such trials. All major relevant topics were discussed by well-known specialists to clarify the points of agreement and disagreement among the members of the group.

In addition to the classic chapters dealing with design of the study, selec-tion of drugs and patients, and evaluation of effectiveness, others deal with the importance of evaluating the effectiveness of the treatments of such meth-ods as computed electroencephalography and positron emission tomogra-phy, procedures that are not used routinely at present.

We know very well that many of the problems are still unsolved, and that no universal consensus was, nor could have been, achieved for so many complex issues. However, we hope that the information in this book will prove useful to scientists who intend to undertake clinical studies of drugs that affect memory.

The Editors

Acknowledgment

The editors thank Smith Kline Beecham S.p.A. for their kind contribution in organizing the Consensus Conference ''Guidelines for Drug Trials in Memory Disorders'' held in Cannes, France on December 6–7, 1991 and for the publication of the proceedings.

Contents

Assessment of Efficacy

Contributors

J. C. Baron, M.D. *INSERM U 320, Centre Cyceron, Boulevard Henri Becquerel, BP 5027, 14021 Caen Cedex, France*

Jose M. Bertolote, M.D., M.Sc., Ph.D. *Senior Medical Officer, Division of Mental Health, Organisation Mondiale de la Santè, 29, Avenue Appia, 1211 Geneve 12, Switzerland*

François Boller, M.D., Ph.D. *INSERM U 324, Centre Paul Broca, 2 Ter, rue d'Alésia, 75014 Paris, France*

Nicola Canal, M.D. *Department of Neurology, University of Milan, Istituto Scientifico H. San Raffaele, Milan, Italy*

Thomas H. Crook, Ph.D. *Memory Assessment Clinics, Inc., 8311 Wisconsin Avenue, Bethesda, Maryland 20814*

Valerie Curran, M.A., Dip. Clin. Psych., Ph.D. *Senior Lecturer, Institute of Psychiatry, London, SE5 8AF, England*

Bonnie M. Davis, M.D. *Department of Psychiatry, Mount Sinai School of Medicine, New York, New York 10029-6574*

David A. Drachman, M.D. *Department of Neurology, University of Massachusetts Medical Center, 55 Lake Avenue North, Worcester, Massachusetts 01655*

Timo Erkinjuntti, M.D., Ph.D. *Memory Research Unit, Department of Neurology, University of Helsinki, Helsinki, Finland*

Steven H. Ferris, Ph.D. *NYU Medical Center, Aging & Dementia Research Center, Millhauser Laboratories HN-314, 550 First Avenue, New York, New York 10016*

C. G. Gottfries, M.D., Ph.D. *Department of Psychiatry and Neurochemistry, University of Göteborg, Mölndals sjukhus, S-431 80, Mölndal, Sweden*

Jordan H. Grafman, Ph.D. *Cognitive Neuroscience Section, Medical Neurology Branch, Building 10, Room 5C422, NINDS, Federal Building, Bethesda, Maryland 20892*

Jane Greenlaw, R.N., J.D. *Director, Division of Medical Humanities, University of Rochester, 601 Elmwood Avenue, Rochester, New York 14642*

Francesco Grigoletto, Sc.D. *Institute of Hygiene, School of Medicine, Università di Padova, Via L. Loredan, 18, 35131 Padova, Italy*

Vladimir C. Hachinski, M.D., F.R.C.P.(C), D.Sc. (Med) *Richard and Beryl Ivey Professor and Chairman, Department of Clinical Neurological Sciences, University Hospital, PO Box 5339, London, Ontario N6A 5A5, Canada*

Robert J. Joynt, M.D., Ph.D. *Vice President and Vice Provost for Health Affairs, Professor of Neurology, University of Rochester, 601 Elmwood Avenue, Rochester, New York 14642*

Amos D. Korczyn, M.D., M.Sc. *Department of Physiology and Pharmacology and Department of Neurology, Sackler Faculty of Medicine, Tel-Aviv University, Ramat-Aviv 69978, Israel*

Malcolm Lader, D.Sc., Ph.D., M.D., F.R.C. Psych. *Professor of Clinical Psychopharmacology, Institute of Psychiatry, London, SE5 8AF, England*

Brian A. Lawlor, M.D., F.R.C.P.I., M.R.C. Psych. *Section on Old Age Psychiatry, Department of Psychiatry, University of Dublin, St. James's Hospital, Dublin 8, Ireland*

Raimond Levy, M.D. *Section of Old Age Psychiatry, Institute of Psychiatry, de Crespigny Park, London, SE5 8AF, England*

Andrea Lippi, M.D. *Department of Neurology and Psychiatry, Università di Firenze, Viale Morgagni, 85, Firenze, Italy*

Richard Mayeux, M.D. *Columbia University, College of Physicians and Surgeons, New York, New York 10032*

Michel Panisset, M.D. *INSERM U 324, Centre Paul Broca, 2 Ter, rue d'Alésia, 75014 Paris, France*

Barry Reisberg, M.D. *Professor of Psychiatry, Department of Psychiatry, New York University School of Medicine, New York, New York 10016*

Sir Martin Roth, M.D., Sc.D. (Hon.), F.R.C.P., F.R.C. Psych. *Trinity College, Cambridge, CB2 1TQ; Addenbrooke's Hospital, Level 9, Hills Road, Cambridge, CB2 2QQ, England*

Andres M. Salazar, Col., M.C. *Department of Neurology, Uniformed Services University of the Health Sciences, 4301 Jones Bridge Road, Bethesda, Maryland 20814-4799*

Bernd Saletu, M.D. *Professor of Psychiatry, Department of Psychiatry, School of Medicine, University of Vienna, Währinger Gürtel 18–20, A-1090 Vienna, Austria*

Mary Sano, Ph.D. *Columbia University, College of Physicians and Surgeons, New York, New York 10032*

Judith Saxton, Ph.D. *Alzheimer Disease Research Center, University of Pittsburgh, Room 400, Iroquois Building, 3600 Forbes Avenue, Pittsburgh, Pennsylvania 15213*

Raimo Sulkava, M.D., Ph.D. *Memory Research Unit, Department of Neurology, University of Helsinki, Helsinki, Finland*

Joan M. Swearer, Ph.D. *Department of Neurology, University of Massachusetts Medical Center, 55 Lake Avenue, North, Worcester, Massachusetts 01655*

Leon J. Thal, M.D. *UCSD Medical Center, Alzheimer Disease Center, 225 Dickinson Street, H-204, San Diego, California 92103*

Peter J. Whitehouse, M.D., Ph.D. *Alzheimer Center, University Hospitals of Cleveland, 2074 Abington Road, Cleveland, Ohio 44106*

G. K. Wilcock, D.M. (Oxon), F.R.C.P. *Department of Care of the Elderly, Frenchay Hospital, Bristol BS16 1LE England*

Aging

VOLUME 39

Guidelines for Drug Trials
in Memory Disorders

Guidelines for Drug Trials in Memory Disorders, edited by N. Canal, et al.
Raven Press, Ltd., New York © 1993.

1

Informed Consent in the Context of Clinical Practice and Scientific Inquiry

Martin Roth

Addenbrooke's Hospital, Cambridge, CB2 2QQ England

THE DEFINITION AND ORIGINS OF INFORMED CONSENT

The concept of "informed consent" in medical care comprises a number of components. It holds that all doctors and other health workers who wish to embark on a procedure in diagnosis, treatment, or in scientific inquiry are under a compelling obligation to explain to the patient what measures will be taken and to provide instruction regarding the ratio of risk to benefit involved in the procedures as compared with alternative procedures and with no form of treatment. In its essence, the origins of the concept can be traced back to ancient philosophical writings. In the present context it is perhaps sufficient to cite a principle expressed in relatively recent years in a case from California (1), in which a patient who underwent translumbar aortography, during the course of which she suffered spinal cord injury, alleged that insufficient information had been given to her beforehand about the procedure. The court ruled that "a physician violates his duty to his patient and subjects himself to liability if he withholds any facts which are necessary to form the basis of an intelligent consent by the patient to the proposed treatment."

Wider considerations have evolved in recent years to provide ethical and philosophical foundations for informed consent. Respect for the autonomy, dignity, and the right to self-determination of the individual are inherent in the contemporary concept. Informed consent has been obtained when the patient is judged to have understood, in the terms cited earlier, the risks entailed as well as the benefits that may accrue, and consents to the treatment proposed.

The principle of autonomy that underlies the obligation to obtain informed consent must be balanced against a second principle that governs the doctor–patient relationship. The doctor has a compelling duty to care for the patient and to use all available knowledge and skill in doing so.

With regard to the first principle, that of informed consent and the autonomy of the individual patient which underlies it, the doctor (or other professional) who undertakes medical treatment without securing proper consent is open, according to some legal authorities, to the charge of "battery" [". . . an act which directly and either intentionally or negligently causes some physical contact with another without that person's consent" (2)]. But breach of the second principle also entails penalties. Failure to provide proper care and treatment leaves the doctor open to a charge of negligence.

These two principles were the main clauses of the draft code of practice published by the "Mental Health Act Commission" in the United Kingdom, which provides guidelines for attempts to secure informed consent to treatment. In its draft document "Consent to Treatment," the Commission sets out a range of circumstances in which consent to treatment, as defined in the Mental Health Act of 1983, can be overridden. The doctor is justified in treating without informed consent such patients as those who have been brought in unconscious or require treatment after a drug overdose or who need an operation after suffering a head injury that impairs awareness and precludes the person from forming a proper judgment concerning the potential risks and benefits of such treatment.

BATTERY IS A CRUDE INSTRUMENT TO PLAY A PART IN THE FORMULATION OF INFORMED CONSENT

Even with these exceptions, however, the concept of battery provides a crude and inappropriate basis for decision-making in clinical practice. In the hurly-burly of the everyday life of psychiatric wards, depressed patients judged to be at risk have to be led away from open windows. Doubly incontinent patients must have nightclothes and bedding changed, sometimes under protest. Failure to do so could lead to the development of bed sores or worse, and might endanger the health of other patients. A demented patient must somehow be prevented from leaving the wards in the middle of the night to go and search for a husband who died 5 years ago. All this can be done by skilled and capable nurses without inflicting harm or loss of dignity. However, it cannot be done without some physical contact, gentle though it may be. It would be a doctrinaire flight from common sense if such management were regarded by the law or by an individual as tantamount to battery, or if every patient requiring help of this nature had to be detained under a section of the Mental Health Act to enable medical and nursing staff to legalize all actions needed to protect patients from harming themselves. It is doubtful whether judges would regard such actions on the part of medical and nursing staff as unlawful. Nevertheless, when guidelines are set forth that make it possible to conceive of such management as approximating to battery, it is probable that sooner or later litigation will result against doctors and nurses engaged in the ordinary tasks of providing humane and proficient care for the very disturbed and confused.

CIRCUMSTANCES IN WHICH DUTY OF CARE TAKES PRECEDENCE

The Mental Health Act Commission in the United Kingdom (5) set out a number of steps which must be taken if duty of care and protection of the patient are to be given precedence over consent to treatment as defined in the Mental Act of 1983. It is recommended that the doctor should consult one or more relatives about the steps in management proposed. However, the opinions of relatives may not be wholly disinterested, and in some cases several relatives may express conflicting views regarding what should be done. A second suggestion is that the physician should consult with representatives of other specialities who are involved in the treatment of the patient. For example, in the case of psychiatrists, the views of physicians, social workers, psychologists, and nurses should be considered, and similar cross-disciplinary consultations are desirable in all branches of medicine. Such practices are already well established in the United Kingdom, where interdisciplinary decisions are usually made at case conferences. Representatives of all professions involved in the care and rehabilitation of the patient participate in decisions about treatment in difficult cases, and particularly for those in which the patient's powers of discrimination, judgment, and self-determination are undermined by a psychiatric or other disorder. It should be noted, however, that the presence of a psychiatric disorder does not necessarily make an individual unable to give informed consent, even when the disorder in question is an early or moderate dementia. A third step recommended is a request for approval of the proposed treatment addressed to a properly constituted ethical committee. A fourth recommendation is already in force as a compulsory measure under Section 58 of the Mental Health Act of 1983 (United Kingdom) in all patients who refuse treatment regarded as essential by the responsible medical officer. A written opinion must be sought from an approved consultant, who in turn must certify that the patient is not capable of understanding the nature and purpose of the treatment or has not consented to it but that ". . . having regard to the likelihood of its alleviating or preventing a deterioration of his condition, the treatment should be given" (2).

RESEARCH IN PATIENTS WITH DEMENTIA, CLOUDING OF CONSCIOUSNESS, AND OTHER SERIOUS MENTAL DISORDERS

The most difficult and refractory problems are posed by the obligation to elicit appropriate consent for scientific investigations in mentally ill or demented adults. There is an implicit obligation for those who engage in psychiatric and medical care to undertake such inquiries. When there is a reasonable hope that the research proposed will improve the methods of treatment available for the alleviation or cure of the disorder from which the patient suffers, and when the inquiry entails minimal risk, no pain or distress, and the patient is competent to provide informed consent and does so in an unambiguous manner, there would be a broad consensus of opinion that the inquiries are ethically justified and are unlikely to come into conflict with the law. To fail to exploit new paths for investigation of the causes or the treatment of a given disease deprives not only the present generation of patients but also future generations of affected individuals of the benefits that might derive from any successes achieved by research. Of course, it is necessary to be certain that consent given by the patient to participate is authentic. It must originate from the patient's independent willingness to participate and must reflect real understanding of what is entailed, rather than merely passive compliance with the perceived intentions and wishes of the investigator.

A sharp line of demarcation has been drawn in some quarters between "therapeutic" research, which would be expected to assist the individual if it succeeded, and "nontherapeutic" research, which would not be directly advantageous. The validity of the distinction is open to question. Although "nontherapeutic" research may not prove directly and immediately advantageous to the patient, a deeper understanding of the origins and causes of the disease or some related disorder would be likely to pave the way for novel approaches to its treatment and management.

The issue that requires further reflection and wider discussion is that posed by the need for research in such patients as those with Alzheimer disease or other forms of dementia. These patients are frequently, although not always, incompetent to give informed consent to participate in research that is harmless and painless but may yield knowledge of value. According to some authorities and official regulatory bodies, all inquiries should be prohibited in such patients. It must be admitted that there is no philosophically impeccable foundation for undertaking research in patients who are unlikely to benefit individually from a given inquiry and who are incapable of understanding the nature and purpose of the procedures in which they will be involved during the course of the research. However, rigid dogmas derived from moral imperatives would put an end to research, not only in Alzheimer disease and other dementias but in many forms of severe mental illness and handicap. They would also bring to a halt many of the most promising lines of investigation into the major psychoses of adult and earlier life. Individuals, their families, communities, and future generations would suffer disadvantage from doctrinaire imperatives.

Nevertheless, further thought and analysis must be given to this difficult area by the professions and by communities. Given the safeguards that have already been mentioned, it is imperative that controlled clinical trials into new forms of treatment, and basic biological research into the dementias and other mental disorders of later life in particular, should be pursued with vigor, imagination, and enterprise. Some clear and valuable guidelines for the conduct of inquiries in such patients have already been set down by the Royal College of Physicians of London (3) among other bodies, and these must be considered in the development of research programs, although available guidelines need to be refined and updated.

In the meantime, investigators should solicit certain consultations before embarking on inquiries in incompetent subjects. Proposals must always be submitted to ethical committees. However, the composition and the decision-making process of these committees should be characterized by greater uniformity and consistency than has emerged from some investigations. In addition to an adequate range of medical disciplines, members of the legal profession and lay members of the community should be included in such committees. Although relatives and other surrogates do not provide the complete answer to the problem of securing consent, they should be fully informed and their permission sought wherever possible. The ultimate responsibility for the investigation, however, lies with the clinician. There is no evidence that improper investigations have been conducted in mentally incompetent patients. Nevertheless, it should be borne in mind, in the light of the increased litigiousness of the general public toward the medical and related professions in recent years, that investigators may in rare instances have to defend both the legality of and the ethical justification for their research. It is perhaps appropriate, in conclusion, to quote from a firm and unambiguous statement by an eminent English legal authority (4) about the difficult problems posed by scientific investigation, one of the main themes of this conference.

"So far as research that involves the invasion of the bodies of such patients are concerned, I believe that English Common Law judges would be willing to adopt as guidance on good practice, the guidelines published by any responsible and authoritative body that they can see to be truly representative of the differing aspects of the public interest in this difficult field, and that they would not be deflected from determining what was acceptable by any dogmatic approach based on rigid rules derived from the supposed requirements of the law of battery."

REFERENCES

1. Salgo v. Leland. Stanford Junior University Board of Trust Pacific Reporter, 2nd ed. Vol. 317:170–820.
2. Mental Health Act 1983, Section 56. Chapter 20. London: Her Majesty's Stationery Office, 1983.
3. Royal College of Physicians of London. *Guidelines on the practice of ethics committees in medical research*. London: Royal College of Physicians; 1984.
4. Brooke H. Consent to treatment or research: the incapable patient. In: Hirsch SR, Harris J eds. *Consent and the incompetent patient: ethics, law and medicines*. London: Gaskell; 1988:20.

Guidelines for Drug Trials in Memory
Disorders, edited by N. Canal, et al.
Raven Press, Ltd., New York © 1993.

2

The Informed Consent

Robert J. Joynt and *Jane Greenlaw

*Department of Neurology; *Division of Medical Humanities, University of
Rochester, Rochester, New York 14642*

The subject of patients' consent for treatment and for research is broad and is becoming more complex. For patients with diminished decision-making capacity, the complexity of consent is amplified. This chapter discusses the history of the development of patient consent, the usual requirements for consent and, finally, the special consideration of consent in patients with memory disorders. We recognize that laws governing patient consent vary from country to country. Our approach necessarily stems from Anglo-American traditions. However, the principles set forward are probably consistent with many systems, because biomedical ethics has evolved with advances in technology and because there is revulsion against coercive research practices stemming from memories of World War II.

For centuries, the patient's role in decision making was embodied in this passage from Hippocrates (1):

> Perform [these duties] calmly and adroitly, concealing most things from the patient while you are attending to him. Give necessary orders with cheerfulness and sincerity, turning his attention away from what is being done to him; sometimes reprove sharply and emphatically, and sometimes comfort with solicitude and attention, revealing nothing of the patient's future or present condition.

The passage summarizes the usual relationship between the patient and physician until fairly recent times. When you engaged the doctor, you also engaged the treatment. Although there may have been explanations for procedures, especially for major surgery, this was widely regarded as the courteous imparting of information rather than a matter of obligation. Indeed, the patient's consent was assumed. This lack or looseness of consent had been questioned on a few occasions. In a frequently quoted court decision, Judge Cardozo in 1914 wrote (2): . . . every human being of adult years and sound mind has a right to determine what shall be done with his own body . . .

Despite the logic of this ruling, actual practice changed very little. However, in the 1950s a new trend began and accelerated: not only should patients be fully informed but they also had a right to make a decision only after the benefits, risks, and alternatives had been explained (3). The enduring respect for physicians in society probably explains the initial reluctance to challenge their role and may well have slowed progress in recognizing the autonomy of the patient.

A landmark decision in the doctrine of informed consent was that written by Justice Bray of the California Court of Appeals in 1957 (4): A physician violates his duty to his patients and subjects himself to liability if he withholds any facts which are necessary to form the basis of an intelligent consent by the patient to the proposed treatment. In closing, Justice Bray wrote: In discussing the elements of risks a certain amount of discretion must be employed consistent with the full disclosure of facts necessary to an informed consent.

Thus, the idea of and the term *informed consent* became firmly fixed in our society. However, in the 34 years since that decision the concept of informed consent has evolved and changed for a number of compelling reasons.

First, medicine and medical technology have changed. Many of the difficult decisions now facing us are a result of these changes. Medications for treatment of neurologic disorders were few and were largely ineffective only a few decades ago. In general, the benefits were slight and the complications were slight. Now, as we develop more effective treatments, both medical and surgical, these treatments must be tested, and side effects and complications are more common. Therefore, information about risks must be provided to the patient.

Second, the understanding between the physician and the patient has changed. What was essentially a convenantal relationship or a bargain of mutual understanding has become a contractual arrangement of reimbursement by the patient for services satisfactorily rendered. The consumer movement, coupled with increased litigiousness, particularly in the United States, has made informed consent a necessity. On the more positive side, physicians are much more responsive to the wishes and needs of their patients, an aspect of the relationship sadly deficient in the past.

Third, increasing costs and decreasing resources have complicated the problem of informed consent. With unrestricted resources and with no consideration of cost, the list of choices available to patients would be extensive. However, in our more restrictive society the alternatives are fewer. For example, renal dialysis and organ transplantation are no longer options for some, even if they could prolong life. Such external influences as the moratorium in the United States on research and use of fetal tissue for transplantation also limit the patients' alternatives.

Fourth, the demographic changes associated with the rapid increase in the number of elderly people and, in particular, the increase in very elderly people, pose a new problem with informed consent. The elderly often have a devalued position in the patient–physician relationship. Furthermore, the growing numbers of elderly people have markedly increased the prevalence of dementia and its attendant problems of informed consent.

The evolution of the concept of patient consent has led to an expanded set of criteria for a valid consent. Indeed, the term informed consent has been criticized as incomplete, because more than information about the treatment or research plan is required (5). Although authorities vary as to exact wording, in general the following are necessary for a valid consent (6): (i) The physician must give sufficient information to the patient. (ii) The patient must not be coerced into making a decision. (iii) The patient must be competent to refuse or accept the treatment or to be a subject for research.

The information imparted to the patient must include risks, benefits, and alternatives. It must be inclusive enough to allow a rational person to make a decision. This does not preclude the physician from making a recommendation. An excellent working rule is for the physician to impart the information that was required to arrive at the particular recommendation. It is also important for the information to be given to the patient in a manner and at a level that is understandable.

There must be no coercion of the patient. In general, coercive measures usually involve undue stress on the potential negative effects of refusing treatment, such that the patient has difficulty in resisting. Coercion can also be positive, e.g., involving promises of reward. This method has been used with prisoner volunteers for experimentation. Federal guidelines specifically preclude benefits accruing to prisoners of such a magnitude that decisions might be unduly influenced (7). Interestingly, the federal government suspended the required need for consent for the use of investigational drugs or biologicals in military personnel during Operation Desert Storm (8). The directive pointed out that it was not feasible to obtain informed consent in times of military combat emergencies.

The third requirement for valid consent is competency. Competency is easier to define than to judge. The essence of competency is the ability to understand and to appreciate the information about the proposed course of action. The phrase "to appreciate" is important, as the patient must be able to take into consideration the circumstances under which the information is being imparted and what the implications are for the decision. The following questions, to be asked of the patient, have been suggested in order to make an objective determination of competency (9):

1. What is your present physical condition?
2. What is the treatment being recommended for you?
3. What do you and your doctor think might happen to you if you decide to accept the treatment?
4. What do you and your doctor think might happen to you if you decide not to accept the recommended treatment?
5. What are the alternative treatments available and what are the probable consequences of accepting each?

There will certainly be a wide variation in responses, ranging from sophisticated answers to no answers. Unfortunately, and particularly in the patient population in whom we are interested, the physician/investigator may not have a clear view of the patient's competency after this test.

Competency is not an all-or-none issue. The courts have established precedents under which competency for wills, contracts, and medical treatment may vary. We might, for example, judge a patient competent to consent or to refuse medical treatment but not competent to drive a car. The fact that a patient can answer your litany of questions for competency correctly but is unable to remember your name may be disquieting but does not negate that patient's ability to consent to or to refuse treatment. In addition, competency may vary: a well-rested patient in a quiet atmosphere may be judged quite differently from the same patient who is fatigued and jangled by noise and competing stimuli.

Competency, the capacity to make a decision, must be differentiated from the quality or rationality of the decision. A person may be competent by the standards we impose but the decision may be quite divergent from usual norms. For example, an 18-year-old patient might refuse antibiotics for a serious infection on the grounds that the treatment may be uncomfortable. We would consider that irrational, knowing the excellent results of such treatment. However, the same decision made by a 75-year-old patient with metastatic carcinoma might be considered quite rational. Therefore, both competency and rationality must be considered for a valid consent.

Although the rationality of patients' decisions can help us to assess their "appreciation" of the relevant facts, physicians, in their role of judging competency and obtaining consent, must guard against paternalism or subverting the patients' autonomy. Paternalism can take several forms, but it can be summed up as "the doctor knows best" and "you may not agree, but you will thank me later." These are roles easily assumed when any question of competency is raised by the patient's condition. Paternalism may even take the form of a narrow definition of competency (e.g., patients are competent if they agree with my recommendation but incompetent if they don't).

Paternalism is a role often assigned to the physician by the patient ("I know you will do the best thing for me, doctor"). This is a responsibility that the physician should not easily assume and it does not obviate the duty to fully inform the patient. Obviously, there are reasons for justified paternalism, such as the unconscious patient requiring emergency treatment who does not have responsible relatives in attendance.

We have examined the evolution of and the mechanism for informed or valid consent. The issue particularly pertinent to our discussion is that of obtaining consent for treatment trials in a population who are often partially competent or are incompetent.

The justifications for research trials involving humans are generally understood to include the following: (i) Full information must be disclosed and valid consent must be obtained. (ii) The risks must be minimal. (iii) Any risks must be reasonable in relation to the potential benefits. (iv) Appropriate and effective therapy must not be otherwise available. In the United States, Institutional Review Boards (IRB) are required to review, approve, and monitor any research on human subjects.

Obtaining a valid consent in an incompetent patient is difficult but not impossible. In a partially competent patient, the consent of the patient, buttressed by the consent of the responsible relative, is often sufficient. A refusal by a partially competent person of treatment or of participation in a study should be respected unless it is irrational by usual standards (5). The ultimate decision should also stand the test of rationality.

A totally incompetent patient cannot make a decision for treatment or for participation in a research trial. In some instances, earlier in the course of the illness the patient may be competent and the possibility of clinical trials at a future date can be discussed. The patient can then make an advanced directive that will guide future participation or nonparticipation. This has been called the Ulysses Contract (10). Ulysses, to save his ship from being lured to destruction on the rocks by the seductive pleading of sea sirens, ordered his crew to tie him to the mast and to ignore his pleadings for release—thus, an advanced directive.

A proxy, usually the next of kin or the responsible relative or guardian, will have the right of consent in most instances. In such situations the doctrine of substituted judgment should prevail. The proxy should act as he or she believes the patient would act in a similar situation, not necessarily as the proxy would act. For example, if there were a question of participation in a clinical trial, the proxy should take into consideration the possible participant's views on medical research, assistance to others, and confidence in the investigator. In some instances the proxy may not be that familiar with the patient, and in such a case must act in the patient's best interests. Although beyond the scope of this presentation, proxies can be legally constituted in several ways, e.g., as durable powers of attorney, guardianship, committee of the person, or health care proxy.

A new approach to consent in incompetent patients without a relative is the volunteer surrogate committee (11). This system is more responsive and more timely then the judicial decisions previously relied on. Experience with this system has been in institutions housing patients with mental retardation who have no relatives. It probably has limited use in the elderly population for whom family members are available.

The consideration of medical treatment that will relieve discomfort in the incompetent, such as a prostatectomy or antibiotic therapy, has greater urgency than a decision to participate in a research study for trial of a new therapeutic agent. Therefore, consent must take into consideration all the other treatment decisions that must be made. Indeed, there is often a certain reluctance to participate in such studies, given the negative aspects of the

history of medical experimentation. Although we must remember the out-
rages of medical experimentation during World War II, we must also remember the sad record of unwarranted experimentation in other societies (12,13).
However, there are still good reasons to carry out suitable supervised clinical
trials in patients with memory and other cognitive disorders. These include:

1. Lack of any other proven therapies.
2. Lack of other appropriate models that can be used for testing.
3. Performance of the trials in the afflicted population is necessary because
   the measurable parameters of the studies, mental and behavioral function, exist only in that population.

The challenge is great from an ethical standpoint, and every possible measure must be taken to preserve the autonomy and dignity of the individual.

REFERENCES

1. Hippocrates. *Decorum,* Vol 2. London: Putnam's Sons, 1923:297, 299. Jones W, translator.
2. Schloendorff V. The Society of New York Hospitals (1914), cited in Ciccone JR. The elderly
   and medicolegal trends in consent to treatment. *NY State J Med* 1986;86:635–8.
3. Katz J. *The silent world of doctor and patient.* The Free Press: New York, 1984.
4. Salgo V. Leland Stanford Jr. University Board of Trustees (1957), cited in ref 3.
5. Bernat J. Ethical issues in neurology. In: Joynt R, ed. *Clinical neurology.* Philadelphia: JB
   Lippincott; 1991:1–105.
6. Culver CM, Gert B. Basic ethical concepts in neurologic practice. *Sem Neurol* 1984;4:1–8.
7. OPPR Reports. Protection of human subjects. 45 CFR 46; rev. March 8, 1983.
8. Federal Register. Informed consent for human drugs and biologics: determination that informed consent is not feasible. 21 CFR 50; December 21, 1990;55:52814–17.
9. Annas GJ, Densberger JE. Competence to refuse medical treatment: autonomy vs paternalism. *U Toledo Law Review* 1984;15:561–96.
10. Treat B. Alzheimer's research: physicians begin to tread in on ethical minefield. *Can Med
    Assoc J* 1989;140:726–9.
11. Sundram CJ. Informed consent for major medical treatment of mentally disabled people.
    N Engl J Med. 1988;318:1368–73.
12. Beecher HK. Ethics and clinical research. *N Engl J Med* 1966;274:1354–60.
13. Romano J. Reflections on informed consent. *Arch Gen Psychiatry* 1974;30:129–35.

Guidelines for Drug Trials in Memory Disorders, edited by N. Canal, et al.
Raven Press, Ltd., New York © 1993.

3

Discussion

Dr. Roth: Informed consent requires that all doctors who wish to embark on a procedure for the purpose of diagnosis or treatment should explain to the patient what is involved and should secure an understanding consent before performance of the procedure. This goes back to ancient philosophical writings, even to the Bible. What has evolved is an entire range of criteria in relation to respect for the individual's autonomy, dignity, and right to self-determination. These are central to the contemporary concept of informed consent. They have been expressed in a number of historical statements, which include the Nuremberg Code and the Helsinki Declaration.

A doctor who fails to obtain informed consent before administering treatment to a patient will offend against a principle clearly enunciated in English law in the following words: "The fundamental principle plain and incontestable is that every person's body is inviolate" (Collins vs. Wilcock, 1984). Failure to respect this principle leaves the doctor open to the charge of "battery." This appears to be an unduly aggressive word. It appears at first sight that we may be charged with "battery" if we try to prevent a psychotically depressed, confused, or paranoid and deluded patient, who has not been compulsorily detained, from going out through the balcony door of a hospital ward and flinging himself over the railings. If we touch such an individual without his consent we might be technically guilty of "battery." This is defined as an act ". . . that directly and either intentionally or negligently causes some physical contact with the person of another without that person's consent."

However, it has been widely recognized by legal authorities that the principle of informed consent and the principle of autonomy that underlies it are in danger of coming into conflict with a second principle, which affirms that a doctor has a compelling duty to heal, care for, and protect the patient and to use all available knowledge in doing so. Failure to provide proper care and treatment leaves the doctor open to the charge of negligence. For this reason, the doctrine of informed consent is associated in the law with a number of exceptional entries. In the light of these exceptions the doctor is justified in treating a patient who is brought in unconscious after a suicidal attempt or who is unconscious for other reasons. The doctor is entitled to deal with any emergency, even though the individual may be unable to give informed consent, and is also entitled to intervene if the patient is in imminent danger of losing his life but is unwilling to consent to measures aimed at keeping him alive. There will be no conflict with the law if a doctor acts in accordance with the instruction to use his utmost skill, ability, and knowledge to discharge his duty of care for his patient, nor would he be culpable if such intervention were judged acceptable in the ordinary conduct of life.

The most difficult and refractory problem, from a philosophical point of view, is that posed by incapable patients: those who are partly conscious, who are very elderly, or who are confused or demented. Those with memory defects and dementia are at the focus of our interest in the present context. They are clearly unable to give informed consent. Although treatment to alleviate pain and distress are admissible, procedures undertaken for the purpose of scientific enquiry alone pose difficult ethical problems.

One solution that has been proposed for dealing with the dilemmas such patients create for us is to seek surrogate permission for all procedures and interventions. This should be a compelling course of action, it is argued, in all interventions no matter how simple, painless, and free from risk. However, such policies are open to criticism for a number of reasons. Relatives may disagree with each other. In other cases their refusal to permit the physician to take some fresh initiative in treatment or to include the patient in a controlled therapeutic trial that entails no risk may not be entirely objective. In practice, it is usually possible to secure consent from relatives to proceed in such situations. However, such consent, even when given by the most disinterested of relatives, has no legal validity, and its ethical basis is also open to question.

The difficulties and dangers posed by rigid rules and regulations for regulating the conduct of scientific research in the field we are discussing can be illustrated by quoting from some documents issued recently by the Mental Health Commission of the United Kingdom. In their Draft Code of Practice (Mental Health Act Commission, 1985) they provide a list of variables they have formulated for the guidance of those who wish to undertake clinical research. It is worth quoting this paragraph in full:

> "Whoever proposes a clinical research programme involving a mental health patient and the ethical committee which considers it must weigh up and balance the many variables including: whether or not the patient is capable of giving a real consent; the likelihood of benefit to the patient; whether the research will actually advance knowledge and experience; whether that knowledge could be obtained by other means; the extent of the experimental intervention; the amount of distress which will or may be caused; whether risks have already been identified and the safety of the patient sufficiently protected. Whether the investigator is adequately experienced and qualified and has the necessary facilities."

These criteria are subsequently developed and enunciated in an inflexible manner. A sharp distinction is drawn between "therapeutic" and "nontherapeutic" research. The validity of this distinction is open to question. Investigations with the aid of a positron emission tomographic scan may identify the receptors involved in the action of drugs used in the treatment of psychiatric disorder and so facilitate refinement of methods of treatment. The experiments that preceded the development of magnetic resonance imaging paved the way for the discovery of new techniques of imaging pathologic changes in the brains of patients during life that had not been possible to visualize with the aid of previous techniques. In each case the types of patient initially studied in these inquiries were to be beneficiaries of the novel forms of therapy and diagnostic investigation of psychiatric disorders that emerged. It would be possible to cite many other examples to illustrate that the antithesis between therapeutic and nontherapeutic research is weak and inadmissible. In its guidelines the Commission concludes that nontherapeutic research is unacceptable in mentally incompetent patients even when they provide consent. Among the safeguards it recommended, the Commission made the following suggestion: "Where non-therapeutic research is proposed, a second opinion should be obtained from a consultant as to the capacity of the patient to consent and the reality of his consent."

These guidelines would virtually preclude all research into patients with psychoses or neuroses such as panic disorders, organic disorders such as the dementias, delirious states and mental handicap, and inquiries into medical and psychiatric disorders of children. Research would in effect be prohibited by such rules even in those quite capable in many cases of providing informed consent, namely, patients with depressive disorders, most neuroses, and those in the early stages of the evolution of dementia. However, in this last group and some others it would be wise to seek additional sanction from a relative on the basis of ethical as well as legal considerations.

It will be evident that guidelines and criteria set down tentatively by official bodies have a way of ossifying into categorical ethical, moral, and legal imperatives. The guidelines cited above would, if implemented, have the effect of retarding or halting scientific inquiry into that large group of cerebral diseases, namely, the dementias, that cause distress and disablement to individuals, families, and societies everywhere. Better solutions than those discussed have to be devised. They should make provision for protecting the dignity and autonomy of individual patients. But they should avoid placing shackles on the investigators who provide the only hope of alleviating the distress and helplessness of those afflicted with cerebral degenerative disease and of the families who shoulder the main burden of caring for them.

Dr. Lader: One point that I want to emphasize has to do with the ethics of the research aspects. At the Institute of Psychiatry we have an Ethics Committee that is probably one of the oldest in the United Kingdom (over 20 years). During that time it must have reviewed over 2,000 research applications, some of which involved people whose informed consent was doubtful or for whom informed consent had to be given by somebody else. Instead of continually reinventing the wheel, we should look at the scientific value of the projects. It is essential that the scientific aspects are assessed and that the ethical aspects are balanced against them. This is a risk–benefit equation we have to solve.

Dr. Joynt: I agree. I believe the scientific value of the study is very important in looking at the risk that we have to take with our patients. It is important to emphasize the risk–benefit ratio over and over again. Every drug has some drawbacks. At the same time, we must remember that we are dealing with a very difficult population, and one that we have not, as yet, really influenced medically. However, we cannot be capricious in the type of testing that we do because this is a population that is not able to give consent. We have to remember the autonomy and the dignity of that population.

Dr. Roth: Bad science is unethical. Good science is likely to be more ethical than bad.

Dr. Korczyn: I wish to add a couple of points to Dr. Joynt's very thorough discussion. One regards what happens in Israel and in many other countries in obtaining permission to perform an autopsy. By definition, autopsy would not help the deceased; it is just for research purposes in the wider sense of the word research. In addition, many emotional and religious implications are involved. We depend almost exclusively on surrogate consent, e.g., next-of-kin or some other relative. If we can perform an autopsy when obviously there is no evidence of any benefit to the deceased person, I can see no reason why we should not take a step back to the time when the person was still alive and perform the study then. My point is that if there is any evidence of benefit, and the risks are acceptable—and I think the IRB is very important in deciding the risk–benefit issues—then having informed consent from a relative or the next-of-kin should suffice. This applies not only to patients who are demented but also to infants and to patients who are in a coma or delirium. With regard to patients with dementia, another issue is that there are benefits derived from participating in a study. This has been our experience in Israel, but I believe many other countries have reported similar findings. Demented patients who participate in such a study whether they are on placebo or in the group receiving the active compound get better treatment than the run-of-the-mill patients, just by adhering to the protocol. This is an advantage for the patients, and we should also consider this aspect.

Dr. Roth: Placebo effects are very striking sometimes, and this needs to be stressed. At times they are so marked that they expose the drug to a very stringent test of its efficacy. The drug has to be truly effective to prove better than the placebo to a statistically significant degree.

Dr. Thal: When a procedure involving a certain degree of risk or a high degree of risk is being offered in a therapeutic setting, should researchers make an attempt to recruit only individuals who are competent or should they allow an individual to endure a trial via a surrogate's judgment? I will give you a specific example. Suppose a procedure is going to involve a brain biopsy along with an experimental treatment for a drug. What level of patient should be allowed to be recruited into such a trial? Should the patient have to have sufficient competency to understand the issues and should the trial be restricted to that cohort of patients, or should one allow patients into such a trial with a substituted judgment?

Dr. Roth: I believe that a brain biopsy—unless there can be benefits to patients that are totally unknown to me—would not be acceptable on a person with a condition such as Alzheimer disease. The person who undertakes such a procedure would be placed in considerable jeopardy, ethically and legally.

Dr. Levy: I agree with the point you raised about brain biopsy, but there are actually even more difficult ones, i.e., exposing a patient in the course of a therapeutic trial to a drug that might be damaging, such as recent trials of drugs that are hepatotoxic. I would have thought that the provisos that apply in relation to brain biopsy would apply equally to that type of situation. There is another issue that has not been addressed and about which there are considerable differences between countries: the question of how the information that is imparted to patients and their relatives is given. should this information, as well as actually the consent be in writing, and should it be witnessed? We have no particular guidance in Britain about this. It has become a habit to impart the information and obtain consent in writing from a mentally competent patient and, if possible, from the patient's relative. But I imagine there must be considerable variability between country to country.

Dr. Roth: A wise clinician puts down that he has sought consent and sets down the precise terms in which it was expressed and the circumstances in which it was obtained. He asks the patient to sign a form or statement only after he has satisfied himself that the patient has understood it.

Dr. Joynt: In the United States (where two and a half lawyers graduate for every doctor), we put everything in writing. Unfortunately, if you read the consent it becomes very complete and death may be a complication. This is like reading the package information on aspirin. You would never take any aspirin if you read it. I believe that any procedure has to be in writing, with a witness if possible.

Dr. McKhann: I'd like to hear comments on the issue of confidentiality and how to handle it, e.g., in terms of diagnosis. In addition, in many studies there is much more information about patients than is usually available. To what extent is that information then available to other people? For example, can it be subpoenaed?

Dr. Joynt: We conducted a recent study in confidentiality at our hospital and it turned out that at least 17 different people had access to that record just in the course of their activity, including the medical insurance representative who came up to see if the treatment was proper. So, confidentiality is something that is very difficult. I would assume that information can be subpoenaed like other medical records.

Guidelines for Drug Trials in Memory Disorders, edited by N. Canal, et al.
Raven Press, Ltd., New York © 1993.

4

Degenerative Disorders

Nicola Canal

*Department of Neurology, University of Milan,
Istituto Scientifico H. San Raffaele, Milan, Italy*

Most of the many diseases with dementia as a symptom [Haase lists more than 60 of these (1)] are degenerative forms, and Alzheimer disease (AD) is definitively the one with highest prevalence (about 50% in the pure form, to which must be added 15% of patients with both degenerative and vascular lesions). The dimensions of the phenomenon can easily be imagined when one combines the high correlation of the disease with increasing age and the increase in mean age of the general population, especially the increase owing to survival of people over 85 years of age (in which group the prevalence of dementia of one type or another has been calculated to range from 20 to 47%).

There is no doubt that if direct treatments for preventing, curing, or retarding the cognitive deficits caused by AD disease were to become available this would be of great advantage to a population that will increase very rapidly in the future. The most important practical way to achieve this goal would be to acquire information about the causes and the pathogenetic mechanisms of the disease. Unfortunately, our acquisitions in this field have been both contradictory and inconsistent. Notwithstanding the great increase in our knowledge in recent decades, there is still profound ignorance about the pathogenesis of degenerative dementia of the Alzheimer type.

This chapter will not detail all the more or less adequate theories that have been proposed in this field, as these are very well known. However, it is worth recalling some points that are especially involved in the theme now under debate, emphasizing what makes it difficult to design good clinical trials for AD.

Several biochemical, pathologic, epidemiologic, and clinical findings suggest that AD might represent only exaggerated aging of the brain (2). One of the most impressive pieces of evidence for this is that screening tests aimed at detecting patients at risk for AD always show a unimodal rather than a bimodal distribution. In other words, there is a continuum between normal aged individuals and early demented patients. This is true for clinical, biochemical, electrophysiologic, psychometric, and bioimaging data (3). On the other hand, it is known that there are clearcut histologic differences between the normal aged brain and the pathologic aged brain, in the density of tangles and senile plaques, in their regional distribution, and in the severity of neuron loss. On the contrary, it appears that amyloid angiopathy is more related to age than to the severity of disease (4), but this is not the case for amyloid deposition in the neuropil and in the plaques.

Although we can postulate that normal and pathologic brain aging are different processes, it is clear that "physiologic" aging strongly interacts with "pathologic" aging of the brain. Both may summate and interact with environmental factors (e.g., toxins and infective agents) to cause the emergence of dementia. Even in our profound ignorance of the primum movens of AD, we can say that abnormal neuron death is the basis of the dementia.

In AD, cholinergic basal forebrain nuclei, hypothalamic nuclei, hippocampal areas, and the noradrenergic locus coeruleus are severely depopulated, probably early in the course of disease. Relatively slight and late alterations are found in the cerebellum, cranial nerve nuclei, and sensory or motor projection areas. The most severe morphologic alterations are seen in the hippocampus, especially in the subiculum and the CA1 region. Here neuron loss is severe, whatever the age of the patient, with plaques and tangles much more dense than in other regions. It is intriguing that this early and severe involvement of the hippocampus leads to a completely different memory deficit in AD than that found in global amnesic syndrome with bilateral destructive hippocampal lesions.

Undoubtedly, several kinds of cell death coexist in AD: (a) Death of neurons due to an underlying (genetically programmed?) basic failure, without appearance of tangles. This is probably the "physiologic" type of neuron death typical of the isocortex. We can postulate that a defect of protein synthesis, based on transcriptional/translational abnormalities in the neurons, leads to decreased activity of the protein synthesis machinery and, eventually, to cell atrophy and death. (b) Death of neurons due to formation of neurofibrillary tangles composed of paired helical filaments. Neurofibrillary tangles may be an unspecific side product of AD pathology. They are found, although at a lower density, in other infectious (postencephalitic parkinsonism, SSPE), degenerative (progressive supranuclear palsy), and toxic (ALS, Parkinson dementia of Guam) brain diseases. It is known that the formation of tangles is triggered by an increased phosphorylation of neurofilament proteins and microtubule-associated proteins, probably mediated by activation of calcium-dependent phosphorylases. We can speculate that "physiologic" neuron death is rather selective and without production of tangles, whereas "pathologic" neuron death is relatively unselective and with production of tangles. (c) Transneuronal anterograde and retrograde death due to death of remote neurons (5). In AD there is a severe reduction of cortical cholinergic and adrenergic innervation. However, cortical neurons that are deafferented because of extensive white matter degeneration, as seen in multiple sclerosis or Biswanger's disease, are not significantly depopulated, probably because they still receive sufficient input from intrinsic neurons. (d) Degeneration of terminal arborization (due to a "toxic" effect of amyloid deposits?) and loss of synaptic and dendritic plasticity (6).

On the basis of the several hints (although with few facts) about pathogenesis of AD, we can list four major approaches for primary and secondary prevention and for treatment of AD:

1. Identification of families at risk for development of AD, to institute genetic counseling.
2. Prevention, retardation, or reversal of amyloid deposition in brains of individuals at risk by use of specific protease inhibitors.
3. Symptomatic treatment, acting on the neurotransmitter systems known to be defective (cholinesterase inhibitors and cholinergic drugs or neuropeptides) or on other interacting systems (nootrophics).
4. Treatment with specific trophic factors that have not yet been identified (7).

Whatever the exact pathogenetic mechanism of AD may be, and although there is still no etiologic treatment, it is indispensable to have a broad understanding of the clinical features of the disease, whether or not there are clinical subtypes, and the natural history of the disease if we want to evaluate the clinical trials that are continually being proposed, based on presumptions that are often purely hypothetical but which might in the future be better grounded.

The definition of AD arrived at by the ad hoc Committee in 1984 (8) requires, among other things, that the dementia be documented "with evidence of deficits in two or more areas of cognition." This definition excludes some forms in which there is selective loss of some symbolic functions and which appear clinically as focal atrophy of cortical areas with specific functions. These forms (some of which have a prevalence that cannot be dismissed as unimportant) should be called non-AD to avoid arbitrary inclusion of such patients in the study population. Obviously, these are problems that can be dealt with only by clinical and/or noninvasive instrumental examinations that do not require cerebral biopsy or by diagnosis only after death at autopsy.

One such syndrome is the *slowly progressing aphasia* (9) that causes decreased ability to use language in the absence of any other cognitive deficits (at least in the early stages). The various cases described in the literature do not have the same clinical pictures, which in some cases includes later development (at differing intervals) of the complete syndrome of dementia. Both the instrumental images and the pathologic findings at autopsy indicate atrophy of the dominant hemisphere, with loss of the large cortical neurons, the astrocytic glia, spongiform degeneration (a characteristic shared by other lobar atrophies) and, sometimes, neurofibrillar tangles and neuritic plaques.

The cases described by Benson et al. in 1988 (10) appear also to have *focal atrophies*. They had ataxia, visual agnosia, disorders of ocular fixation, agraphia, and acalculia, and the imaging and pathologic features revealed atrophy predominately in the parieto–occipital lobes, with loss of cortical neurons and, in some but not all cases, with neurofibrillar tangles.

Two other syndromes of lobar atrophy are characterized by selective involvement of the frontal lobes. *Pure frontal dementia* has been described by groups in Manchester and in Lund (11). The clinical picture consists of changes in personality characteristic of frontal syndrome (bulimia, stereotypic behavior, appearance of archaic reflexes), confirmed by neuropsychological tests. There is relative sparing of visuospatial functions and a progressive impoverishment of speech. The neuropathologic examination shows atrophy of the frontal and temporal lobes, with gliosis and cortical and subcortical spongiosis. No neurofibrillar tangles or denditric plaques have been reported, but 20% of the cases have balloon cells and neuronal inclusion bodies of the type described for Pick disease. Complete details of this last form of disease are yet to be determined, but it appears to be distinctly different from AD.

The relationship of AD to extrapyramidal pathology is of particular interest in view of the frequency with which (a) the clinical picture of AD is complicated by extrapyramidal signs and symptoms and (b) Parkinson-type lesions are found along with the pathology typical of AD. A representative form of this double pathology is *cortical Lewy body dementia*. This anatomic and clinical (12) entity has the following neuropathologic characteristics:

1. Loss of cortical neurons and neurons in the subcortical nuclei.
2. Widespread presence of Lewy bodies (which can be stained with anti-ubiquitin immunoserum) in the neurons of the neocortex and of the subcortical nuclei (substantia nigra, nucleus basalis).
3. Spongiform changes in the temporal lobe.
4. Senile plaques in the cortex, with the same distribution as the Lewy bodies.
5. In a few cases only, neurofibrillar degeneration.

The clinical picture consists of impairment of cognitive functions such as attention, verbal fluency, writing, and visuospatial performance. At the same time there is extrapyramidal symptomatology with bradykinesia, hypomimia, and tremor. There is still no consensus as to whether this is a distinct subtype of AD or a form of Parkinson disease (PD) in which the neuropathologic lesions (i.e., the Lewy bodies) are dispersed in the neocortex.

Other questions arise about the relationship between AD and classical PD. Epidemiological studies have found the prevalence of cognitive impairment in PD to vary widely, from the 93% reported by Pirozzolo et al. in 1982 (13) to the 10.9% reported by Mayeux et al. in 1988 (14), who used the more restrictive criteria of DSM-III for primary degenerative dementia. If we look at the total of the most homogeneous studies, abnormalities are found in 20% of the cases and milder changes in about 60%. For the frequency of parkinsonian symptoms in AD, the various reports have cited 20–30%, and this has been confirmed by neuropathologic studies. According to some investigators (15), the coexistence of PD and AD is found in a subtype with more rapidly progressive AD. The levels of neurotransmitters in the brain have been studied, and several investigators have found that patients with PD plus dementia exhibit not only a decrease of dopamine in the caudate and frontal cortex but also a decrease in choline acetyltransferase in the nucleus basalis.

One of the principal aims in studying AD is to find a marker that can be used for early diagnosis. Biologic abnormalities (blood, cerebrospinal fluid), neurophysiologic abnormalities, and those that can be seen by conventional imaging (computed tomography and magnetic resonance imaging) have not yet revealed anything sufficiently specific or detectable early enough to be used for this purpose. A method that is hypothetically sensitive enough to detect metabolic changes in discrete brain areas, to be correlated with the clinical picture and the neurophysiological abnormalities as the disease progresses, is positron emission tomography (PET) of regional cerebral glucose and oxygen metabolic rates.

Since the first investigations by the group of Frackowiack, begun in the 1980s (16), there have been several direct studies of the metabolic changes that accompany the impairment of cognitive function in AD. Particular attention has been given to determining: (a) whether in AD there are metabolic deficits localized in specific cerebral areas; (b) whether these metabolic changes precede or are concomitant with the cognitive deficits; and (c) the correlation between the metabolic impairment and the progression of the disease.

Scouring the literature, we can see that despite the considerable variability from patient to patient there is a reasonably constant pattern. The most constant finding for the distribution of metabolic changes is that the decreased metabolic rates for glucose and oxygen are more marked in the cerebral cortex than in the subcortical areas (thalamus, basal ganglia). This decrease is also more marked in the parietotemporal areas than in the prefrontal area, although there are exceptions to this. This metabolic deficit is often not symmetrical in the two hemispheres. This asymmetry has a clinical correlate: subjects with left hemisphere abnormalities of metabolism have a greater language deficit and those with predominately right hemisphere abnormalities have greater deficits of visuospatial functions. Although this pattern is variable, it has been confirmed in many laboratories, including ours. In the longitudinal studies, the metabolic abnormalities worsened as the disease progressed, in parallel with the neuropsychological impairment.

According to some investigators, the metabolic deficit precedes the neuro-psychological impairment.

This last observation makes it possible to discuss a concept that in theory should be of great importance. Can we consider that a change in metabolic pattern detected by a PET scan, in the absence of cognitive impairment, is really indicative of the initiation of the dementia process? Obviously, this a crucial issue when a treatment strategy must be chosen, because it would permit treatment to be initiated in a very early phase of the disease, when any type of treatment should, in theory, be more effective. It is easy to see the methodological difficulties that complicate establishing this type of research program.

In conclusion, we have attempted to suggest and to offer for discussion some points that may be of importance in the correct selection of cases to be included in therapeutic trials and in the selection of objective parameters to be used in evaluating the possible beneficial effects of treatment.

REFERENCES

1. Haase GR. Diseases presenting as dementia. In: Wells CE, ed. *Dementia*. Philadelphia: FA Davis, 1971.
2. Editorial. Senile dementia of Alzheimer's type—normal ageing or disease? *Lancet* 1989;1: 476–7.
3. Berg L. Does Alzheimer's disease represent an exaggeration of normal aging? *Arch Neurol* 1985;42:737–9.
4. Yamada M, et al. Cerebral amyloid angiopathy in the aged. *J Neurol* 1987;234:371–6.
5. Hertz L. Is Alzheimer's disease an anterograde degeneration originating in the brainstem and disrupting metabolic and functional interactions between neurons and glial cells? *Brain Res Rev* 1989;14:335–53.
6. Hamos JE, et al. Synaptic loss in Alzheimer's disease and other dementias. *Neurology* 1989;39:355–61.
7. Hefti F, Weiner WJ. Nerve growth factor and Alzheimer's disease. *Ann Neurol* 1986;20: 275–81.
8. McKhann G, et al. Clinical diagnosis of Alzheimer's disease: report from the NINCDS-ADRDA Work Group under the auspices of Department of Health and Human Services Task Force on Alzheimer's disease. *Neurology* 1984;34:939–44.
9. Mesulam MM. Slowly progressive aphasia without generalized dementia. *Ann Neurol* 1982; 11:592–8.
10. Benson DF, et al. Posterior cortical atrophy. *Arch Neurol* 1988;45:789–93.
11. Neary D, et al. Dementia of frontal lobe type. *J Neurol Neurosurg Psychiatry* 1988;51: 353–61.
12. Kosaka K, et al. Lewy body disease with and without dementia: a clinico-pathological study of 35 cases. *Clin Neuropathol* 1988;7:299–305.
13. Pirozzolo FJ, et al. Dementia in Parkinson's disease: a neuropsychological analysis. *Brain Cogn* 1982;1:71–81.
14. Mayeux R, et al. An estimate of the prevalence of dementia in idiopathic Parkinson's disease. *Arch Neurol* 1988;45:260–3.
15. Mayeux R, et al. Heterogeneity in dementia of the Alzheimer type: evidence for subgroups. *Neurology* 1985;35:453–61.
16. Frackowiack RSJ, et al. Regional cerebral oxygen supply and utilization in dementia: a clinical and physiological study with oxygen-15 and positron tomography. *Brain* 1981;104: 753–78.

Guidelines for Drug Trials in Memory
Disorders, edited by N. Canal, et al.
Raven Press, Ltd., New York © 1993.

5

Vascular Disorders

Vladimir C. Hachinski

*Department of Clinical Neurological Sciences, University of Western Ontario,
London, Ontario, Canada*

Memory disturbances are the most common and ubiquitous of adult cognitive disorders. At one time the view prevailed that the most common cause was vascular. Although we no longer believe that narrowing of cerebral arteries leads to chronic cerebral ischemia, vascular etiologies continue to cause or contribute to a sizable proportion of memory disorders. Vascular problems are particularly important because some are treatable and many are preventable.

VASCULAR PROBLEMS AS A CAUSE OF MEMORY DISORDERS

Memory depends on so many brain interconnections that any major cerebral lesion is likely to affect it to some degree. However, pure memory disorders are most likely to arise from disruption of the components of the limbic system (1). The main mechanisms are listed in Table 1.

Ischemia

Global Ischemia

Caronna and Finkelstein (2) described a post–cardiac arrest amnesic syndrome characterized by severe anterograde amnesia, variably retrograde amnesia, and preservation of immediate and remote memory, resembling Korsakoff's syndrome. Twelve of their 16 patients recovered within 7–10 days and all recovered by a month. Presumably the disorder was caused by bilateral injury to the hippocampus, one of the areas of the brain essential for memory and susceptible to ischemia.

TABLE 1. *Vascular causes of amnesia*

Ischemic
  Global
    Cardiac arrest
  Focal
    Transient global amnesia
    Amnestic stroke
    Thalamic infarction
    Multi-infarct dementia
    ? Leukoaraiosis
Hemorrhagic
  Aneurysms, especially of the anterior communicating artery
  Arteriovenous malformations
  Intracerebral hemorrhage

Transient Global Amnesia

This is a well-recognized syndrome of sudden impairment of recent memory, lasting for hours. The etiology is probably multifactorial, although the leading cause is likely to be vascular because of the increased risk for stroke (3) and the observation that some patients have nystagmus, suggesting ischemia of the brainstem in the vertebrobasilar system, which also supplies the hippocampi, the presumed site of the memory disorder (4).

Amnesic Stroke

Bechterew (5) described a patient with severe memory loss whose autopsy years later showed infarction of both hippocampi and of the lingual, fusiform, and hippocampal gyri. Since that time, amnesia resulting from infarcts in the posterior circulation has become a well-recognized entity (6). What remains at issue is whether bilateral hippocampal damage is necessary to produce amnesia.

Thalamic Amnesia

Thalamic amnesia can result from bilateral or, occasionally, left thalamic infarction. Infarcts usually occur in the "polar" (anteriobasal) region of the thalamus irrigated by the polar artery, which usually arises from the middle of the posterior communicating artery and accounts for about two-thirds of the thalamic blood supply. If the polar artery is absent, its territory is taken over by the paramedian branches of the posterior communicating artery. The polar artery also supplies the hypothalamic nuclei, the columns of the fornix, and the caudal part of the mammillothalamic tract. Thalamic amnesia probably depends more on white matter than on nuclear lesions. Interruption of the ventral mammillothalamic tract disrupts the connection of the medio-dorsal nucleus and its neocortical projection sites, and damage to the ventral part of the lamina medullaris interna interferes with the amygdothalamic connections, all of which are important for memory (7).

Multi-infarct Dementia

Because multi-infarct dementia is the result of various lesions of diverse etiologies, the constellation of cognitive impairment is variable. Because most infarcts occur in the carotid circulation (8) and most memory disorders arise from lesions in the vertebrobasilar system, memory impairment is not as prominent nor as constant a feature as it is in other dementias, such as Alzheimer disease.

Leukoaraiosis

Although leukoaraiosis has been associated with the degree and progression of cognitive impairment (9,10) a clear relationship between white matter changes and memory disorders has not yet been established.

Hemorrhage

Berry Aneurysms

Rupture of a berry aneurysm, particularly of the anterior communicating artery, can lead to an amnestic syndrome (11).

Arteriovenous Malformations

Arteriovenous malformations can cause memory impairment either by direct involvement of memory related structures or by remote hemodynamic effects (12).

Intracerebral Hemorrhage

Spontaneous intracerebral hemorrhage due to hypertension, amyloid angiopathy, and other causes can cause amnestic syndromes similar to those produced by ischemia. Thalamic hemorrhages are a particularly well-recognized cause of amnestic problems.

TREATMENT AND PREVENTION OF VASCULAR MEMORY AND OTHER COGNITIVE DISORDERS

Until relatively recently, neurology was characterized by diagnostic precision and therapeutic helplessness. Neurologists were admired for their ability to localize lesions in the nervous system, to classify the disorder, and to attach an eponym to it. Despite the considerable advances in treatment and prevention, particularly in cerebrovascular disorders, some of this thinking persists. Historically, there was not much that could be done to treat or prevent stroke, so the emphasis in studying cognitive disorders was on the consequences and not the cause. There is rich literature in the description of type, subtypes, and variants of all types of cognitive disorders. By contrast, little has been written about the etiological classification of vascular cognitive disorders.

A further reflection of static taxonomic thinking is the concept of dementia. At the time when nothing could be done about any of the dementias, irreversibility was an important part of the definition. In addition, global intellectual impairment was originally considered to be a hallmark of this condition. Now we know that one or two strategically placed lesions can produce a clinical picture that may meet criteria for a dementing disorder. The problem with all definitions of dementia as applied to vascular disorders is that they emphasize a late stage in the evolution of these disorders, when the least can be done. It makes much more sense to consider vascular memory disorders along with other types of problems that arise from vascular causes and to provide a classification that emphasizes treatment and prevention, offering opportunities for clinical trials (Table 2). The most effective measures can be taken for high-risk individuals at the time when they have no cognitive impairment ("brain at risk" stage). When the patient has become symptom-

TABLE 2. *Treatment and prevention of vascular dementia*

Brain at risk stage
    The aged
    Hypertensives
    Smokers
    Diabetics
    Atrial fibrillators
    Cardiac patients
Predementia stage
    Patients with transient ischemic attack
    Patient with stroke
    Patient with subtle cognitive impairment
    Patient with silent cerebral infarctions
Dementia stage
    Cardiac embolism
    Atherosclerotic cerebrovascular disease
    Hypertensive cerebrovascular disease

TABLE 3. *Potential therapies for vascular dementia*

Brain at risk stage
  Smoking cessation
  Exercise (prevention and management of diabetes)
  Diet (control of diabetes, hyperlipidemias, obesity)
  K^+ supplementation (vascular protective effect)
  Antihypertensives (ACE inhibitors and Ca^{2+}-channel blockers may be particularly suitable)
  Lipid-lowering agents
  Anticoagulants (for atrial fibrillation)
  Aspirin (for selected patients at high risk)
Predementia stage
  Carotid endarterectomy (symptomatic patients with carotid stenosis of 70–99%)
  Anticoagulants
  Aspirin
  Ticlopidine
  Agents that interfere with amyloid deposition in vessels
  Ca^{2+}-channel blockers (pretreatment to attenuate effect of infarcts)
Dementia stage
  Antidepressants
  Antihypertensives
  Cholinergics
  Aspirin
  Ticlopidine

ACE, angiotensin-converting enzyme.

atic, with or without cognitive impairment, the opportunities for treatment and prevention are still considerable ("predementia" stage) and the least can be done when the patients manifest major cognitive problems ("dementia" stage). Even in this phase the mechanism of the cerebral lesions can be addressed, and measures can be taken to prevent further damage (Table 3). At each of these stages, certain therapeutic interventions are likely to be most applicable or effective. Table 3 lists some of these potential therapies.

CONCLUSION

Of all the causes of amnestic syndromes and vascular dementia, none are more amenable to treatment and prevention than those arising from vascular causes. Two conceptual barriers are hampering progress in these areas. One is the tendency to pigeonhole patients into categories that emphasize consequences and not causes. Which particular syndrome a patient presents with is less important than the underlying cause. A number of vascular mechanisms can now be treated or prevented from causing harm. A second problem is that by insisting on strict criteria for cognitive impairment the emphasis tends to be on patients identified at a late stage, when little can be done. We must try to escape our taxonomic prisons and to shift the emphasis from obscure vascular syndromes to broad etiologic categories and from late-stage thinking to early preventive therapy for those at high risk. Of the many measures now available to prevent cognitive and vascular damage to the brain, very few are being used systematically. It is time to act.

ACKNOWLEDGMENT

Dr. Vladimir Hachinski is a Career Investigator with the Heart and Stroke Foundation of Ontario.

REFERENCES

1. Mesulam M-M. *Principles of behavioral neurology*. Philadelphia: FA Davis, 1985.
2. Caronna JJ, Finklestein S. Neurological syndromes after cardiac arrest. *Stroke* 1978;9: 517–20.
3. Kushner MJ, Hauser WA. Transient global amnesia: a case-control study. *Ann Neurol* 1985;18:684–91.
4. Longridge NS, Hachinski VC, Barber HO. Brain-stem dysfunction in transient global amnesia. *Stroke* 1979;10:473–4.
5. Bechterew WWV. Demonstation eines Gehirns mit Zerstörung de vorderen und inneren Thiele der Hirnrinde beider Schlafenlappen. *Neurol Zentbl* 1990;19:990–1.
6. Benson DF, Marsden CD, Meadows JC. The amnesic syndrome of posterior cerebral artery occlusion. *Acta Neurol Scand* 1974;50:133–45.
7. von Cramon DY, Hebel N, Schuri U. A contribution to the anatomical basis of thalamic amnesia. *Brain* 1985;108:993–1008.
8. Hachinski VC, Norris JW. *The Acute Stroke*. Philadelphia: FA Davis, 1985.
9. Mirsen TR, Lee DH, Wong CJ, et al. Clinical correlates of white-matter changes on magnetic resonance imaging scans of the brain. *Arch Neurol* 1991;48:1015–21.
10. Diaz JF, Merskey H, Hachinski VC, et al. Improved recognition of leukoaraiosis and cognitive impairment in Alzheimer's disease. *Arch Neurol* 1991;48:1022–5.
11. Alexander MP, Freedman M. Amnesia after anterior communicating artery aneurysm rupture. *Neurology* 1984;34:752–7.
12. Hachinski VC, Norris JW, Cooper PW, Marshall J. Symptomatic intracranial steal. *Arch Neurol* 1977;34:149–53.

Guidelines for Drug Trials in Memory Disorders, edited by N. Canal, et al.
Raven Press, Ltd., New York © 1993.

6

Traumatic Brain Injury

Andres M. Salazar and *Jordan H. Grafman

*Department of Neurology, Uniformed Services University of the Health Sciences,
Bethesda, Maryland 20814-4799; and *Cognitive Neuroscience Section, Medical
Neurology Branch, National Institute for Nervous Disorders and Stroke,
Bethesda, Maryland 20892*

Traumatic brain injury (TBI) is the leading cause of death and disability in young adult Americans today (1). The incidence of TBI requiring hospitalization is about 200/100,000; each year, about 75,000 persons die and another 75,000 are permanently disabled. Largely because it affects the young and can result in a lifetime loss of earnings, the total economic cost of TBI in America has been estimated at over $25 billion per year. Although TBI is not commonly thought of in the context of Alzheimer dementia, the two conditions do share some common ground. In particular, there may be an etiologic link between some forms of progressive dementia and repeated TBI, and both can result in cognitive and especially memory disorders (2,3). Obvious differences include the relative youth of the TBI population, the multiplicity of pathologic findings in TBI, and the dynamic nature of TBI, with its nadir in the first few days after injury and a natural history of improvement or compensation.

We would like to emphasize a number of underlying themes in the following discussion of TBI, particularly in relation to the insights that a study of this problem can give us for the design of drug trials for Alzheimer disease (AD). First, it must be recognized that TBI represents a spectrum of disorders with regard to the mechanism of injury (penetrating vs. closed head injury), the severity of injury, and the pathology (see below). This chapter will generally be referring to moderate and moderately severe uncomplicated closed head injury, for which a relatively consistent cognitive and behavioral syndrome can be described and which is probably most relevant to the subject at hand. Second, TBI is a dynamic process. The acute evolution of secondary cell injury and brain swelling in the first hours after trauma offers a therapeutic window of opportunity that is the subject of intense study and rapid development in the field at present. After the acute stage, the natural history of TBI is one of recovery, often to a remarkable degree in young adults. This natural compensation stresses the importance of proper controlled study design in the evaluation of post-acute pharmacologic or rehabilitation treatments, studies that have been sadly lacking in TBI. Third, it is important to remember that in TBI, as in AD, "outcome" is a summation of a variety of factors, including not only physical and cognitive recovery but also behavioral and psychosocial reintegration. It is misleading, for example, to emphasize improvement in memory function at the expense of behavior change. In most societies, successful return to gainful employment may be one of the best single measurements of outcome after TBI, but this may not be practical in the older AD population. Fourth, preinjury status is a major determinant of final outcome after TBI; this has been reemphasized in a recent study showing that preinjury intelligence was the single most important determinant of cognitive performance in a large cohort of head-injured Vietnam veterans (4). Finally, unlike AD, the cause of TBI is known, and prevention remains the simplest and most powerful "therapeutic" option.

This chapter briefly reviews our current understanding of the pathogenesis of TBI, with some comments on current experimental treatment. It also discusses the cognitive and psychosocial outcome after head injury and the potential relevance of the TBI experience to the design and selection of end points in therapeutic drug trials for degenerative brain disease, particularly AD.

CLOSED HEAD INJURY PATHOGENESIS

Given that TBI results in a spectrum of pathologies, all of which can affect the outcome, it is relevant to review briefly our current understanding of the various components. Over the past decades we have moved from conceptualizing the pathology of closed head injury (CHI) in terms of hematomas and "coup–contrecoup" contusions to a four-component classification (5). Three parallel components were initially identified: focal injury, diffuse axonal injury (DAI), and superimposed hypoxia/ischemia. More recently (4), diffuse microvascular injury with loss of autoregulation has been implicated as playing an important role in the acute stage of moderate and severe head injury. All of these pathologic features have been reproduced in animal models of angular acceleration without impact. With the possible exception of diffuse axon injury, all are also features of penetrating head injury (PHI) (6)

Focal Injury

Focal tissue disruption, swelling, contusions, or hematomas at the site of impact or penetration result in focal cortical neurologic deficits referable to that area (e.g., aphasia, hemiparesis), but by far the most common location for contusions after acceleration injury is in the orbitofrontal and anterior temporal lobes, where the brain lies next to bony edges. Therefore, a relatively typical pathologic picture is seen in most CHI, and among its most troubling clinical sequelae are attention, memory, and behavior abnormalities which may be referable to the frontal and temporal lobe injury. Subdural hematomas are most common with rapid decelerations such as occur with impact after a fall, especially in the aged, and are usually due to rupture of bridging veins; they appear to be much less common after penetrating head injury. Recent studies suggest that delays longer than 4 h in the surgical management of hematomas significantly worsen the prognosis. Delayed hematomas, as well as bleeding into contusions, are particularly important in the so-called "talk and die" patient, who may initially appear to be at low risk but then deteriorates unexpectedly (7).

Another important aspect of hematoma or free blood in the brain relates to delayed cell injury and the role played by iron in the metabolism of the oxygen free radical and the process of lipid peroxidation (see below). The demonstrated relationship of hematomas and free iron to posttraumatic epilepsy may also be related to the production of oxygen free radicals (8).

Diffuse Axon Injury

DAI is one of the most important causes of prolonged coma and persistent severe neurologic deficit in CHI. Originally described as a "shearing" injury of axons, it was characterized by axon "retraction" balls microscopically in the hemispheric white matter, corpus callosum, and brainstem (9,10) Recent work with mild to moderate fluid-percussion injury in animal models, however, shows that the typical light microscopic histopathology of DAI showing axon shear may not emerge until 12–24 h after injury. The only early abnormality is a relatively subtle focal intraaxon disruption seen on electron microscopy, with an intact axon sheath. This leads to a disturbance of axon flow, accumulation of transport material with axon ballooning proximal to the injury, and eventually delayed severing of axons 12–24 h later (11,12). The role of alterations in calcium metabolism at the injured site on the axon may be particularly important. One obvious clinical implication of these findings is that that there may be a potential 12–24 h window of therapeutic opportunity after injury during which treatment may prevent total axon disruption. Another important conclusion is that DAI can be demonstrated after even "minor" head injury, even in the absence of morphopathologic change in any other vascular, neural, or glial elements. This confirms earlier uncontrolled pathologic studies in humans and makes such axon damage a possible organic basis for the "post-concussion syndrome" and perhaps for the cumulative effects of repeated concussion, as seen in some boxers (13).

Interestingly, the major feature of the pathology of dementia pugilistica is the presence of neurofibrillary tangles (NFTs). NFTs in AD and in other conditions such as Guam amyotrophic lateral sclerosis (ALS) have been postulated to result from abnormalities in axon flow, in the latter case probably related to aberrant calcium metabolism (14). Similarly, although classic Alzheimer plaques are not seen in this condition, recent studies have shown plaque-like structures which stain with monoclonal antibody to the β-amyloid precursor protein (APP), both chronically in boxers and acutely after severe head injury (15–17). It is unknown whether repeated trauma might alter the secretion, metabolism, or structure of the APP in such a way as to lead to plaque and NFT formation or whether the oxygen free radical or lipid peroxidation (see below) may play a role in this process.

Hypoxia–Ischemia

The classic pathology of hypoxia–ischemia, involving mainly the hippocampus and the vascular border zones of the brain, is frequently superimposed on the other pathologic features that are more specific for TBI. The traumatized brain is particularly sensitive to hypoxia–ischemia, and the relationship is probably more than merely additive (18). When present, such pathology, including the concomitant hippocampal necrosis, can obviously become a major determinant of ultimate clinical outcome, particularly with regard to posttraumatic memory disorders. Recent improvements in the survival of the TBI patient have largely resulted from recognition of the importance of this component and its prevention, especially through the development of emergency resuscitation and transport systems.

Microvascular Change

Diffuse microvascular damage has also been recently implicated as a major component of both closed and penetrating TBI. Depending on the severity of the trauma, early physiologic changes include an early loss of cerebrovascular autoregulation, with a decreased response to changes in CO_2 and perfusion pressure, and an initial transient systemic hypertension (probably related to release of catecholamines) (19,20). The loss of autoregulation makes the brain particularly susceptible to fluctuations in systemic blood pressure. For example, systemic hypertension can increase the risk of vascular dilatation with hyperemia and brain swelling, or otherwise tolerable hypotension can result in ischemic damage. In addition, altered vascular sensitivity to circulating catecholamines or acetylcholine can lead to vasoconstriction and further focal ischemia or reperfusion injury ("no-reflow" phenomenon).

The pathology appears to be biphasic, with an early, transient alteration of the blood–brain barrier (BBB), and a more delayed (>6 h) endothelial change (21,22). Diffuse perivascular damage with astrocyte footplate swelling is a prominent feature at both the light and the electron microscopic level within minutes after high-velocity gunshot wounds and after acceleration injury in nonhuman primates. The basic cause of this swelling was initially thought to be a break in the endothelial BBB, but recent studies have demonstrated an increased pinocytotic transfer of horseradish peroxidase marker with intact endothelial tight junctions (23). The astrocyte swelling is usually maximal at 30–60 min and is much reduced by 6 h after injury; it is thought to represent an initial reaction to the altered transport across the BBB. It should be emphasized, however, that the classic concept of BBB breakdown and cerebral edema after TBI is undergoing radical revision, particularly in the absence of evidence for increased brain water after either uncomplicated PHI or CHI (24). Cerebral edema per se may become more of a factor when hypoxia and/or ischemia complicate the injury.

The second microvascular phase is one of endothelial change, including formation of intraluminal microvilli or blebs, which then break to form endothelial craters. This peaks at about 6 h after injury but usually persists as long as 6 days. Although the clinical significance of these changes is still not known, they are probably related to the altered microvascular sensitivity to circulating neurotransmitters, to the loss of autoregulation, and perhaps to secondary brain swelling.

Recent studies have shown an associated loss or inhibition of various endothelial hormones, including endothelium derived relaxing factor (EDRF). EDRF was first described almost a decade ago and has recently been identified as nitric oxide (25). Inhibition of EDRF may be responsible for prolonged vasoconstriction and perhaps the so-called "no-reflow" phenomenon leading to secondary focal ischemia, whereas loss of other factors may have the opposite effect. One of the principal inhibitors of EDRF in TBI appears to be the superoxide radical, which has also been shown to have a vasoconstrictive effect in experimental models (26,27). Importantly, application of free radical generators (such as xanthine–xanthine oxidase) to the intact pial surface of nontraumatized animals reproduces endothelial blebs and craters that are very similar to those seen after TBI (28,29). Superoxide dismutase (more so than indomethacin, catalase, or mannitol) prevents or reverses this vascular hyperreactivity under experimental conditions, suggesting that the vasoconstrictive effect is mediated by the superoxide radical itself.

SECONDARY TISSUE INJURY

The picture of a TBI patient who is initially relatively stable and awake or in light coma and then deteriorates and dies is all too common. Although some of these cases represent delayed hematoma amenable to surgery, most are probably related to an uncontrolled brain swelling that does not respond to conventional management. Over the past decade, delayed secondary in-

TABLE 1. *Traumatic brain injury–contrast with Alzheimer dementia*

Young population
Relatively focal frontotemporal injury
Dynamic process with its nadir in first days after injury
Natural history of improvement/compensation
Multifactorial determinants of outcome
Potential etiologic link

jury at the cellular level has been recognized as a major contributor to this phenomenon and to the ultimate tissue loss after TBI. Understanding of the pathogenesis of secondary injury is therefore particularly important to the management of the head-injured patient. As suggested above, a cascade of biochemical and physiologic events is set into motion in injured tissue. This includes changes in arachidonic acid metabolites such as the prostaglandins and the leukotrienes (30), the formation of oxygen free radicals (19), changes in neuropeptides (31), in electrolytes such as calcium and magnesium (32), in neurotransmitters such as glutamate and acetylcholine (33,34), in lactic acid (35), in various kinins, and the appearance of a leukocyte response with release of lymphokines such as interleukin-1 (Table 1) (36). These products can cause progressive secondary injury to otherwise viable brain tissue through a number of mechanisms [e.g., by altering vascular reactivity and producing further ischemia, by producing brain swelling (hyperemia and/or edema), by injuring neurons and glia directly or activating macrophages that result in such injury, or by establishing conditions favorable to secondary infection]. In other words, much of the ultimate brain loss after PHI may be due not to the injury itself but to an uncontrolled vicious cycle of biochemical events set into motion by the trauma.

Oxygen Free Radicals and Lipid Peroxidation

Perhaps the most important cause of cell injury in TBI involves oxygen free radicals. These are produced early in ischemic and traumatic tissue injury, both in the central nervous system (CNS) and elsewhere (19,37,38). The superoxide radical (O_2^*) is formed through a variety of mechanisms, including normal mitochondrial respiration, the xanthine oxidase and arachidonic acid pathways, and by activated leukocytes (Fig. 1). Receptor-mediated phospholipase activation may play an important role in the initial release of arachidonic acid after both trauma and ischemia.

The superoxide radical causes tissue injury in its own right through its effect on the microvasculature. However, when combined in the presence of free iron with its own metabolite, hydrogen peroxide, it forms the hydroxyl radical (OH*). This reacts with the abundant lipids in brain in the process of lipid peroxidation, with further release of arachidonic acid and a vicious

Traumatic Brain Injury

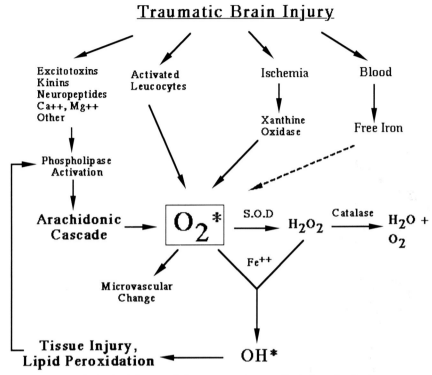

FIG. 1. Traumatic brain injury and the oxygen free radical: hypothetical sequence of events. O2*, oxygen free radical; OH*, hydroxyl radical; SOD, superoxide dismutase.

cycle in which more free radicals are produced through the cyclooxygenase pathway (along with prostaglandins), overwhelming natural free radical-scavenging mechanisms. Recent clinical studies in severely head-injured patients have confirmed a fourfold rise in jugular venous thiobarbarbituric acid-reactive substance (TBRS, a lipid peroxidation marker) as early as 2 h after injury and lasting at least 5 days. This confirms the ongoing nature of delayed secondary cell injury in the postacute period, as well as the possibility that the postinjury "therapeutic window of opportunity" may be considerably longer than has previously been believed. Furthermore, TBRS was shown to correlate with $AVDO_2$, a commonly used marker of cerebral blood flow after head injury (39).

Two mechanisms in particular may account for the destructiveness of free radicals in brain. Given the abundance of lipids in brain cells, the self-perpetuating process of lipid peroxidation, along with the concomitant inflammatory response that it invokes, probably plays an important role in secondary injury (40). In addition, the effect of oxygen free radicals on the microvasculature, as discussed above, may play a crucial role on the loss of autoregulation. This, in turn, may lead to hyperemic brain swelling, with the uncontrolled rise in intracranial pressure that is associated with most fatal cases, or to vasoconstriction with "reperfusion" injury and subsequent infarction.

Pharmacologic intervention to reduce the formation of free radicals and/or to scavenge those already formed would therefore be expected to reduce ultimate tissue injury. Animal models have confirmed this potential benefit in several systems. Because free radicals are formed through a number of biochemical pathways, a variety of drugs or drug combinations may be useful to control them. These include steroids to inhibit lipid peroxidation and the release of arachidonate (megadose methylprednisolone and especially the nonglucocorticoid 21-aminosteroids or "lazaroids") (41); α-tocopherol (vitamin E) and its analogues (42,43); cyclooxygenase inhibitors to block prostaglandin formation; xanthine oxidase inhibitors such as allopurinol (44,45); iron chelators such as desferroxamine (46); enzymes such as superoxide dismutase and catalase (29,47); and various other free radical scavengers such as mannitol and dimethyl sulfoxide (DMSO).

Superoxide dismutase (SOD) may be a particularly attractive form of therapy, since it scavenges all superoxide radicals regardless of their source. A beneficial effect of SOD has been shown in myocardial ischemia, kidney ischemia (48,49), cerebral ischemia, and cerebral trauma (50). CNS closed head-injury models have also demonstrated a beneficial effect of SOD in controlling the trauma-associated microvascular injury (29). In a particularly relevant model that used intracranial balloons in dogs to mimic subdural hematoma, SOD in doses equivalent to those being used in current clinical pilot trials practically eliminated BBB breakdown and postdecompression pathologic change when compared with conventional therapies, and decreased mortality from 80% to zero (47). Clinical pilot studies are now under way with bovine SOD conjugated to polyethylene glycol (PEG–SOD) as well as recombinant human SOD (r-hSOD) in severely head-injured patients. Preliminary results suggest a marked improvement in useful survival for PEG–SOD-treated patients, but final conclusions must await a larger controlled study (50a).

OUTCOME

A surprisingly good overall outcome can be seen in many young, moderately to severely injured patients, a finding that probably reflects compensation for lost functions more than recovery of the injured tissue itself. Thus, "floating" or dynamic end points can be identified in the post-TBI course: resolution of coma, return to orientation, resolution of posttraumatic amnesia, resolution and duration of retrograde amnesia, number of significant deficits identified on initial neuropsychological testing, number of significant deficits identified on the last neuropsychological evaluation, and the steep-

TABLE 2. *Elements of outcome after TBI*

Preinjury status
Neurologic
Motor, visual fields, epilepsy
Cognitive
Attention, memory, language
Behavioral
Fatigue, apathy, aggression, violence
Psychosocial
Activities of daily living, employment, community adjustment, social cognition

ness of the recovery slopes. Nevertheless, an important milestone yet to be reached in the TBI field is the development of reproducible, universally accepted measurements of function and long-term outcome with which to compare the value of various interventions (1). As suggested above, final outcome is a composite of a number of elements, including preinjury, neurologic, cognitive, behavioral, and psychosocial function, all of which may interact differently in each individual patient (Table 2). When the efficacy of a given therapy is evaluated, it is necessary to study all of these elements in the context of outcome as a whole; any evaluation battery should therefore include at least some measurement of each. It is misleading, for example, to use improvement in a particular overlearned memory task as a measurement of outcome. On the other hand, one must maintain some level of flexibility of end points between TBI therapeutic trials; that is, one must be prepared to learn from each trial and to modify end points appropriately for the next.

Although there may not be any ideal surrogate or summary measurement of outcome, return to gainful employment may be a useful one in most TBI populations. We have had the opportunity to study the disabilities which impact on return to work in a large cohort ($n = 520$) of head-injured Vietnam veterans. A 1-week, standardized multidisciplinary outcome evaluation was completed on each of them. Some 15 years after injury, 56% of these men were gainfully employed compared with 82% of an uninjured Vietnam veteran control group (51). The occupational distribution of those who were working was essentially no different from that of normal uninjured young American males (52). After exclusion of severe aphasic or triplegic patients, none of whom worked, a multistage statistical analysis of these data, including factor and multiple logistic regression analyses, identified seven specifically defined disabilities that significantly affected the ability to return to work. These were posttraumatic epilepsy, hemiparesis, visual field loss, verbal memory loss, visual memory loss, psychological problems, and violent behavior. Interestingly, these seven items were found to be relatively equipotent, so that a simple sum of any of them could yield a "disability score" that predicted return to work (Fig. 2). Patients were able to compensate relatively well for up to three of these impairments in any combination, but

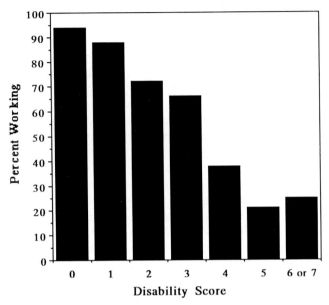

FIG. 2. Vietnam Head Injury Study: employment rates some 15 years after penetrating head injury in relation to disability score (see text).

beyond that there was a sharp drop in work rates. Other factors that contributed significantly to return to work included preinjury intelligence, total brain volume loss on computed tomography scan, and education after injury. This experience is a further reminder of the importance of considering outcome as dependent on a set of functional skills, rather than identifying one or two disabilities as the only target of experimental therapies. It also suggests that, in the absence of a single summary outcome measurement for the AD population (such as employment), it may be useful for therapeutic studies to construct a composite score that reflects various functional domains in that group.

Cognitive and Behavioral Aspects of Outcome: Attention, Memory, and Personality

Given the mix of pathologies that could affect outcome in TBI, it may seem surprising that a relatively typical syndrome of cognitive and behavioral change can be described. Although some TBI patients may present striking deficits in language, perception, and visuospatial processing, the more typical picture post-TBI emphasizes deficits in memory, attention, personality, and social cognition.

Memory problems include a rather striking deficit in explicit retrieval of new information presented after injury (posttraumatic amnesia), along with a more modest period of retrograde amnesia for events preceding the injury (53). However, immediate recall and older memories are usually intact, as are implicit or automatic memory processes. The deficit therefore appears to be primarily in the "consolidation" of new episodic memory. These memory problems are usually accompanied by slowed information processing (slowed reaction times), an attentional deficit, and an impaired ability to divide cognitive resources. Related to this is a deficit in concept formation with an inability to shift mental set, manifested by perseveration on tasks such as the Wisconsin Card Sorting (WCS) test.

Perhaps the most impressive problem (usually reported by family members) is a change in mood and personality (54,55). The patient may be disinhibited, behave irrationally, have mood swings, ignore social convention, and not care about the future consequences of current actions. A few may also manifest aggressive or even violent behavior for months or years after the injury. This aggressive behavior can be either directed or nondirected, and may be accompanied by an often explosive autonomic and emotional response. Some of these "episodic discontrol" events are believed to represent a subtle form of temporal lobe epilepsy, particularly because they often appear to respond to anticonvulsant drugs such as carbamazepine.

The most likely neuropathologic basis for these behavior disorders seems to be damage to the prefrontal cortex, including the orbitofrontal region. Damage to the temporal lobes (especially the hippocampus) may be responsible for the anterograde and retrograde amnesia. In addition, damage to the basal forebrain (BFB) in the proximal orbitofrontal lobe may contribute to the episodic memory deficit as well to the slowed reaction times and attention deficits. In our long-term study of head injured Vietnam war veterans, we have found that BFB-injured men differed from their non–BFB-injured matches only in having a longer loss of consciousness after injury, episodic memory deficits, and poorer performance on the WCS test (56,57). The basal forebrain lesions alone, however, were not sufficient to produce dementia. The role of diffuse axon injury in the genesis of traumatic memory disorders is less clear; it is probably most relevant to the long-term residual cognitive deficits seen in more severely injured patients.

Neuropsychological Assessment

The neuropsychological assessment of TBI can begin at a very early stage. The Galveston Orientation and Amnesia Test (GOAT) can be used with the disoriented patient and is designed for repeated administration (53). It enables the investigator to evaluate the duration and severity of posttraumatic amnesia as well as the duration of retrograde amnesia. A more detailed retrograde amnesia test can supplement the GOAT. Other tests that make minimal demands on the patient, such as simple and choice reaction time tasks, picture naming, verbal fluency, and letter cancellation can aid the investigator in establishing the acute recovery slope and determining when more extensive neuropsychological testing can be attempted.

The more formal neuropsychological evaluation should incorporate standard clinical measures such as the Wechsler Adult Intelligence Scale-Revised, Wechsler Memory Scale-Revised, and the neurobehavioral rating scale. Other more experimental tests of memory, attention, personality, and social cognition are used in TBI, but none have emerged as specific for TBI, and a full review is beyond the scope of this chapter. The specific battery used in a given hospital is often dependent on the particular interests of the attending neuropsychologist (53,58).

TBI patients are usually evaluated at least three times in the postacute recovery period. To chart the slope of cognitive recovery, it is important to include some repeatable tests in the evaluation that are relatively resistant to test–retest or "practice" artifact. Repeatable tests may be clinical tests that have different versions equated for difficulty, or information processing tests on which stimuli can be randomly selected for presentation and the dependent measure reflects the subject strategy rather than the particular stimuli used. Examples are various versions of the selective reminding test and of choice reaction-time tests.

Long-term recovery is usually assessed by evaluating the rate of improvement, preferably with at least three testing points and over at least 1 year after injury. In addition to the neuropsychological measures, other indices of recovery, such as functional independence in activities of daily living, employability, school performance, family and community adjustment, and other social functions, become more important at this stage.

In addition to the clinical utility of neuropsychological evaluations in conjunction with drug studies, the study of TBI patients may provide insights into basic mechanisms of attention, memory, and social cognition. For example, acute retrograde amnesias can be ideally studied in TBI, and the frequency of frontal lobe injury also makes TBI a good population to study executive function deficits. Modern brain-imaging techniques lend a particularly exciting structure-function dimension to such studies.

Postacute Management of the TBI Patient: Rehabilitation

One of the most encouraging aspects of TBI rehabilitation is the amazing ability of the young adult brain to compensate naturally for many aspects of injury. Over the past two decades, however, we have come to realize that most TBI patients would also benefit from some level of TBI-specific rehabilitation. The field of TBI rehabilitation has grown exponentially over this time, but the exact form and intensity of rehabilitation indicated for a given patient remains hotly debated. Multiple therapeutic strategies, including coma stimulation, reality orientation, cognitive therapy, speech therapy, occupational therapy, recreation therapy, and music therapy, have been applied to the TBI patient. Although selected elements of many of these will undoubtedly prove useful in the TBI setting, there has been a paucity of scientific validation for these sometimes expensive interventions (including comparison with minimal-care supportive models). If progress is to be made in this area, rehabilitation modalities must be subject to the same scrutiny for indications, dosage, duration of treatment, and efficacy as are other medical treatments, including drugs. As in AD, the ultimate goal of therapy should be the independence and community reintegration of the patient within his or her limits, rather than the specialized treatment of specific deficits simply because they are there. All too often, scarce resources available to the patient are used up in the early acute and postacute phases on evaluation and therapy of deficits that will improve anyway or which are relatively unimportant to the ultimate goal of independence. Some programs may be actually counterproductive by fostering continued dependence. Relatively cost-effective interventions such as training in specific community reintegration skills (e.g., decision making) and certain forms of behavior modification may end up being omitted because the limited funds available were used up in earlier less relevant therapies.

Although cognitive rehabilitation has yet to fulfill its promise by submitting to careful group and case-series analyses, the reality is that most TBI patients will receive some form of cognitive rehabilitation during their postinjury course. In fact, some drug therapies may potentially be most effective when used in conjunction with cognitive remediation programs. Therefore, the possibility of rehabilitation–drug interactions when drug effects on independent variables are evaluated must be addressed in pharmacologic studies by, at a minimum, categorizing the type, frequency, and duration of remediation. More sophisticated studies can adopt both therapy and agent as dependent factors.

Pharmacologic Intervention

The pharmacologic management of TBI patients is yet in its infancy, and has been concentrated mostly on symptomatic management of the behavioral changes, particularly agitation and aggression (Table 3). Even that remains controversial, and behavior control is often best achieved through nonpharmacologic intervention. In theory, cholinergic, noradrenergic, and dopaminergic drugs tend to activate or increase aggression in TBI patients, whereas serotoninergic (fluoxetine, trazadone) and GABA-ergic (benzodiazepines, valproate) drugs tend to decrease it. In practice, however, pharmacologic management of symptoms in a given individual remains largely empirical.

TABLE 3. *Postacute drug treatment of head injuries*

Behavioral disorders	Cognition
Carbamazepine (episodic dyscontrol)	Cholinergic drugs
Propranolol, lithium	Physostigmine/lecithin, others
Sedating antidepressants (amitriptyline)	Amphetamines/methylphenidate
Activating antidepressants (fluoxetine)	Gangliosides
Bromocriptine, amantadine	Others
Others	

Among other drugs used to control aggression and agitation are lithium, tricyclic antidepressants, β-adrenergic blockers such as propranolol, and buspirone. "Activating" antidepressants such as amantadine, bromocriptine, desipramine, and fluoxetine may be useful in patients who are generally underaroused with only occasional episodes of agitation. Antipsychotics such as haloperidol should be used sparingly in TBI patients because of their potential adverse effect on cognitive recovery (59).

One intriguing facet of the problem of aggression is the phenomenon of episodic dyscontrol, in which the patient manifests periods of explosive and irrational aggression, often followed by remorse or amnesia. This condition often responds effectively to phenytoin or carbamazepine, but its potential relationship to temporal lobe epilepsy remains hotly debated, especially in the absence of other ictal or electroencephalographic (EEG) abnormalities.

Recent unconfirmed clinical and animal studies have suggested that the combination of dextroamphetamine with physical therapy in the early phases of rehabilitation can permanently improve ultimate motor scores, whereas the use of other agents such as haloperidol will inhibit recovery (59–61). The most interesting features of these findings are that it is the combination of the two modalities that is crucial for the effect, that it is not merely an additive phenomenon, and that the intervention must be made soon after injury. It is unknown whether such a combined effect might also occur in the cognitive arena, although anecdotal reports suggest a positive effect of methylphenidate and amphetamine on attention and cognition in TBI survivors (62). Similarly, involvement of the basal forebrain region in TBI patients suggests that, as in AD, their memory deficits may be particularly aggravated by medication with an anticholinergic effect, such as amytriptyline, or benefited by cholinergic drugs. However, preliminary trials have not demonstrated a significant benefit for physostigmine/lecithin treatment (63). In addition, cholinergic agents may actually aggravate the behavior problem by increasing aggression. These studies in TBI also suggest that a similar strategy, combining pharmacologic stimulation with memory training, could also be of use in the AD population. In any case, these findings have given new life to the study of the role of neurotransmitters in structural neural recovery.

"MILD" HEAD INJURY

One group of patients that has been frequently mismanaged in the past is that with so-called "mild" head injury. As noted above, however, not only has diffuse axon damage been demonstrated in animal models of concussion but magnetic resonance imaging (MRI), positron emission tomography (PET), and power-spectral EEG have repeatedly shown structural, metabolic, and functional changes in humans with "mild" head injury. The most important element in the management of these cases is the recognition that there is usually an organic, pathologic basis for their complaints, at least in the early postinjury period, and that it usually resolves over a few months. If mishandled, however, these patients often develop an overlying neurosis which makes evaluation and management infinitely more difficult. There is nothing more frustrating to the intelligent minor head injury victim than to be told by his physician, his family, and his employer that there is "nothing wrong." Proper counseling should therefore include not only the patient but also the family, school, or employer. MRI and specialized electrophysiologic and specific neuropsychologic tests, such as choice reaction time early in the course, can help to delineate the deficits (58,64,65). One important research challenge in this area is better defining the anatomic, physiologic, and behavioral criteria for recognizing and measuring the severity of minor head injury.

The basic elements of the postconcussion syndrome are cognitive, somatic, and affective. Clinically significant neuropsychological impairments have been documented repeatedly even after minor "dings" without loss of consciousness (66). The most frequent somatic complaints in one large recent study were headache (71%), decreased energy or "fatigue" (60%), and dizziness (53%); these had all markedly improved at three months (67). The proper management of the "fatigue" element (which may relate to orbitofrontal injury) is a major factor in recovery, and requires the cooperation of the school or employer (68). We suggest a graded return to full work load over a period of 4–8 weeks.

SUMMARY

We live in exciting times for the field of TBI. Our understanding of the complex pathogenesis of acute TBI, of the pivotal role played by delayed secondary brain injury and of its cellular basis has been growing exponentially over the past two decades. Although present management remains essentially symptomatic and empirical, the lessons of the laboratory are beginning to find their way into the clinic, to include the realization of the importance of early, intensive medical management in severe cases. The aggressive management of acute hypoxia and shock and of elevated intracranial pressure has been one of the most significant recent clinical advances. Among the more promising medical therapies now entering clinical trials are the management of nutrition and metabolism, the control of lipid peroxidation with 21-amino steroids, and the control of oxygen free radicals with SOD.

By the same token, the postacute management and rehabilitation of the TBI patient are undergoing rapid change. We have come to understand that most TBI patients have a relatively reproducible syndrome of neurological, attention, memory, and behavior deficits, all of which contribute to final outcome, and that it is usually inappropriate to rehabilitate them in settings developed for stroke, dementia, mental retardation, or psychiatric illness. Nevertheless, the intense debate over the exact nature and intensity of TBI rehabilitation required for an individual patient will be resolved only with properly controlled randomized studies that consider the multiple facets of outcome in their design. One useful summary measurement in the TBI population is return to gainful employment. For the older AD population, other less stringent measurements of functional independence must be found or composite measurements must be constructed.

A potential etiologic link between TBI and AD is suggested by the entity of dementia pugilistica as well as by some epidemiologic studies, and the study of the pathogenesis of TBI may yet hold some clues for AD. Yet, on a more immediately practical level, they have in common certain elements of attention, memory, and behavior symptoms that may be amenable to similar pharmacologic interventions. Although their long-term natural histories differ, the design of experimental therapeutic studies in both conditions is also likely to overlap considerably.

REFERENCES

1. HHS. Interagency Head Injury Task Force Report. Washington, DC: Department of Health and Human Services; 1989.
2. Mortimer J, van Duijn C, Chandra V, et al. Head trauma as a risk factor for Alzheimers disease: a collaborative reanalysis of case-control studies. *Int J Epidemiol* 1991;20:S28.
3. Corkin S, Rosen J, EV S, Clegg R. Penetrating head injury in young adulthood exacerbates cognitive decline in later years. *J Neurosci* 1989;9:3876–83.
4. Grafman J, Jonas B, Martin A, et al. Intellectual function following penetrating head injury in Vietnam veterans. *Brain* 1988;111:169–84.
5. Hume Adams J, Graham DI, Gennarelli TA. Contemporary neuropathological considerations regarding brain damage in head injury. In: Becker DP, Povlishock JT, eds. *Central nervous system trauma status report.* Bethesda, MD: NINCDS, NIH;1985:65–77.
6. Gennarelli T, Thibault L. Biological models of head injury. In: Becker D, Povlishock J, eds. *Central nervous system trauma status report—1985.* Bethesda, MD: NINDS, NIH; 1985:391–404.
7. Marshall L, Toole B, Bowers S. The National Traumatic Coma Data Bank, Part II. Patients who talk and deteriorate: implications for treatment. *J Neurosurg* 1983;59:285–8.
8. Willmore L. Post-traumatic epilepsy: cellular mechanism and implications for treatment. *Epilepsia* 1990;31(suppl 3):S67–73.
9. Strich S. The pathology of brain damage due to blunt head injuries. In: Walker A, Caveness

W, Critchley M, eds. *The late effects of head injury*. Springfield, IL: Charles C Thomas; 1969:501–26.

10. Gennarelli T, Thibault L, Adams J, Graham D, Thompson C, Marcincin R. Diffuse axonal injury and traumatic coma in the primate. *Ann Neurol* 1982;12:564–74.

11. Povlishock J. The morphopathologic responses to head injuries of varying severity. In: Becker D, Povlishock J, eds. *Central nervous system trauma status report*. Washington, DC: NINCDS, NIH;1985:443–52.

12. Povlishock J, Coburn T. Morphopathological change associated with mild head injury. In: Levin H, Eisenberg H, Benton A, eds. *Mild head injury*. New York: Oxford University Press; 1989:37–53.

13. Oppenheimer D. Microscopic lesions in the brain following head injury. *J Neurol Neurosurg Psychiatry* 1968;31:299–306.

14. Gajdusek D. Hypothesis: interference with axonal transport of neurofilament as a common pathogenetic mechanism in certain diseases of the central nervous system. *N Engl J Med* 1985;312:714–9.

15. Roberts G, Allsop D, Burton C. The occult aftermath of boxing. *J Neurol Neurosurg Psychiatry* 1990;53:373–8.

16. Clinton J, Ambler M, Roberts G. Post-traumatic Alzheimer's disease: preponderance of a single plaque type. *Neuropathol Appl Neurobiol* 1991;17:69–74.

17. Roberts G, Gentleman S, Lynch A, Graham D. Beta A4 amyloid protein deposition in brain after head trauma. *Lancet* 1991;338:1422–3.

18. Ishige N, Pitts L, Hashimoto T, Nishimura B, Bartkowski H. Effect of hypoxia on traumatic brain injury in rats: Part 1. *Neurosurgery* 1987;30:848–54.

19. Kontos H, Wei E. Superoxide production in experimental brain injury. *J Neurosurg* 1986; 64:803–7.

20. Proctor H, Palladdino G, Fillipo D. Failure of autoregulation after closed head injury: an experimental model. *J Trauma* 1988;28:347–52.

21. Maxwell W, Irvine A, Adams J, Graham D, Gennarelli T. Response of cerebral microvasculature to brain injury. *J Pathol* 1988;155:327–35.

22. Allen I, Kirk J, Maynard R, Cooper G, Scott R, Crockard A. An ultrastructural study of experimental high velocity penetrating head injury. *Acta Neuropathol* 1983;59:277–82.

23. Povlishock J. Experimental studies of head injury. In: Becker D, Gudeman S, eds. *Textbook of head injury*. Philadelphia: WB Saunders; 1989:437–50.

24. Carey M, Sarna G, Farrell J. The effect of an experimental missile wound to the brain on brain electrolytes, regional cerebral blood flow and blood brain barrier permeability. In: US Army Medical R&D Command, Annual Report DAMD 17-83-C-3145, 1987.

25. Palmer R, Ferige A, Moncada S. Nitric oxide release accounts for the biological activity of endothelium-derived relaxing factor. *Nature* 1987;327:524–6.

26. Ward P, Maldonado M, Moreno M, Gunther B, Vivaldi E. Oxygen derived free radicals mediate the cutaneous necrotizing vasculitis induced by epinephrine in endotoxin primed rabbits. *J Infect Dis* 1990;161:1020–2.

27. Lawson D, Mehta J, Nichols W, Mehta P, Donnelly W. Superoxide radical-mediated endothelial injury and vasoconstriction of rat thoracic aortic rings. *J Lab Clin Med* 1990;115: 541–8.

28. Lamb F, King C, Harrell K, Burkel W, Webb R. Free radical mediated endothelial damage in blood vessels after electrical stimulation. *Am J Physiol* 1987;252:H1041–6.

29. Wei E, Kontos H, Dietrich W, Povlishock J, Ellis E. Inhibition by free radical scavengers and by cyclooxygenase inhibitors of pial arteriolar abnormalities from concussive brain injury in cats. *Circ Res* 1981;48:95–103.

30. Ellis E, Wright K, Wei E. Cyclooxygenase products of arachidonic acid metabolism in cat cerebral cortex after experimental concussive brain injury. *J Neurochem* 1981;37:892–6.

31. Faden A. Neuropeptides and CNS Injury. *Arch Neurol* 1986;43:501–4.

32. McIntosh T, Faden A, Yamakami I, Vink R. Magnesium deficiency exacerbates and pretreatment improves outcome following traumatic brain injury in rats. *J Trauma* 1988;5: 17–31.

33. Faden A, Demediuk P, Panter S, Vink R. The role of excitatory amino acids and NMDA receptors in traumatic brain injury. *Science* 1989;244:798–800.

34. Hayes R, Pechura C, Katayama Y, Povlishock J, Giebel M, Becker D. Activation of pontine

cholinergic sites implicated in unconsciousness following cerebral concussion in the cat. *Science* 1984;233:301–3.

35. Suguru I, Marmarou A, Clarke G, Andersen B, Fatouros P, Young H. Production and clearance of lactate from brain tissue, CSF, and serum following experimental brain injury. *J Neurosurg* 1988;69:736–44.

36. Giulian D, Chen J, Ingeman J, George J, Noponen M. The role of mononuclear phagocytes in wound healing after traumatic injury to adult mammalian brain. *J Neurosci* 1989;9: 4416–29.

37. Demopoulos H, Flamm E, Seligman M, Pietronigro D. Oxygen free radical in central nervous system ischemia and trauma. In: Autor A, ed. *Pathology of oxygen.* New York: Academic Press, 1982:127–55.

38. Ikeda Y, Long DM. The molecular basis of brain injury and brain edema: the role of oxygen free radicals. *J Neurosurg* 1990;27:1–11.

39. Bochicchio M, Latronico N, Zani D, et al. Free radical induced lipoperoxidation and severe head injury. A clinical study. *Intensive Care Med* 1990;16:444–7.

40. Hall E, Braughler J. CNS trauma and stroke. II. Physiological and pharmacological evidence for the involvement of oxygen radicals and lipid peroxidation. *Free Radical Biol Med* 1989;6:303–13.

41. Hall E, Yonkers P, McCall J, Braughler J. Effects of the 21-aminosteroid U74006F on experimental head injury in mice. *J Neurosurg* 1988;68:456–61.

42. Hall E. Intensive antioxidant pre-treatment retards motor nerve degeneration. *Brain Res* 1987;413:175–8.

43. Yoshida S. Brain injury after ischemia and trauma: the role of vitamin E. *Ann NY Acad Sci* 1989;570:219–35.

44. Taylor M, Palmer G, Callahan A. Protective action by methylprednisolone, allopurinol and indomethacin against stroke-induced damage to adenylate cyclase in gerbil cerebral cortex. *Stroke* 1984;15:329–35.

45. Manning A, Coltart D, Hearse D. Ischemia and reperfusion-induced arrhythmias in the rat: effect of xanthine oxidase inhibition with allopurinol. *Circ Res* 1984;55:545–8

46. Willmore L, Hiramatsu M, Kochi H, Mori A. Formation of superoxide radicals after Fe^{Cl3} injection into rat isocortex. *Brain Res* 1983;277:393–6.

47. Schettini A, Lippman H, Walsh E. Attenuation of decompressive hypoperfusion and cerebral edema by superoxide dismutase. *J Neurosurg* 1989;71:578–87.

48. Hansson R, Jonsson O, Lundstam S, Pettersson S, Schersten T, Waldenstrom J. Effects of free radical scavengers on renal circulation after ischemia in the rabbit. *Clin Sci* 1983; 65:605.

49. Paller M, Hoidal J, Ferris T. Oxygen free radicals in ischemic acute renal failure in the rat. *J Clin Invest* 1984;74:1156.

50. Levasseur J, Patterson J, Ghatak N, Kontos H, Choi S. Combined effect of respirator-induced ventilation and superoxide dismutase in experimental brain injury. *J Neurosurg* 1989;71:573–7.

50a. Muizelaar JP, Marmarou A, Young HF, et al. Improving the outcome of severe head injury with the oxygen radical scavenger polyethylene glycol-conjugated superoxide dismutase: a phase II trial. *J Neurosurg* 1993;78:375–82.

51. Schwab K, Grafman J, Salazar A, Kraft J. Residual impairments and work status fifteen years after head injury: a report of the Vietnam Head Injury Study. *Neurology [in press]*.

52. Kraft J, Schwab K, Salazar A, Brown H. Occupational and educational achievements of head injured Vietnam veterans at 15-year follow-up. *Arch Phys Med Rehab* 1993 (in press).

53. Levin H, Goldstein F. Neurobehavioral aspects of traumatic brain injury. In: Rita BY, ed. *Traumatic brain injury.* New York: Demos, 1989:53–72.

54. Lezak M. Living with the characterologically altered brain injured patient. *J Clin Psychol* 1978;39:592–8.

55. Brooks N, Campsie L, Symington C, Beattie A, McKinlay W. The five year outcome of severe blunt head injury: a relative's view. *J Neurol Neurosurg Psychiatr* 1986;49:764–70.

56. Salazar A, Grafman J, Vance S, Weingartner H, Dillon J, Ludlow C. Unconsciousness and amnesia following penetrating head injury: neurology and anatomy. *Neurology* 1986;36: 178–87.

57. Salazar A. Penetrating war injuries of the basal forebrain: neurology and cognition. *Neurology* 1986;36:459–65.

58. Levin H, Amparo E, Eisenberg H, et al. Magnetic resonance imaging and computerized tomography in relation to the neurobehavioral sequelae of mild and moderate head injuries. *J Neurosurg* 1987;66:706–13.
59. Feeney D, Gonzalez A, Law W. Amphetamine, haloperidol and experience interact to affect rate of recovery after motor cortex injury. *Science* 1982;217:855–7.
60. Feeney D, Westerberg V. Norepinephrine and brain damage: alpha noradrenergic pharmacology. *Can J Psychol* 1990;44:233–52.
61. Sutton R, Hovda D, Feeney D. Amphetamine accelerates recovery of locomotor function following bilateral frontal cortex ablation in cats. *Behav Neurosci* 1989;103:837–41.
62. Evans R, Gualtieri C, Patterson D. Treatment of chronic closed head injury with psychostimulant drugs—a controlled case study and an appropriate evaluation procedure. *J Nerv Ment Dis* 1987;175:106–10.
63. Levin H, Peters B, Kalisky Z, et al. Effects of oral physostigmine and lecithin on memory and attention in closed head injury patients. *Cent Nerv Syst Trauma* 1986;3:333–42.
64. Gronwall D. Cumulative and persisting effects of concussion on attention and cognition. In: Levin H, Eisenberg H, Benton A, eds. *Mild head injury*. New York: Oxford University Press;1989:153–62.
65. Eisenberg H. Mild to moderate brain injury clinical diagnosis. In: Levin H, Eisenberg H, Benton A, eds. *Mild head injury*. Cambridge: Blackwell;1989:95–105.
66. Barth J, Alves W, Ryan T, et al. Mild head injury in sports. In: Levin H, Eisenberg H, Benton A, eds. *Mild head injury*. New York: Oxford University Press, 1989:257.
67. Levin H, Mattis S, Ruff R, et al. Neurobehavioral outcome following minor head injury: a three-center study. *J Neurosurg* 1987;66:234–43.
68. Wrightson P. Management of disability and rehabilitation services after mild head injury. In: Levin H, Eisenberg H, Benton A, eds. *Mild head injury*. New York: Oxford University Press, 1989:245–56.

Guidelines for Drug Trials in Memory Disorders, edited by N. Canal, et al.
Raven Press, Ltd., New York © 1993.

7

Discussion

Dr. McKhann: At a previous meeting in Milan 2 years ago (the forerunner for this meeting), the focus was on Alzheimer disease and the issues of therapeutic options. In the course of that meeting it became clear that if you wanted to explore the issue of drugs and memory disorders, then maybe starting with Alzheimer disease was starting with the most difficult problem. Alzheimer disease is a multifaceted problem; it's not just a dementia, it clearly has behavioral components, and it may not be a single entity. A question raised at the previous meeting was: What about other disorders of memory? Perhaps some of these were simpler. Perhaps some of these are the right prototype to use for looking at medications. And, if so, which ones?

The following discussion concerns the problems of Alzheimer's versus aging, the criteria for diagnosis, the parameters for change in such people, and whether there are other parameters in just clinical issues that can be examined in terms of evaluation, as well as the issue of degenerative disorders that leads to dysfunctions of memory, and the difficult area of vascular disorders, what their criteria are, and how do we distinguish them. Normally we wouldn't think about the problems of patients who have had an acute problem leading to a memory disorder, but in some ways this is the purest population to deal with. The head injury population is complicated; however, patients who have an acute anoxic episode may not be as complicated in terms of therapeutic opportunities.

Dr. Ferris: Dr. Canal, do you have as yet any longitudinal data on the success of PET scans over time, validating the possibility that metabolic changes may precede some cognitive changes?

Dr. Canal: A PET scan is very expensive and is rather invasive, because an arterial puncture is involved and not every patient wants to undergo this procedure. We have not done a systematic study on this type of follow-up of patients.

Dr. Levy: With regard to the issue of the lack of discontinuity between normal aging and Alzheimer disease, I think there has been too ready acceptance of this question of lack of bimodality in studies that have attempted to look at this problem—there is no ready solution. For instance, the studies that had been published have included only patients over the age of 75 years and have not had the power to detect bimodality. That's only the epidemiologic side; on the neurobiologic side there are now a number of variables that seem to be different in Alzheimer disease and in normal aging, such as the suggestion that the abnormally phosphorylated tau protein may be different. There are also others; the plate changes that have been described first by Zubenko and others seem to go in a direction opposite to that of normal aging.

Dr. Canal: I'm convinced that as soon as we can go from epidemiologic studies to more basic studies to find some marker, we will solve this problem, or will have a more precise result.

Dr. Thal: Patients who have the Lewy body disease is an area in which we have been very interested. We have seen these patients for many years and they were clearly inappropriately recognized neuropathologically as no one described the cortical Lewy bodies until fairly recently. Yet these patients have had these symptoms for many years. When these patients are examined very early, they are indistinguishable from other patients with Alzheimer disease. During their illness they develop a different constellation of symptoms, however, and their disease can be recognized clinically. We cannot recognize them clinically if they present to us extremely early, during the very, very earliest phases of their dementia. It is clear from the pathologic studies that we have performed that the majority of these patients do indeed have all of the neuropathologic features that patients with Alzheimer disease have; namely, they have plaques and many of them have tangles. Indeed, they also have cortical Lewy bodies. We also see other patients who have only cortical Lewy bodies, so it is clear that Lewy bodies alone, without plaques and tangles, are sufficient to cause dementia.

Dr. Canal: If there is doubt that a patient has Lewy body disease, would it be suitable to perform a biopsy?

Dr. Thal: No, I believe that we can now diagnose these patients ante mortem if they are not in the earlier stages of dementia. Whether they should be included or excluded from clinical drug trials is a more difficult question to decide because their biochemistry is different from that of patient's with classic Alzheimer disease.

Dr. Canal: I believe they should be excluded.

Dr. Thal: That's another issue, and they form a very substantial proportion (about one-third) of the Alzheimer patients that we see at our center.

Dr. Roth: This is a very important phenomenon. The Lewy body dementia syndrome seems to be a significant issue in relation to genetic research into Alzheimer disease and especially in families in which a single autosomal dominant gene is responsible for transmission of the disease. There could be much confusion in research into Alzheimer disease unless this issue is clarified. In a recently reported isoleucine–valine substitution, a mutation described by Goate et al. (Goate A, et al. Segregation of a missense mutation in the amyloid precursor protein gene with familial Alzheimer's disease. *Nature* 1991;349:704–6) in some slides shown at meetings was suggestive of Lewy body dementia rather than Alzheimer disease. In a recent communication on familial Alzheimer disease, one kindred who showed the phenomenon of Dutch familial hemorrhagic amyloidosis was described as having Alzheimer disease. Because there are no plaques or tangles in the brains of patients with this syndrome, they are not demented in life, and they die of cerebral hemorrhage, this diagnosis is incorrect. If these cases are diagnosed as Alzheimer disease, we will complicate the problem of heterogeneity of Alzheimer disease to the detriment of genetic and other research in this field.

Dr. Gottfries: Dr. Hachinski, you divided the dementias into global vascular dementia and focal vascular dementia. According to the findings in our institute there is too little emphasis on the global forms. We autopsied a number of cases. In the first 22 cases only one, or possibly two, had the focal form, and the others had general disturbances of the brain, which could be assumed to be due to vascular factors. I must emphasize that I'm working at a psychiatric unit, and, therefore, that may explain some of these differences. We believe that the list of factors causing global vascular dementia should include not only cardiac arrest, as you had, but also arrhythmias, blood pressure falls, sleep apneas, and even anesthesia. Do you think that these more global vascular dementias possibly are underestimated and not diagnosed, and that in some cases the stroke attacks are more end points without any etiologic importance for the dementia, for the cognitive impairment?

Dr. Hachinski: I agree that additional mechanisms such as arrhythmias, hypotension, and anesthesia should be added to the list of factors causing global vascular dementia. In fact, I believe that there are a number of cognitive changes with anesthesia. Some of them are hemodynamic, some of them are probably chemical, but it's a problem that I believe is larger than we estimate. I would welcome the additional etiologic factors that you have mentioned, because many of them are potentially treatable.

Dr. Gottfries: What do you think about the prevalence of global vascular dementias?

Dr. Hachinski: The problem is one of sampling. In my hospital, if I wanted to find the largest proportion of people with vascular dementias, I would go to the cardiology and cardiovascular service: the people who had cardiac operations, the patients who have had heart attacks, myocardial infarcts and sudden silent infarcts of the brain, people with subtle deficits, and also the patients who have had strokes. Usually patients with vascular dementias do not come to a neurologist or even to a psychiatrist. They are probably in the general wards.

Dr. Roth: I believe that etiology is being confused with pathogenesis, which refers to the final common pathway to the production of clinical features. Early studies in collaboration with Tomlinson showed that there was a very close relationship between measures of dementia and the volume of infarction. The correlations were of a highly significant order. Where there were exceptions, one could explain them in terms of concomitant Alzheimer change in most cases. One can differentiate patients with dementia of mixed etiology because no patient with dementia due to vascular disease becomes demented after the first stroke. If a patient suffers a short transient cerebral ischemia and after recovery manifests severe cognitive impairment, there has usually been a previous degenerative process most often of the Alzheimer type that has been aggravated by the subsequent stroke.

I agree with you that the process of diagnosing dementia should be studied, but threshold effects do occur. There are increasing encroachments on the brain's reserve capacity beyond a certain level before mental impairment appears; in Newcastle it was estimated that about 75 to 100 cc of brain tissue had to be destroyed before a process of increasing mental impairment is initiated. A diagnosis of dementia implies a prediction of progressive decline of cognitive and personality functioning as distinct from a circumscribed neurological lesion. Although we cannot arrest the progression, there are methods of treatment that are immensely important and we have to take note of them. Perhaps when the process can be identified in the preclinical stage, cautious preventive measures with anticoagulants should begin before brain pathology has caused definite clinical changes, followed by increasing global mental deterioration. The concept of dementia cannot be dismissed because, even with all the tests available worldwide, dementia will remain a clinical diagnosis.

I recently had a patient, a Cambridge academic, who came to my office and performed brilliantly in cognitive tests and then went out of the room and emptied his bladder in the corridor. It was not until I had interviewed his wife that I became aware of the manner in which this individual's personality had fallen apart. Dementia is not a matter of cognitive impairment alone. I am in favor of cognitive tests, but they should be an adjunct. There is no substitute for a clinical history and developmental history together with thorough psychiatric and neurological examination. Although you have provided an outstanding conspectus of all the etiologic factors, this does not mean that the classification that is based on brain pathology should be dismissed, particularly when there is such a high and impressive correlation between the quantitative estimate of brain pathology and the quantitative estimate of mental impairment and the forecase of growing decline in Alzheimers disease and in multiple infarct cases.

Dr. Hachinski: I believe that the only way we will learn more about dementia is by doing careful clinical, radiologic, and pathologic studies. That is fundamental. With regard to the other two points, I believe that the paper by Tomlinson and yourself is one of the classics. In retrospect, however, one could be critical of the selection factors, methodology, and some of the correlates. Empirically, one could render a person totally demented and totally incapable by withdrawing 5 or 10 cc of brain tissue from the left angular gyrus, the lateral part of the frontal hornes, and a part of the hippocampi. Contrariwise, one could take 10 cc parallelly from a person's frontal lobe in a particular area, and there would not be a detectable difference. So clearly it is not only volume but also site. I believe that with MRI, for example, that we have the means for quantitating volume. A number of factors are involved: site and size; side, right versus left; and tempo, because clearly if you have multiple lesions in a short time that has a different effect than if they are spread over time. In terms of dementia, it's a question of time. We should begin with the things that matter to individuals, and should take into account cultural aspects. In Western Africa the first sign of a dementia is when a fisherman can no longer fish. In Southern France one of the earliest signs of impairment is when a person cannot make telephone calls. I believe that the history is tremendously important. And when I was asking for some core cognitive assessment meant to imply behavioral assessments as well. If one agrees to do it by history and examination, that's fine, but please include these too, so we can review some of the information and not simply rely on someone's clinical impression. At an NIH workshop on vascular dementia, when I suggested that they dismiss the term "dementia" I was almost physically attacked. I have no quarrel with those who want to retain the term, but I believe that it should be described empirically. If at a particular stage someone is diagnosed as demented, the evidence on which that judgment is based should be given.

Dr. Korczyn: In your article you mentioned alcohol in reference to its protective effect. You did not mention alcoholism when you mentioned the brains at risk among hypertensives, smokers, diabetics, and so on. Also, you discussed the nosology and the etiopathology of vascular dementia and then you went on to the prevention of strokes, almost implying that every patient who had a stroke is likely to develop vascular dementia as a random process. We don't know that this is true. We don't know what the risk factors are that would put a patient who had a stroke or is likely to develop a stroke at the risk of developing vascular dementia. In Tel Aviv, we are doing a prospective study on patients who had had their first stroke and who left the hospital nondemented. We are finding that they develop dementia at a rate of about 10% a year, and the presentation of dementia is not acute but gradual. We would have thought in most of the patients that this was a primary degenerative dementia rather than vascular dementia. We have been able to identify some of the risk factors that would make patients who have had a stroke more susceptible to develop dementia. I believe these are the issues that we should study to try and find out what makes patients with stroke more susceptible to development of dementia.

Dr. Hachinski: In terms of alcohol use, in little doses it may be protective, but in high doses it's certainly harmful and increases the risk of strokes. I certainly wouldn't advocate someone taking up drinking for that reason. I do say that people at risk for any stroke are also at risk of multiinfarct dementia, but I recognize also that there may be other factors and that, in particular, we should look at the interaction. We know that the coincidence of Alzheimer disease and infarcts is very common. It is said that lesions in the brain do not add up, they multiply. Probably there is an individual threshold. But given a particular change in an aging brain, all you need is two or three infarcts with a particular volume. We should start from basic principles and not on previous assumptions.

Dr. Ferris: Dr. Hachinski, I believe that your breakdown of the white matter lesions or leukoaraiosis into three categories is intriguing. I'm particularly curious about the "aging alone" subtype, whether it is a subtype or whether it's perhaps on a continuum with either of the other two categories. Do you really believe that there is no pathology when various volumes and locations of white matter show these effects on scanning techniques? You talked about there being no apparent clinical consequences, and yet evidence of motor function changes correlated with aging is beginning to emerge. Certainly, with sophisticated measurement of fine motor function and motor control one can distinguish between normal elderly with and without these changes. In addition, there is the issue of size and location of these regions.

Dr. Hachinski: When I alluded to a category in which there was no clinical correlate, I meant no detectable clinical correlates. I'm not aware of any longitudinal study that details whether and when they merge into the other two types. One of the most intriguing findings of the study that I mentioned was that 11% of our controls had white matter changes. They had subtle intellectual impairment, and a minority of them had focal neurogical impairments.

Dr. Salazar: With regard to the issue of brain reserve, Corkin et al. have described a phenomenon that was called "exacerbated decline" following penetrating brain wounds in World War II veterans. What is interesting about that phenomenon, as opposed to, for example, dementia pugilistica where there may be some etiologic progression, is that these patients suffered low-velocity wounds, which are essentially like ablative experiments. The loss of brain tissue in those cases was probably limited to the lesion seen on CT scan. Those men, when examined in the 1980s, showed much more rapid cognitive decline than a control group with peripheral nerve injury, presumably because of the loss of brain reserve.

Dr. Joynt: What about the temporal lesions? We tend to forget the momentum of the lesion. If you have a patient with a multinfarct dementia with a number of different lesions that develop at different times, versus a patient who suddenly has a shower of biembolia, as might happen after cardiac bypass, there is a difference in those patients. There is an issue of momentum of lesion.

Dr. Hachinski: I totally agree. A good clinical example would be a huge tumor with mild symptoms, which implies that it has developed over a very long time, in contrast to the fact that even a small infarct in the thalamic area causes a major disturbance.

Dr. Reisberg: Dr. Salazar, an article that appeared in *Science* about a decade ago titled "Do We Really Need a Brain?" showed a CT scan of a young man with severe hydrocephalus. The scan showed a sliver of a brain unilaterally; the patient's IQ was given as 120. This article was very interesting and I'd like your comments on it with regard to the issue of compensation.

Dr. Salazar: Like the patient you describe, the Vietnam veterans whom we studied were also young men and had a remarkable capacity to compensate. However, they were normal preinjury. By the time an Alzheimer patient is diagnosed, the brain's compensation capacity has probably already been reached. In other words, there may not be a significant "brain reserve" that we can tap in their management.

Dr. Boller: Dr. Salazar, I think everybody in this room is aware of the importance of what you would call brain reserve, but it seems that you and other people involved in head-injury studies are talking about behavioral, cognitive, or psychiatric changes much more than other people. Is it greater awareness on your part or is it the particular site of lesions that occur in Alzheimer disease or in Lewy body disease? Which of these factors do you think is more important in bringing out these considerably important behavioral changes as opposed to what we see in Alzheimer disease? Not that they are not present, but certainly in head injuries they are seen to be more prominent.

Dr. Salazar: It is probably mainly the diffuseness and progressive nature of the lesion in Alzheimer disease as opposed to trauma.

Dr. McKhann: We have a rehabilitation unit for children who have had head injuries, and an amazing number of these children have had preinjury hyperactive behavior that probably led them to having the head injury.

Dr. Salazar: The head injury, if it's a frontal lobe injury, produces additional behavioral problems, and combined with their attention disorders makes compensation even more difficult.

Dr. Roth: I found it very interesting to observe the contrast and the comparison you made between Vietnam veterans and patients with dementia pugilistica. You've had these remarkable results in the Vietnam veterans. You attribute the good capacity for recovery to their youth. There was a difference between the young population of patients and the population with dementia, and you compared the related features of both to the Alzheimer system. There is a marked difference between the two. That patient you described in whom there was a loss of the brain had suffered a limited, circumscribed loss. He didn't have a diffuse brain degenerative disease—most of his brain was intact and was able to regenerate. In patients with dementia pugilistica there is a diffuse damage of the brain; repeated blows give rise to lesions in many parts. You drew attention to the amyloid printing. I question your extrapolation to Alzheimer disease because in elderly people there are masses of β-amyloid protein in the neuropil, cerebellum spinal cord, and corpus striatum, without any damage to neurons. Surprisingly, there are plaques and tangles, tangles in abundance, in patients with dementia pugilistica. In contrast to your patients—who 15 years later are better—in patients with dementia pugilistica after a several-year interval, depletion of their brain reserve adds up to perhaps 10 years of aging.

Dr. Salazar: We believe that dementia pugilistica is the result of a pathologic process that is set into motion by multiple concussive blows, a pathologic process that has something in common with Alzheimer's progressive dementia. One of the interesting things about the young men in Vietnam who sustained head injury is that most of them had little or no loss of consciousness at the time of the injury. A number of men with fragments in their brains stayed in battle, and they could tell us in detail what happened. We deduce from this that their lesions were quite focal, in contrast to most closed-head injuries or concussions.

Dr. Erkinjuntti: These minor brain injuries may also be a confounding factor in clinical trials. At a young age the brain is able to compensate for these injuries. It is obvious that in normal aging, there is a decline in the compensation or in the compensatory capacity. As a consequence of this phenomenon, these minor brain injuries that occurred in young age (biopsies don't have any clear-cut clinical history of that) may be clinically relevant in old age. They may be even a contributing factor to these progressive diseases in older age. Therefore, can brain injuries contribute or cause Alzheimer disease?

Dr. Salazar: Epidemiologic studies have been equivocal on that point. According to Dr. Corkin's study, patients who had static focal brain lesions with nothing else to produce a progressive dementia, appear to lose cognitive functions faster as they become older than do patients who did not have any loss of brain, as opposed to the dementia pugilistica in whom the repeated trauma induces a progressive disorder.

Dr. Erkinjuntti: How should you treat this confounding factor in clinical trials? For example, should you exclude those cases from trials because this can be a contributing factor to the cognitive process?

Dr. Salazar: I'm not sure that we need to, except in the most obvious cases of severe injury.

Dr. Joynt: In dendritic morphometry studies, even in Alzheimer disease, there is some effort at compensation by the brain. Has anyone done dendritic morphometry studies in head injury to see if there is any effort of this injured brain to make new connections?

Dr. Salazar: Yes, these studies have been done, and these neurons do reestablish connections. Of course, one of the problems is to reestablish the correct connections. Misdirected regeneration might exacerbate behavioral problems and other symptoms, particularly in the case of limbic and temporal circuits.

Dr. Hachinski: How well was Dr. Corkin's study controlled? Many veterans have a number of other habits, such as drinking, that can contribute to intelligence decline. If they have neuropathy they are more likely to be alcoholics. How normal are the controls in whom we account for deterioration on some other factors?

Dr. Salazar: Dr. Corkin was not able to account for the decline based on other factors. But of course, we are talking about a population that was identified after injury in World War II, which was studied in the 1950s and studied again in the 1980s. That's a long follow-up period, and much can happen along the way. She still has had almost 100 patients in the cohort, about 50 head injured controls and about 30 or 40 peripheral nerve injury controls. I'm sure there were other factors that could be accounted for. Her conclusion was that it was the loss of brain tissue that accounted for the accelerated decline.

Dr. Drachman: In relation to the question of size, site, the pace of the injury, and the age of the individual, we did a study on primary brain tumors, all on the left side of the brain. The results of this study showed that, with relation to the degree of aphasia developing, the only factor that was highly significant was age; the size of the tumor, the exact location of the tumor, and the histology of the tumor failed to correlate.

Dr. McKhann: How are we going to design therapeutically open-ended clinical studies. With regard to degenerative diseases, are there ways of doing this by other than clinical parameters? The use of PET is one approach, but there are other approaches, such as the use of CSF.

Dr. Gottfries: At our institute we think that especially the primary degenerative disorders in Alzheimer disease are very heterogeneous. We investigated CSF to see if we could find markers for subgroups. We began by studying the monoamine metabolites. There has been a discussion of whether homovanilic acid and hydrolacetic acid are reduced in Alzheimer patients. Comparing the results of more than 100 controls and more than 100 patients, we found definitely reduced concentrations of monoamine acids in Alzheimer patients. However, they cannot be used as diagnostic tools because there is such a great overlap with controls that you can only identify some types of neurotransmitters disturbances. We did find that GM1 was reduced in brain material for these patients; therefore our laboratory has designed a method for determining GM1 in CSF. In a recently published article we showed that GM1 is significantly increased in CSF in early onset Alzheimer dementia, whereas it's not increased in vascular dementia and late onset Alzheimer dementia. These preliminary data indicate that the determination of GM1 may delineate a subgroup that we call early onset Alzheimer dementia or pure Alzheimer dementia. We also are studying the determination of sulfatides because sulfatides are a component that could be a marker of vascular dementia. Again, preliminary data indicate that vascular dementia patients have increased concentrations of sulfatides in CSF. Degeneration of synapses is a very important factor in Alzheimer-type dementia. At present, we are studying synaptic facin, chromogranin and ubiquitin in CSF, because they could be markers for synapse degeneration. There is one other thing I'd like to mention. We also are investigating a rather small subgroup of Alzheimer-type dementia patients, less than 20%, who seems to possess antibodies against epitopes of the cholinergic neurons. Whether this will eventually provide any diagnostic markers is still unknown.

Another finding that could be of interest is that we have also taken up a method for determining vitamin B_{12} levels. When we investigated senile dementia of Alzheimer type with late onset, we found that 23% of those patients had pathologically low vitamin B_{12} levels in serum. We found that there is a subgroup of those who at present are diagnosed as senile dementia of the Alzheimer type, who have lower ratios between CSF B_{12} and serum B_{12}. They have a reduced transport of vitamin B_{12} into the brain. The preliminary data seem to indicate that it is elderly men with dementia who have this reduced level of vitamin B_{12} in CSF. Whether this has any importance for the dementia we still do not know, however, reduced B_{12} may be a risk factor. We believe that the senile dementia of the Alzheimer type is a very heterogeneous disorder for which you have to find the risk factors: aging is certainly one. But vitamin B_{12} and vascular factors certainly are other risk factors that should be investigated.

Dr. Wilcock: We have about 25 people in the elderly age group with low vitamin B_{12} who we thought had Alzheimer disease. We treated them over a period of time, and have noted little improvement in the intellectual cognitive function or in other aspects.

Dr. Hachinski: Dr. Gottfries, it's quite encouraging to see that GM1 seems to be a marker for early Alzheimer disease and that sulfatides are increased in vascular dementia. Although we know that the concentration of any given compound is related to the CSF flow which, in turn, is influenced considerably by the activity of the patient, how do you compensate for the confounding factor of patients' activity, and therefore increased turnover, when you do these chemical studies?

Dr. Gottfries: The most confounding factor is the length of the spinal cord if you have gradients, and that you have in all the CSF metabolites. We always take our spinal taps in the morning after a night of rest. We don't think that the movement or the activity of patients is of great importance. But we have checked it very carefully and we know that the gradients have to be checked here. There were no gradients for sulfatides or GM1. We have measured that in different portions of the CSF taps.

We have carefully investigated Alzheimer patients and have found that in those with late onset Alzheimer dementia there are significantly more vascular factors, as marked by increased albumin ratio in CSF, compared to the early onset. If we rate vascular factors, we find more vascular factors in the old age group than in the early onset group. We also find white matter low attenuations to a greater extent, which we think cannot be explained only by the age factor. What we presume is that the leukoareiosis you see in the group called Alzheimer dementia is due to their combinations with vascular factors. But we have significant differences between early and late onset. Dr. Hachinski, what is your opinion of this?

Dr. Hachinski: With regard to pure Alzheimer disease, we postulate that there is deposition of amyloid in blood vessels, mainly in the meningeal and cortical vessels. We know that once the amyloid penetrates the brain, even if the pathology is on the surface, it affects the deep white matter. We also know that there is loss of cells in areas such as the locus coeruleus, which has to do with the blood–brain barrier and with cerebral vessels. Compared to aged controls, the blood vessels in Alzheimer patients are denuded. Therefore, one can presume that cerebral autoregulation is impaired. Contrary to popular belief, the most sensitive cells to ischemia in the brain are not the neurons but the oligodendroglia. If this is correct, then the autoregulation is impaired. In healthy individuals blood pressure changes are normally compensated for. However, in the elderly, who are more prone to hypotension and who have more cardiac arrhythmia, blood pressure changes can cause multiple damage that will impair oligodendroglia, and thus cause loss of white matter, which will account for leukoaraiosis. We have some preliminary evidence to suggest that in fact there is impaired autoregulation. A study performed in our laboratory using CT scan and xenon showed that Diamox can increase the blood flow considerably, almost double, in normal controls, but not in patients with leukoaraiosis. Therefore, I believe there is a vascular component in Alzheimer disease and that indeed they interact.

Dr. Gottfries: You suggest that infarcts could be avoided in the elderly by intensive antihypertension treatment. By reducing the blood pressure in the elderly to such an extent, aren't you concerned that this may facilitate the development of dementia or a general disturbance of the brain?

Dr. Hachinski: Yes, but safeguards can be implemented so that someone monitors the results and therefore harm in patients would be stopped, and then we could answer that question empirically. It could be correct for certain patients. But I suspect that the ones who would be harmed are not the ones who have vascular risk factors, hypertension and so on, because they have intact autoregulation. The ones who might be harmed are the Alzheimer type who may have an impairment in autoregulation.

Dr. Erkinjuntti: One of the limitations in analyzing leukoaraiosis was that it has been treated as absent or present. We know that white matter changes should be analyzed with regard to the type, location, and extent. For example, with regard to the location, there may be differences in risk factors and causes of these white matter changes located in the periventricular area compared with those in the centrum semiovale or in the deep subcortical white matter. In Alzheimer patients, we analyzed those diffuse changes extending to the deep white matter, which are more in the centrum semiovale type of white matter changes. We found that Alzheimer patients who had these changes were more older and their disease seemed to progress faster. They had more frequent changes in the blood–brain barrier, and this may be a vascular factor. But if you look at the tiny white matter changes in the subcortical white matter they don't necessarily correlate with these vascular risk factors. We should be careful in analyzing the white matter changes with regard to the extent, type, and location, not only as present or absent.

Guidelines for Drug Trials in Memory Disorders, edited by N. Canal, et al. Raven Press, Ltd., New York © 1993.

8

Introduction

Minimal Pharmacologic Requirements for Drug Selection

C. G. Gottfries

Department of Psychiatry and Neurochemistry, University of Göteborg, S-431 80 Mölndal, Sweden

It is well known that extensive preclinical studies are undertaken before a drug is allowed to be used in human evaluations. The clinical drug evaluation is usually divided into different stages (Fig. 1).

This chapter discusses which preclinical considerations have to be made before drugs are used in main therapeutic studies in memory disorders. Which requirements must govern the selection of drugs for clinical evaluation in memory disorders?

Because the selection of drugs for clinical use is a complex issue, this is a matter for a multidisciplinary team approach. Very often it is not sufficient to obtain the opinion of a chemist or a clinical pharmacologist. Therefore, laboratory personnel, clinicians, and experts on regulatory matters must participate in the selection of such drugs.

GENERAL REQUIREMENTS

Safety

An important rule in medicine is "primum non nocere," and this is also true in the evaluation of new drugs. Careful studies of potential toxic effects must be performed in animal models before a drug is used in humans. Because the population used in early studies consists of healthy volunteers, for whom the benefit-to-risk ratio is in the direction of no benefit and only risk, extreme caution must be taken in the early studies. The toxicology of the drug should be tested so that "vulnerable organ" and side effects can be anticipated in the clinical trials.

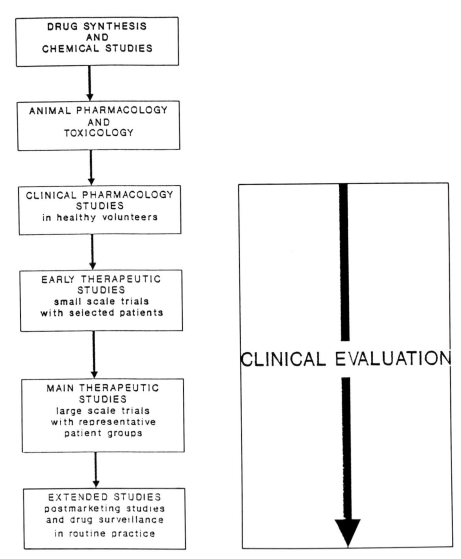

FIG. 1. Clinical drug evaluation.

Pharmacological Properties

The pharmacokinetics and the pharmacodynamics of the drug should be determined to the extent possible before it is used in clinical studies. For example, a drug presumed to influence neurotransmitter metabolism must be shown to penetrate the blood–brain barrier (BBB). The effect of the drug on the functions of different neurotransmitters should also be evaluated. In addition, it is highly desirable to have available a laboratory assay that can determine or estimate the concentration of the new drug in, e.g., plasma and CSF.

SPECIFIC REQUIREMENTS

Drugs can be classified either from a pharmacologic standpoint or from a clinical standpoint. The word *nootropic* is sometimes used to describe drugs intended to improve attention, cognition, and memory in patients suffering from symptoms of aging or dementia. The term is then used in its broad clinical sense. In some countries, however, this term is used only in a narrower and strictly pharmacologic sense. The nootropics comprise a group of drugs that either belong to the piracetam family or have similar pharmacologic effects.

At present there is no common name for drugs that improve cognitive functions. Moreover, it can be assumed that memory disturbances are complex processes caused by derangements in more than one system of the brain. Therefore, several types of drugs may have effects on memory.

Reference Drugs

When a new drug is synthesized, it is usually compared to a reference drug with known clinical effects. However, thus far there are no reference drugs concerned with treatment of memory disorders. The development of new drugs must therefore follow other strategies.

Animal Models

Biologic models are helpful in the development of new therapeutic agents. At present, great efforts are being directed toward development of an animal model for the largest groups of dementias, Alzheimer disease/senile dementia of the Alzheimer type (AD/SDAT) and vascular dementia (VAD). However, as yet there is no known animal disease comparable to these dementias. In the animal models presently used, attempts are made to produce a state of memory defect, and in the pharmacologic testing these defects should be either prevented or reversed by the test drug. Such models include, for example, brain lesions, electroconvulsive shock, genetic models, hypoxia, drug-induced deficit models, and the use of aged animals (1). Experiments on normal animals have also been done in screening of new drugs. The passive avoidance test is often used to determine the antiamnesic activities of a drug. Data from these experiments are not always clear, and their relevance to clinical problems remains to be demonstrated.

Other complex animal models attempt to address memory-related functions more specifically, e.g., the radial maze, the Morris water maze, and models of delayed response. Aged animals exhibit reduced ability to perform these tests. The results obtained, particularly in aged monkeys, suggest that the drugs used at present have only minimal effects in memory enhancement.

Obviously, testing in animals can delineate only disturbances of one component of memory function and not disturbances of other cognitive functions. In several investigations drugs have been used in clinical studies based on the fact that they have produced some improvement in animal models. In the phase 2 and phase 3 testing of such drugs, some minor but significant differences have been shown in comparison to the responses to placebo. On the basis of these findings, these drugs have been introduced for treatment of the elderly and of patients with dementia. Hydergine, piracetam, vinpocetine, and cinnarizine are examples of drugs now in common use, although the clinical effects are still questionable. The widespread use of these drugs is based more on the great need for such drugs than on convincing pharmacologic and clinical effects.

Studies on Human Volunteers

In phase 1 and 2 studies the pharmacokinetics of a new drug are investigated in human subjects. It is, of course, possible to extend phase 2 studies to include experimental psychometric studies when drugs with a presumed effect on memory functions are tested. However, as in animal experiments this is possible only when valid models exist. Therefore, subjects are studied under conditions of hypoxia or mental stress. Certain drugs (e.g., scopolamine) can also induce memory deficits. Healthy elderly subjects with memory deficits can be used to study the capacity of such drugs to prevent deficit when administered prophylactically or to improve deficit after it occurs. Assessment of the effects can be made either behaviorally or by electroencephalographic (EEG) recording.

Such pilot studies in volunteers are, in my view, useful for evaluating the effect on cognitive functions of a new drug that has previously been tested only in animals. The results of the pilot study cannot scientifically prove an effect on memory, but if the pilot study demonstrates no effect it can then be questioned whether testing should proceed to phase 3 studies.

Pathophysiology of Cognitive Disorders

The pathophysiology of several cognitive disorders has now been delineated to some extent. On the basis of these neurochemical findings, pharmacologic strategies can be formulated. From a historical point of view, the most well known strategy is the use of vasodilators. Some decades ago it was assumed that the development of arteriosclerosis in the elderly was caused by a reduction in the supply of blood to the brain. Drugs that could improve the cerebral blood flow (CBF) were therefore hoped to achieve beneficial effects. However, this assumption has been called into question, and during the last two decades it has been presumed that the primary etiology for VAD stems from brain tissue infarcts. The dementia was therefore called *multi-infact dementia* (MID). The use of vasodilators has been abandoned. However, it should be pointed out that recent findings indicate that other factors than thromboembolism may be of importance in VAD. Not only arteriosclerosis, hyalinosis, and amyloid angiopathy but also disturbance of systemic circulation, disturbed regulation of cerebral blood flow, and hyperviscosity may cause dysfunction of the brain (2). The effect of vasodilators therefore may still be of value in subgroups of VAD. A reliable diagnosis of the disorder must be made for the effect of vasodilators to be correctly evaluated.

Nootropic drugs have elicited new interest because they are believed not only to increase blood flow but also the rate of brain metabolism, especially the rate of glucose utilization. These drugs are presumed to normalize or stabilize impaired homeostatic functions within central nervous system (CNS). However, the mechanism of these drugs is obscure, and it is obvious that their effects observed in animal models cannot be reproduced in clinical investigations on human subjects.

On the basis of findings of morphologic and neurochemical deficits in the human brain, it is presumed that disturbances in neurotransmitter systems lead to memory impairment. A simple cause–effect model has been applied. In the Alzheimer type of dementia, a severe derangement of the cholinergic system is evident. Because clinical experiments with anticholinergic drugs have shown that these drugs cause impairment of memory function, the hypothesis has been formulated that the memory disturbances in AD/SDAT are caused by a defect in the cholinergic transmitter system (3). On the basis of this hypothesis, several "cholinergic" drugs have been selected for clinical evaluation. Again, however, attempts to improve memory functions by administration of these drugs have been largely unsuccessful. Drugs that influence acetylcholine (ACh) metabolism both pre- and postsynaptically have been used. There may be several reasons for the failure of effectiveness of cholinergic drugs. One reason may be, of course, that we still do not have a cholinergic drug that is at the effector site. This hypothesis has still not been fully tested. Another reason may be that in this type of replacement therapy the cholinergic system becomes flooded with the neurotransmitter or a receptor agonist. This may be the correct strategy in a system that controls tonus. However, memory is based on an information system that depends on impulses, and in such a system overenhancement of cholinergic activity may fail.

It is obvious that the cholinergic hypothesis is an oversimplification. Memory is a very complex process which is dependent on the normal functioning of several neurotransmitter systems. In AD/SDAT it is well documented that there are multiple disturbances in neurotransmitter functions within the brain. Therefore, it might not be sufficient to supplement only one of these systems.

When the strategy of supplementing the cholinergic system is used, it is necessary to delimit homogeneous clinical groups in the treatment trials. It is obvious that at present the antemortem clinical diagnostic methods are insufficient. A number of data indicate a heterogeneity of AD/SDAT (4).

The cholinergic treatment strategy was formulated on the basis of known or assumed pathophysiology. There are several similar approaches in the treatment of AD/SDAT. Drugs with effect on monoamines and on neuropeptides have been used. Of interest is that the use of selective 5-hydroxytryptamine reuptake blockers has produced effects on intellectual functions (5). In general, the effect of monoaminergic drugs on memory has not been impressive.

Prevention, retardation, or reversal of the accumulation of β-amyloid protein are strategies under discussion at present. These approaches are based on the assumption that the accumulation of β-amyloid in brain tissue in AD/SDAT has a primary role in the memory disturbance seen in this disorder.

There is some evidence that aluminum is accumulated in brain tissue of patients with AD/SDAT. Treatment with aluminum chelating agents has therefore been tried, but thus far no data have been presented on the effect of such treatment.

Trophic Factors

The discovery of nerve growth factor (NGF) has been of great interest in the study of nerve cell differentiation and nerve growth. Gangliosides are especially enriched in the synaptosomes of the CNS. They are assumed to give stability to the plasma membrane and are also of importance for the maturing and plasticity of neurons. Together with NGF, gangliosides influence the survival of neurons and neuron sprouting. As atrophic processes dominate in brains with AD/SDAT, especially of the synapses, the use of trophic factors is of theoretical interest and such trials are presently in progress. It is obvious, however, that in parenteral administration of GM1 ganglioside to AD/SDAT patients this agent is unable to penetrate the BBB (6). It can be assumed that NGF also will not easily penetrate this barrier. One way to overcome this is by intrathecal administration.

CONCLUSION

The minimal pharmacologic requirements for drug selection in the treatment of cognitive disorders are the following: the drug must be safe; it must penetrate the BBB; it must be proven effective in animal models and in phase 1 and 2 clinical studies; and the drug must have pharmacologic properties that are assumed to have a beneficial effect on the pathophysiology of the disorder.

In the United States, the Food and Drug Administration has stated that to be registered for the indication of treatment of dementia a drug must have a proven effect on memory impairment. I do not agree with this approach. Dementia syndromes include a variety of symptoms in addition to memory impairment. This is not surprising, as in AD/SDAT, for example, several neurotransmitter systems are impaired. Because the complex process of memory is dependent on the normal functions of several neurotransmitter systems, drugs that affect functions such as mood, drive, attention, and emotional disturbances may be of great value in dementia syndromes.

It is possible that treatment of memory disturbances and other impaired cognitive functions will require a combined pharmacologic treatment strategy. Preliminary data indicate that the combined use of noradrenergic and cholinergic drugs seems to have a greater effect on memory than the separate use of these drugs.

REFERENCES

1. Amaducci L, Angst J, Bech P, et al. Consensus conference on the methodology of clinical trials of "nootropics," Munich, June 1989. *Pharmacopsychiatry* 1990; 23:171–5.
2. Wallin A. *Vascular dementia—pathogenetic and clinical aspects*. Doctoral thesis. Medical Faculty of University of Göteborg, Sweden, 1989.
3. Cowburn RF, Hardy JA, Roberts PJ. Neurotransmitter deficits in Alzheimer's disease. In: Davies DC, ed. *Alzheimer's disease: towards an understanding of the etiology and pathogenesis*. London: John Libbey; 1989:9–32.
4. Blennow K. *Heterogeneity of Alzheimer's disease*. Doctoral thesis. Medical Faculty of University of Göteborg, Sweden, 1990.
5. Nyth AL. A controlled clinical multicentre study of citalopram and placebo in elderly patients with depression with or without concomitant dementia. (Submitted.)
6. Svennerholm L, Gottfries CG, Blennow K, et al. Parenteral administration of GNM1 ganglioside to presenile Alzheimer patients. *Acta Neurol Scand* 1990:81:48–53.

Guidelines for Drug Trials in Memory Disorders, edited by N. Canal, et al.
Raven Press, Ltd., New York © 1993.

9

Selection of Drugs for the Treatment of Memory Disorders

David A. Drachman and Joan M. Swearer

Department of Neurology, University of Massachusetts Medical Center, Worcester, Massachusetts 01655

The identification and selection of drugs for the treatment of memory disorders presents an important and difficult challenge to physicians, pharmacologists, and pharmaceutical manufacturers. Unlike many other areas in which drugs are under development, such as antibiotics, sedatives, and cancer chemotherapeutic agents, there are at present no drugs that improve memory at a clinically useful level in the vast majority of memory disorders. The classic methods of pharmacologic development, in which molecular modifications of drugs of known usefulness are designed to enhance activity or limit toxicity, may not be applicable here. There are, however, a few exceptions: conditions that impair memory in which treatments *have* been effective in at least some patients. These few exceptions are diseases of known etiology, in which we are able to treat the underlying etiology of the memory impairment directly and either to remove the cause (e.g., temporal lobe epilepsy) or to prevent irreversible damage from taking place (e.g., *Herpes simplex* encephalitis).

This emphasizes the fact that impairment of human memory can be caused by a wide variety of underlying disorders (Table 1). The selection of candidate therapeutic agents requires a clear understanding of the underlying cause, as it would be unlikely that the memory impairment of Korsakoff's syndrome and that due to Creutzfeld–Jakob disease would respond to the same treatment. Even if the range of memory disorders were narrowed to the dementias, or even merely to Alzheimer disease (AD), this would mean addressing multiple etiologies and multiple pathogenetic mechanisms for memory loss.

This chapter will discuss a strategy for selecting drugs to be considered for the treatment of memory disorders. The strategy consists of four distinct steps:

TABLE 1. *Etiologies of memory disorders*

Alzheimer disease
Age-associated memory impairment
Other dementias (e.g., multiinfarct dementia; Lewy body dementia; Creutzfeldt–Jakob
  disease)
Parkinsonism
Head trauma
Anoxia/ischemia
Korsakoff's syndrome
Herpes simplex encephalitis
Temporal lobe epilepsy
Drug intoxications
Strokes
Brain tumors (third ventricle)
Post temporal lobectomy

1. Deciding on the rationale for considering a particular drug.
2. Assessing the preliminary observations for relevance to the pathologic
   condition, and the promise of success.
3. Avoiding the traps and pitfalls that lead to misinterpretation of both
   experimental and clinical studies.
4. Setting the standard for the type and extent of benefit that would be
   acceptable for a given form of treatment.

RATIONALES FOR CONSIDERING A THERAPEUTIC AGENT

In general, four quite different rationales may suggest the use of a candidate drug for the treatment of a memory disorder. These are *intervention, substitution, facilitation,* and *serendipity.* How each rationale leads to consideration of certain therapeutic agents will be illustrated below; much of the consideration will be directed to identifying possible drugs for AD or age-associated memory impairment (AAMI).

To appreciate the differences between the first two rationales, it is necessary to consider the difference between the etiology of a disease that causes memory impairment and the pathogenesis of the memory impairment itself. Etiology describes the underlying cause of the disease, whereas pathogenesis refers to the mechanism by which memory is impaired. To illustrate this point, in *Herpes simplex* encephalitis the etiology is infection of the brain by a specific virus, and the pathogenesis of the memory impairment is the bilateral destruction of the hippocampal complexes.

An intervention targets the specific etiology of the disorder to prevent, arrest, or reverse the progress of the underlying disease process. At present we do not know the etiology of AD (or, more correctly, the etiologies of AD) but we have a long list of possibilities (Table 2). It is clear that AD must have more than one etiology, because some cases are familial whereas others

TABLE 2. *Etiologies of Alzheimer disease*

Abnormal amyloid precursor protein gene	Viral disorder
Other genetic abnormality	Lack of nerve growth factor
Amyloid toxicity	Immune disorder
Endogenous excitotoxins	Lack of estrogen (women)
Protein conformational change	Head trauma
Aluminum toxicity	Cosmic radiation

are sporadic (1). Among those that are dominantly inherited, a few are due to a missense mutation in the amyloid precursor protein (APP) gene (2), others are linked to chromosome 21 outside the APP gene domain (3), and still others are not linked to chromosome 21 but the site of the abnormality is unknown (4). The sporadic AD cases are presumably due to a nongenetic mechanism, which may be any of those listed.

Interventions can be designed to interfere with many of the possible etiologies of AD. If, for example, amyloid is itself toxic (5), then pharmacologic strategies might be effective if they could prevent the "clipping" of the APP molecule to form amyloid (6), degrade amyloid, or antagonize its putative toxicity (e.g., ? substance P) (7). If deposition of aluminum causes AD (8), then chelation by the use of ethylenediaminetetraacetic acid (EDTA) or desferrioxamine (9) might be useful. If a deficiency of estrogen leads to AD in elderly women, then administration of estradiol might be of value (10). Other intervention strategies would depend in each case on the hypothesized etiology of AD; it is worth noting that if the theory is wrong these treatments would fail. Such strategies would, of course, be of no use in the treatment of other memory disorders, such as those caused by Creutzfeld–Jakob disease and multi-infarct dementia.

The strategy of substitution attempts to compensate for structural or functional losses that result in memory impairment by providing replacements for the critical losses. This strategy is far more likely to succeed when there is a single deficit, or at least a single *locus minoris resistentiae* (site of least resistance), whose loss accounts for the memory impairment, rather than multiple areas of deficiency. The most successful neurologic model of an effective substitution strategy has been parkinsonism, in which levodopa replacement of the function of lost substantia nigra dopaminergic neurons has been highly effective (11,12).

Structural losses causing memory disorders may be partial or complete. Minor losses of neurons may be clinically inapparent because of the "safety factor" built into most brain structures and the plasticity of the nervous system (13). As the brain is a postmitotic structure in which all the neurons that will be available throughout life are present at birth, it is teleologically appropriate to have a surplus of neurons available in crucial structures to serve as replacements for those that may be lost. Until the losses reach some critical threshold, therefore, the effects of minor losses are not behaviorally evident, as sufficient neurons remain to carry out normal function. A second compensatory mechanism for the partial loss of neural structures is plasticity, in which remaining neural elements take over extra functions, in part as the result of axon growth (sprouting) in surviving neurons.

In AD, major neuronal losses are found in the entorhinal cortex, with loss of the perforant pathway and synapses in the outer molecular layer of the dentate gyrus (14), in the subiculum, in area CA1 of the hippocampus (15), in the amygdala (16), in the nucleus basalis of Meynert (17), in the locus coeruleus (18), and in widespread cortical association areas, especially in the temporal and parietal lobes (19,20).

Significant losses of neurons can be approached therapeutically by efforts to achieve functional substitution or facilitation, or by structural replacement by means of "brain transplants" (21). If some neurons remain, for example, facilitation of neurotransmission can be attempted by providing an excess of neurotransmitter precursors (22) or by blocking the enzymatic hydrolysis of released transmitters (see below) (23). Another substitution strategy attempts to provide "new parts for old" by transplanting either fetal brain tissue (24) or genetically engineered fibroblasts that may provide a critical substance such as nerve growth factor (NGF) (25). Although studies in experimental animals have shown preliminary success with these techniques, their practical application to human medicine remains for the future (26).

Functional losses may entail decreased signaling or memory capability among surviving neurons or actual loss of some (but not all) neurons involved in critical memory processes. A large proportion of the pharmacologic studies and trials in AD to date have attempted to amplify or substitute for declining neurotransmission involving one or more pharmacologic systems of the brain. Drugs designed to enhance function in cholinergic (27–36), catecholaminergic (37–41), serotoninergic (42–46), and peptidergic (47,48) neural systems have been tried in AD with little benefit to date (Table 3).

Facilitation of memory function can be approached with a strategy analogous to putting high-test gasoline in an old car. There are two main strategies: nonspecifically increasing brain metabolism in general and specifically increasing those processes known to be essential to memory formation.

Nonspecific increases in brain metabolism have been approached with several classes of drugs: "nootropics" such as piracetam, which are thought to increase brain metabolism, often in poorly understood ways (49); cerebral vasodilators or rheologic agents, such as cyclandelate and pentoxyfylline (50); and vasodilation/metabolism enhancers, such as Hydergine (dihydroergotoxin mesylates) (51). Although many studies have been carried out, these drugs have never shown a significant improvement in memory function in controlled trials of patients with AD.

The strategy of specific facilitation of underlying biochemical processes essential for memory formation has only occasionally been tried, perhaps

TABLE 3. *Drugs to enhance neurotransmitter function*

Category	Agent	Reference
Cholinergic	Choline	27
	Lecithin	28
	Acetyl-L-carnitine	29
	Physostigmine	30
	Tetrohydroaminoacridine	31
	Pyridostigmine	32
	Arecoline	33
	RS-86	34
	Bethanecol	35
	Nicotine	36
Catecholaminergic	Levodopa	37
	Memantine	38
	Clonidine	39
	Quantacine	40
	L-Deprenyl	41
Serotoninergic	Tryptophan	42
	Alaproclate	43
	Zimeldine	44
	m-Chlorophenylpiperazine	45
	THIP	46
Peptidergic	Vasopressin analogues (LVP, DDAVP, DGAVP)	47
	ACTH analogues (ACTH 4–9, ACTH 4–10)	48

because of the wide gulf between basic scientific studies of neuronal memory in simple organisms and their application to clinical situations.

Although much work has been done on the mechanisms of memory, we will only briefly mention the basic studies on short-term memory (STM) and long-term memory (LTM) that have been carried out by Kandel and his colleagues on *Aplysia* (52). In studying the limited array of neurons involved in the gill-withdrawal reflex, they have demonstrated that STM involves facilitated release of transmitter, whereas LTM involves synthesis of new proteins.

In STM a complex mechanism is initiated by the interaction of a transmitter such as serotonin with a neuronal surface receptor. The activation of adenylyl cyclase by interaction with G-protein produces cyclic adenosine monophosphate (cAMP) which binds to cAMP-dependent phosphokinase. This phosphorylates (and thereby blocks) potassium channels, facilitating the influx of calcium into the neuron, which results in an increase in the releasable pool of transmitter and the release of transmitter.

LTM is facilitated when protein kinase A, which is also increased by neurotransmitter–receptor interaction, enters the neuron nucleus and phosphorylates transcriptional activators that bind to a cAMP-regulatory element (CRE). This then activates two genes: one that encodes a synaptic protein that increases the number of synapses and enlarges the active zone of synapses, and another that deactivates a protein kinase regulator, thus keeping the protein kinase active.

This "Rube Goldberg" mechanism (which may be somewhat simpler than the human counterpart) provides many steps at which pharmacologic facilitation might take place. It is not known which of these steps might be normally rate-limiting, or whether in AD or AAMI facilitation of a rate-limiting step in the formation of memories might be effective. Trials of 4-aminopyridine (a potassium channel blocker) (53,54) magnesium pemoline (an RNA enhancer) (55), and bovine cortical phosphatidylserine (BC-PS, a presumed neuron membrane component) (56) have been carried out, with some optimistic preliminary findings with BC-PS. Exploration of additional possible areas of facilitation based on this strategy may be a fruitful area for future study.

PRELIMINARY OBSERVATIONS

Once a candidate drug has been selected, the question often arises as to what results of preliminary investigations would clearly indicate the value of proceeding with further major development efforts, including full-scale human drug trials. The answer must be somewhat conjectural, because no drug has yet been shown to produce clinically significant improvement in memory disorders, especially in AD. (On March 18, 1993 an FDA panel recommended approval of tacrine for the treatment of AD.) Nevertheless, a critical analysis of both experimental animal and human studies is a necessary prelude to further development.

Experimental Animal Studies

The translation of experimental animal studies that assess the effects of drugs on memory requires considerable caution. Species differences, differences in brain anatomy, the lack of an animal model for AD (57), differences in drug dose effects and toxicity, and the problems in comparing human versus animal behavior paradigms all add uncertainty to both the design and the interpretation of experimental animal drug studies (58). Table 4 lists some of the variables in these experiments.

TABLE 4. *Memory treatments: experimental animal studies*

Animal species
  Rat, mouse, primate
Disordered memory model
  Aged, scopolamine, other (e.g., APP transgene)
Treatment
  Drug, etc.
Behavior task
  Conditioned avoidance (go–no go)
  Mazes
    T-maze, water maze, radial-arm maze
  Discrimination
  Delay tasks
    Position (WGTA), matching from sample,
    Nonmatching from sample

Rats, mice, and primates have been utilized most extensively in experimental studies of memory. Because in experimental animals language cannot be used for instructions, they must learn a task in order to demonstrate formation and persistence of memory. It is difficult then to differentiate between those aspects of the task involving pure memory storage, and those that require additional learning ability; and the precise nature of the learning tasks only approximately represents the human operations they are intended to parallel. In rats, for example, conditioned avoidance tasks (59) are often used as a simple learning/memory model. The rat is trained to avoid a conditioned stimulus, often by moving on a signal to another chamber in a shuttle-box apparatus, to avoid a shock. The response latency after training (i.e., the time it takes the animal to leave the initial chamber) is considered a measure of the strength of learning. Although this reflects one important aspect of the task, learning to escape the negative reinforcement quickly also depends on a number of other features in addition to the ability to remember, such as perception of the association, general activity level, and response to aversive stimuli. Learning of a radial-arm maze by mice (60) and of a water maze by rats (61) is considered a less confounded task.

In general, the experimental animal paradigm that most closely simulates a human short-term memory task is learning of a nonmatching to sample task by a primate (62). Retention of the behavior (e.g., savings in relearning) is a reasonable approximation of long-term memory.

There are at present no close animal models of AD (57). The decline in learning in very old animals is an approximate model (63), but is questionably relevant to AD, for the same reasons that the memory impairment of AAMI is thought to differ from that of AD. Moreover, although aged subhuman primates develop cerebral senile plaques and some deposits of amyloid with advanced age (64), only certain very aged bears have been shown at autopsy to develop neurofibrillary tangles in addition to senile plaques and amyloid deposits (65). Experimental models of AD based on central muscarinic cholinergic deficits have included the use of animals given scopolamine (66) and animals with lesions of the nucleus basalis of Meynert (67). Recent promising attempts to create a better animal model of AD have utilized a genetic modification strategy, producing transgenic mice that overexpress the amyloid precursor protein (unpublished data), or have tried direct injection of amyloid intravenously or intracerebrally (7).

Preliminary Human Studies

Before a major drug trial in AD or other memory disorders is undertaken, what small-scale studies should be done to reduce the likelihood of failure? We believe that pilot studies are valuable as an initial step. Even though they take time, and cannot provide definitive answers, they can either support or

TABLE 5. *Traps and pitfalls of therapeutic trials*

Size of study; power	Multiple outcome measures
Positive and negative	Requires Bonferroni or other correction
Use of subgroups of "responders"	Post hoc selection
Inverted U-shaped curve	Subgroup of patients
Multiple drug doses, single placebo	Subset of test battery improves
Validity of outcome measure	Crossover study
Floor, ceiling effects	Carryover effect; withdrawal effect
Nonlinearity of scores	
Loss of double-blind	
Toxic drug, inert placebo	

discourage embarking on a far more time-consuming and costly study with the power to evaluate a potentially useful drug definitively. Pilot studies of drugs with a presumptive direct and rapid effect on memory and cognitive functions are simpler to carry out than studies on drugs intended to alter the course of a disease process over years. In brief, drugs should show some reasonable evidence of effectiveness in experimental animal and human pilot trials before a large-scale commitment to a multicenter definitive study is made.

Avoiding the Traps and Pitfalls of Therapeutic Trials

There are many reasons why the design and interpretation of drug trials for the treatment of memory and cognitive disorders are difficult (Table 5). For the most part, errors arise when extraordinary efforts are made to establish the significance of a marginal and/or inconsistent benefit, in some subset of patients who improve to a small extent on a specially designed test with a carefully adjusted drug dosage (68). We will discuss here a few of the more common problems seen in human drug trials to determine the effectiveness of candidate drugs in improving memory or other cognitive function.

DESIGN OF CLINICAL DRUG TRIALS

Size of Study and Power

The ability of a study to compare the effect of an active drug with that of a placebo is determined by a number of variables, including the size of the sample, the expected magnitude of the differences between treated and untreated groups, the variability of the outcome measure, and the significance level. A very large study is often required to find a small but statistically significant improvement in a fraction of the patients (69); whether this is of clinical value or trivial is determined by medical judgment. When drug trials are designed, it is crucial to decide on the magnitude of a meaningful benefit. The power of the test, given the extent of improvement anticipated and the proportion of patients expected to show such an effect, must then be calculated to avoid inappropriately negative conclusions (70). For example, a therapeutic study of 200 patients showing a statistically significant 2-point increase in the Wechsler Memory Quotient (71) is of trivial value, whereas the observation that "none of 10 patients showed liver toxicity" is clinically misleading, because the null hypothesis could not be rejected with so few patients.

Use of Subgroups of Responders

AD is a disorder of heterogeneous etiology (see above), and it is widely assumed that only a subgroup of AD patients will therefore respond to a given drug (72). Although this may be true, the response heterogeneity should be concordant with the etiologic differences among patients, and it is an error to regard the upper end of a normal distribution of variability in test performance as "responders" to a given drug. If, in comparison with baseline or placebo scores on a psychometric test, some individuals subsequently obtain higher scores, some the same, and some lower after drug administration, one cannot conclude that the drug has been effective in a sensitive subgroup of responders. Proof of the efficacy of the drug would depend on replication of the study in this selected subgroup to demonstrate repeatability of the finding.

Misuse of the Inverted U-shaped Curve

In principle, many drugs may be beneficial only over a dosage midrange (73), which varies from individual to individual. At either dosage extreme they may be useless or harmful. The use of many trials of a drug at different doses versus a single trial of placebo to identify a "best dose" can produce an apparent benefit at *some* drug dose merely by chance. This should be accepted only when the improvement is considerably greater than the variability of the test or when the result is replicated using the selected drug dose in a single comparison with placebo.

Validity of Outcome Measures

A multitude of psychometric tests are available for assessing memory and other cognitive functions (74). Some tests have been well studied, whereas others have not been shown to have reliability (numerical repeatability), linearity over a wide range of performance, or validity in measuring what they purport to assess. Test scores that vary widely on repetition make differences between baseline and treatment conditions unreliable, and possible drug effects must be questioned. Failure of linearity (equivalent changes of score for equal changes in performance over a range of baseline performance), and the issues of "floor" and "ceiling" effects limit the range of comparability of a psychometric test. Many psychometric tests used to evaluate drug effectiveness suffer from these limitations.

INTERPRETING THE RESULTS OF CLINICAL DRUG TRIALS

Loss of Double-Blind

When a drug with clearly apparent side effects is compared with an inert placebo, the double-blind status of the study may be broken. Both the patient and the physician will know that the "blinded" drug is active if it causes nausea or diarrhea (as anticholinesterases may) (75); the physician will be aware if liver enzymes are elevated [as with tetrahydroaminacridine (THA)] (76). Knowledge of the treatment may bias the outcome.

Multiple Outcome Measures

One of the most common faults in AD drug trials is often the consequence of using multiple tests of memory or cognitive function. If uncorrected statistics (such as Student's t test) are used to determine significance of improvement after treatment, the probability of finding a statistical difference increases with the number of outcome measures tested. Many standard statistical methods give the result as the chance that a drug treatment group differs from a placebo group on a test measure; significance at the $p < 0.05$ level indicates less than one chance in 20 that the two groups are the same. If 20 tests are done, however, the odds become 2:1 that at least one test will show a significant difference at $p < 0.05$ (70)! When multiple tests are used, a correction (such as the Bonferroni correction) (77,78) must be made, adjusting the odds downward appropriately.

Post Hoc Selection

After a drug trial, subsequent selection of outcome measures or patient subgroups can falsely produce the appearance of improvement. If a large battery of tests has been administered, post hoc selection of only those that showed improvement as being the designated "outcome measures" falsely elevates the significance of any improvement, which may have been due to chance variation. This problem is especially troublesome when authors fail to report the large number of tests that were actually carried out. Similarly, the investigators may designate those patients who showed improvement after treatment as a "subset of responders." Although it is possible that there are subsets of responders, these must be confirmed either by advance (rather than post hoc) prediction, based on a particular characteristic, or by replication of the study using only those subjects.

Interpretation of Crossover Study Design

In a crossover drug study design, each subject is given either placebo or drug first, then the other treatment randomly chosen. This design for drug studies is appealing because it uses each subject as his/her own exact control and it reduces the total number of subjects needed, as compared with a parallel design (one group receives drug, the other placebo). A crossover design can provide an accurate measure of drug effect, however, only if two conditions are met: first, that the drug is completely washed out between the drug and placebo periods; and second, that the disease does not worsen during the treatment period (79). If drug treatment is not completely washed out, either a "carryover" or a "withdrawal" effect may overlap the placebo phase, and if the disease itself worsens, this may obscure or exaggerate the drug effect, depending on the sequence. An unexpected variant of these problems may arise when a trial is initiated with a titration phase to determine the "best dose" of drug; here, too, the issues of washout, carryover, and worsening of disease over time may contaminate the expected outcomes.

SETTING THE CRITERIA FOR EXTENT OF BENEFIT

In addition to the validity of the experimental design and the statistical analysis used, the predetermined criteria for "success" in a clinical drug trial are important in determining the clinical usefulness of the results. Problems in interpretation arise primarily when the investigator is willing to accept a very small increment in performance as evidence of drug effectiveness. Three levels of improvement will be considered.

Slight Improvement

No investigator wishes to waste years of effort evaluating a drug, only to find that it produces no significant effect. To avoid such failures, the sample size can be increased excessively to detect small yet statistically significant changes in performance. Caution must be exercised in interpreting such results, especially when the change in performance is so small that it is within the variability of the test. The criteria for success should be explicitly stated before the study is begun. We believe that acceptance of clinically ineffective and barely measurable "improvements" on psychometric tests as the criterion for improvement inappropriately encourages efforts to "prove" that there was indeed a drug effect, although it may be of no clinical value.

Modest Improvement

Modest improvements are those that are beyond the variability of the outcome measure but are below a clinically meaningful level. Some have argued that this situation may occur when the duration of the clinical trial is insufficient to detect clinical differences between treated and untreated groups (80). Small but real drug effects may be of value when they represent an effect on the underlying cause of the disease, rather than an alteration of symptoms; the analogy to chemotherapeutic agents used in *combination* in leukemia is appropriate, and suggests that converging therapeutic strategies may be of value.

Large Improvement

Substantial increments in performance uniformly observed in all patients, comparable to the effect of penicillin in pneumonia, obviate many of the traps and pitfalls that occur in imperfect study designs and inappropriate analytic methods. This is, of course, the goal of treatment, but no candidate drugs with this level of effectiveness have as yet been suggested for the treatment of AD.

CONCLUSIONS

The selection of drugs for the treatment of memory disorders, and especially AD, remains uncertain at present, because no drugs have been shown to be clinically useful in AD. Nevertheless, there are four rationales that are useful in selecting candidate treatments: intervention, based on interfering with the underlying etiology of the disease process; substitution, which replaces lost or missing structural or functional components of the memory-forming components of brain; facilitation, which nonspecifically or specifically increases brain function or memory processes; and serendipity, which searches for some treatment with a less clear rationale.

Full-scale investigation of a candidate drug is a major investment, and both experimental animal, and preliminary human pilot studies should be carried out before a large human drug trial is undertaken. The design of such studies and their interpretation are complex, however, with many opportunities for statistical error. The degree of drug effect to be accepted as "successful'' is a particularly important decision and avoids acceptance of clinically meaningless (but statistically significant) changes induced by experimental drugs.

ACKNOWLEDGMENT

This research was supported by NIA Grant 2-P50-OAG05134, Alzheimer's Disease Research Center, by the Sterling Morton Charitable Trust, and by the Stanley and Harriet Friedman Fund.

REFERENCES

1. Kay DWK. Heterogeneity in Alzheimer's disease: epidemiological and family studies. *Trends Neurosci* 1987;10:194–5.
2. Goate A, Chartier–Harlin MC, Mullan M, et al. Segregation of a missense mutation in the amyloid precursor protein gene with familial Alzheimer's disease. *Nature* 1991;349:704–6.
3. St. George–Hyslop P, Tanzi R, Polinsky R, et al. The genetic defect causing familial Alzheimer's disease maps on chromosome 21. *Science* 1987;235:885–90.
4. St. George–Hyslop P and the FAD Collaborative Study Group. Genetic linkage studies suggest that Alzheimer's disease is not a single homogeneous disorder. *Nature* 1990;347:194–7.
5. Yankner BA, Dawes LR, Fisher S, Villa-Komaroff L, Oster–Granite ML, Neve RL. Neurotoxicity of a fragment of the amyloid precursor associated with Alzheimer's disease. *Science* 1989;245:417–20.
6. Yankner BA, Duffy LK, Kirschner DA. Neurotrophic and neurotoxic effects of amyloid β protein: reversal by tachykinin neuropeptides. *Science* 1991;250:279–82.
7. Kowall NW, Beal MF, Busciglio S, et al. An *in vivo* model for the neurodegenerative effects of β amyloid and protection by substance P. *Proc Natl Acad Sci USA* 1991;88:7247–51.
8. DeBoni V, Crapper McLachlan D. Biochemical aspects of SDAT and aluminum as a neurotoxic agent. In: Crook T, Gershon S, eds. *Strategies for the development of an effective treatment for senile dementia*. New Canaan, CT: Mark Powley; 1981:215–30.
9. Crapper–McLachlan D, Dalton A, Kruck T, et al. Intramuscular desferrioxamine in patients with Alzheimer disease. *Lancet* 1991;337:1304–8.
10. Fillit H, Weinreb H, Cholst I, et al. Hormonal therapy for Alzheimer's disease. In: Crook T, Bartus R, Ferris S, Gershon S, eds. *Treatment development strategies for Alzheimer's disease*. Madison, CT: Mark Powley; 1986;311–36.
11. Cotzias GC, Papavasilious PS, Gellene R. Modification of parkinsonism—chronic treatment with L-dopa. *N Engl J Med* 1969;280:337–45.
12. Hornykiewicz O. Dopamine and brain function. *Pharmacol Rev* 1966;18:925–64.
13. Coleman PD, Rogers KE, Flood DG. Neuronal plasticity in normal aging and deficient plasticity in Alzheimer's disease: a proposed intercellular signal cascade. *Prog Brain Res* 1990;86:75–87.
14. Hamos JE, DeGennaro LJ, Drachman DA. Synaptic loss in Alzheimer's disease and other dementias. *Neurology* 1989;39:355–61.
15. Ball MJ, Hachinski V, Fox A, et al. A new definition of Alzheimer's disease: a hippocampal dementia. *Lancet* 1985;1:14–6.
16. Herzog AG, Kemper TL. Amygdaloid changes in aging and dementia. *Arch Neurol* 1980;37:625–9.
17. Doucette R, Fisman M, Hachinski VC, Mersky H. Cell loss from the nucleus basalis of Meynert in Alzheimer's disease. *Can J Neurol Sci* 1986;13:435–40.
18. Bondareff W, Mountjoy CQ, Roth M. Selective loss of neurones of origin of adrenergic projection to cerebral cortex (nucleus locus coeruleus) in senile dementia. *Lancet* 1981;1:783–4.

19. Hansen LA, DeTeresa R, Davies P, Terry RD. Neocortical morphometry, lesion counts, and choline acetyltransferase levels in the age spectrum of Alzheimer's disease. *Neurology* 1988;38:48–54.
20. Terry RD, Peck A, DeTeresa R, Schechter R, Horoupian DS. Some morphometric aspects of the brain in senile dementia of the Alzheimer type. *Ann Neurol* 1981;10:184–92.
21. Madrazo I, Garcia L, Torres C, et al. Initial neurotransplants in humans. In: Koller WC, Paulson G, eds. *Therapy of Parkinson's disease*. New York: Marcel Dekker; 1990:473.
22. Bierkamper G, Goldberg A. Effect of choline on the release of acetylcholine from the neuromuscular junction. In: Barbeau A, Growdon J, Wurtman R, eds. *Nutrition and the brain*. New York: Raven Press; 1979.
23. Koelle GB. Anticholinesterase agents. In: Goodman LS, Gilman A, eds. *The pharmacological basis of therapeutics*. 4th ed. 1970:442–65.
24. Gage F, Bjorklund A. Cholinergic septal grafts into the hippocampal formation improve spatial learning and memory in aged rats by an atropine sensitive mechanism. *J Neurosci* 1986;6:2837–47.
25. Rosenberg M, Friedman T, Robertson R, et al. Grafting genetically modified cells to the damaged brain: restorative effects of NGF expression. *Science* 1988;242:1575–7.
26. Phelps CH, Gage FH, Growdon JH, et al. Potential use of nerve growth factor to treat Alzheimer disease. *Neurobiol Aging* 1989;10:205–7.
27. Smith C, Swash M, Exton–Smith A, et al. Choline therapy in Alzheimer's disease [Letter]. *Lancet* 1978;2:318.
28. Little A, Raymond L, Chuaqui–Kidd P, et al. A double-blind, placebo-controlled trial of high dose lecithin in Alzheimer's disease. *J Neurol Neurosurg Psychiatry* 1985;48:736–42.
29. Passeri M, Cucinotta D, Bonati PA, et al. Acetyl-L-carnitine in the treatment of mildly demented elderly patients. *Int J Clin Pharm Res* 1990:75–9.
30. Mitchell A, Drachman DA, O'Donnell B, et al. Oral physostigmine in Alzheimer's disease. *Neurology* 1986;36(suppl):295.
31. Eagger SA, Levy R, Sahakian B. Tacrine in Alzheimer's disease. *Lancet* 1991;337:989–92.
32. Molloy DW, Cape RDT. Acute effects of oral pyridostigmine on memory and cognitive function in SDAT. *Neurobiol Aging* 1989;10:199–204.
33. Christie J, Shering A, Fergusen J, et al. Physostigmine and arecoline: effects of intravenous infusions in Alzheimer presenile dementia. *Br J Psychol* 1981;138:46–50.
34. Wettstein A, Spiegel R. Clinical trials in Alzheimer's disease (AD) and senile dementia of the Alzheimer type (SDAT) with the cholinergic drug RS-86. *Psychopharmacology* 1984; 84:572–3.
35. Harbaugh R. Intracerebroventricular bethanechol chloride administration in Alzheimer's disease. *Ann NY Acad Sci* 1988;531:174–9.
36. Newhouse P, Sunderland T, Tariot P, et al. Intravenous nicotine in Alzheimer's disease: a pilot study. *Psychopharmacology* 1988;95:171–5.
37. Adolfsson R, Brane G, Bucht G, et al. A double-blind study with levodopa in dementia of Alzheimer type. In: Corkin S, Davis K, Growdon J, Usdin E, Wurtman R, eds. *Alzheimer's disease: a report of progress*. New York: Raven Press; 1978:469–74. (Aging series, Vol 19).
38. Fleischhacker W, Buchgeher A, Schubert H. Memantine in the treatment of senile dementia of the Alzheimer type. *Prog Neuropsychopharmacol Biol Psychiatry* 1986;10:87–93.
39. McEntee W, Mair R. Memory enhancement in Korsakoff's psychosis by clonidine: further evidence for a noradrenergic deficit. *Ann Neurol* 1980;7:466–70.
40. Frith C, Dowdy J, Ferrier L, et al. Selective impairment of paired associative learning after administration of a centrally-acting adrenergic agonist (clonidine). *Psychopharmacology* 1985;97:490–3.
41. Tariot P, Sunderland T, Weingarten H, et al. Cognitive effects of L-deprenyl in Alzheimer's disease. *Psychopharmacology* 1987;91:489–95.
42. Smith D, Stromgren E, Petersen H, et al. Lack of effect of tryptophan treatment in demented gerontopsychiatric patients. *Acta Psychiatr Scand* 1984;70:470–7.
43. Dehlin O, Hedenrud B, Jansson P, et al. A double-blind comparison of alaproclate and placebo in the treatment of patients with senile dementia. *Acta Psychiatr Scand* 1985;71: 190–6.
44. Cutler N, Haxby J, Kay A, et al. Evaluation of zimeldine in Alzheimer's disease. *Arch Neurol* 1985;42:744–8.

45. Lawlor B, Mellow A, Sunderland T, et al. A pilot study of serotoninergic system responsivity in Alzheimer's disease. *Psychopharmacol Bull* 1988;24:127–9.
46. Mohr E, Bruno G, Foster N, et al. GABA agonist therapy for Alzheimer's disease. *Clin Neuropharmacol* 1986;9:257–63.
47. Durso R, Fedio P, Brouviers P, et al. Lysine vasopressin in Alzheimer's disease. *Neurology* 1982;32:674–7.
48. Branconnier R, Cole J, Gardos G. ACTH 4-10 in the amelioration of neuropsychological symptomatology associated with senile organic brain syndrome. *Psychopharmacology* 1979;61:161–5.
49. Giurgea C. *Fundamentals to a pharmacology of the mind.* Springfield, IL: Charles C Thomas; 1980.
50. Yesavage J, Hollister L, Buriane E. Vasodilators in senile dementia. A review of the literature. *Arch Gen Psychiatry* 1979;36:220–4.
51. McDonald R. Hydergine: a review of 26 clinical studies. *Pharmacopsychiatr Neuropsychopharm* 1979;12:407–22.
52. Kandel ER. Cellular mechanisms of learning and the biological basis of individuality. In: Kandel ER, Schwartz, JH, Jessell TM, eds. *Principles of neural science.* New York: Elsevier; 1991:1009–32.
53. Wesseling H, Agoston S, Van Dan G, et al. Effects of 4-aminopyridine in elderly patients with Alzheimer's disease. *N Engl J Med* 1984;310:988–9.
54. Davidson M, Zemishland Z, Mohs R, et al. 4-Aminopyridine in the treatment of Alzheimer's disease. *Biol Psychiatry* 1988;23:485–90.
55. Eisdorfer C, Conner JF, Wilkie, FL. The effect of magnesium pemoline on cognition and behavior. *J Gerontol* 1968;23:283–8.
56. Amaducci L, SMID Group. Phosphatidylserine in the treatment of Alzheimer's disease: results of a multicenter study. *Psychopharmacol Bull* 1988;24:130–4.
57. Price DL, Cork LC, Struble RG, et al. Neuropathological, neurochemical, and behavioral studies of the aging nonhuman primate. In: David RT, Leathers CW, eds. *Behavior and pathology of aging in rhesus monkeys.* New York: Alan R Liss; 1985:113–35. (Monogr Primatol, Vol 8.)
58. Collerton D. Cholinergic function and intellectual decline in Alzheimer's disease. *Neuroscience* 1986;19:1–28.
59. Bolles RS. Specific defense reactions. In: Rovert BF, ed. *Aversive conditioning and learning.* New York: Academic Press; 1971.
60. Olton DS. The radial arm maze as a tool in behavioral pharmacology. *Physiol Behav* 1987; 40:793–7.
61. Wishaw IQ. Cholinergic receptor blockade in the rat impairs locale but not taxon strategies for place navigation in a swimming pool. *Behav Neurosci* 1985;99:979–1005.
62. Mishkin M, Delacour J. An analysis of short-term visual memory in the monkey. *J Exp Psychol Anim Behav Processes* 1975;1:326–34.
63. Presty SK, Bachevalier J, Walker L, et al. Age differences in recognition of memory of the rhesus monkey (Macaca mulatta). *Neurobiol Aging* 1987;8:435–40.
64. Selkoe DJ, Bell DS, Podlisny DL, et al. Conservation of brain amyloid proteins in aged mammals and humans with Alzheimer's disease. *Science* 1987;235:873–6.
65. Cork LC, Powers RE, Selkoe DJ, et al. Neurofibrillary tangles and senile plaques in aged bears. *J Neuropathol Exp Neurol* 1988;47:629–41.
66. Bartus R, Johnson H. Short-term memory in the rhesus monkey: disruption from the anticholinergic scopolamine. *Pharmacol Biochem Behav* 1976;5:39–46.
67. Aigner TG, Mitchell SJ, Aggleton JP, et al. Effects of scopolamine and physostigmine on recognition memory in monkeys with ibotenic-acid lesions of the nucleus basalis of Meynert. *Psychopharmacology* 1987;92:292–300.
68. Drachman DA, Swearer JM. Alzheimer's disease. In: Porter RS, Schoenberg BS, eds. *Controlled clinical trials in neurological disease.* Boston: Kluwer; 1990:361–92.
69. Meinert C, Tonascia S. *Clinical trials: design, conduct and analysis.* New York: Oxford University Press; 1986. (Monographs in Epidemiology and Biostatistics, Vol 8).
70. Kirk R. *Experimental design: procedures for the behavioral sciences.* 2nd ed. Belmont, CA: Brooks/Cole; 1982.
71. Wechsler D. A standardized memory scale for clinical use. *J Psychol* 1945;19:87–95.

72. Davis K, Mohs R. Enhancement of memory by physostigmine. *N Engl J Med* 1979;301: 946.
73. Davis J, Erickson S, Dekirmenjian H. Plasma levels of antipsychotic drugs and clinical response. In: Lipton M, DiMascio A, Killam K, eds. *Psychopharmacology: a generation of progress*. New York: Raven Press; 1978.
74. Lezak M. *Neuropsychological assessment*. 2nd ed. New York: Oxford University Press; 1983.
75. Smith C, Semple S, Swash M. Effects of physostigmine on responses in memory tests in patients with Alzheimer's disease. In: Corkin S, Davis K, Growdon J, Usdin E, Wurtman R, eds. *Alzheimer's disease: a report of progress*. New York: Raven Press; 1982. (Aging series, Vol 19).
76. Chatellier G, Lacomblez L. Tacrine (tetrahydroaminoacridine; tacrine) and lecithin in senile dementia of the Alzheimer type: a multi-center trial. *BMJ* 1990;300:495–9.
77. Dunn O. Multiple comparisons among means. *J Am Stat Assoc* 1961;56:52–64.
78. Tukey J. Some thoughts on clinical trials, especially problems of multiplicity. *Science* 1977; 198:679–84.
79. White BG. Initial statistical consideration. In: Porter RJ, Schoenberg BS, eds. *Controlled clinical trials in neurological disease*. Boston: Kluwer; 1990:17–28.
80. Stern Y, Sano M, Mayeux R. Long term administration of oral physostigmine in Alzheimer's disease. *Neurology* 1988;38:1837–41.

Guidelines for Drug Trials in Memory Disorders, edited by N. Canal, et al.
Raven Press, Ltd., New York © 1993.

10

Phase 1 Studies

Malcolm Lader and Valerie Curran

Institute of Psychiatry, London SE5 8AF, England

Classical phase 1 studies comprise the first introduction of a new drug for human use. The subjects are usually normal, healthy volunteers, but patients may be used on occasion. After initial cautious dose-determination studies and preliminary pharmacokinetic estimations in relatively few subjects, detailed observations are made to detect some hint of an appropriate therapeutic action and also to uncover any unexpected toxicity. Therefore, some prediction of therapeutic profile of the new chemical entity must be made on the basis of the preclinical studies so that the search for pharmacodynamic actions can progress on a rational rather than a haphazard basis.

This chapter reviews the usefulness of phase 1 studies in predicting therapeutic efficacy in memory disorders. It does not deal with either the pharmacokinetic aspects or the detection of toxicity, as these topics are no different for memory enhancers than for any other medication. (The obvious point is that these areas must be carefully explored in the elderly and the infirm elderly.)

DIVERSE ACTIONS

There is a danger of narrowing the focus of interest to only those compounds dubbed "cognitive enhancers" or "nootropics." Much of this is wishful thinking on the part of the pharmaceutical industry, which senses a yawning void of therapeutic futility with current remedies for memory disorders. A separate class of compounds has been created on dubious scientific grounds. The mode of action of these compounds remains obscure and many dispute the existence of such an artificial entity. In turn, this leads to one of the major problems in this area, the lack of a credible, comparator, benchmark compound. The efficacy of all current compounds is marginal, so that putative new cognitive enhancers (NCEs) cannot be calibrated. In many countries, drugs such as piracetam are either unlicensed or ignored, reflecting

TABLE 1. *Approaches to the treatment of memory disorders*

Neurotransmitter systems	Disorders postulated to involve these systems	Proposed drugs
Acetylcholine	Alzheimer disease	Physostigmine
		Lecithin
		Choline
	Alcoholic dementia	THA
		RS-86
Dopamine	Dementia with behavioral disturbance	Antipsychotics
Norepinephrine	Alzheimer disease	Clonidine
	Behavioral disturbance	MAO inhibitors
		Propranolol
Serotonin	Alzheimer disease	Antidepressants
GABA	Behavioral disturbance	Chlormethiazole
	Insomnia	
Peptides	Alzheimer disease	ACTH
		Vasopressin
		CRF
		TRH
		Opioid antagonists
Antiviral agents	Creutzfeld–Jakob disease	Amantadine
Antihypertensive agents	Multi-infarct dementia	Various

the skepticism of medical practitioners. Nor are cerebral vasodilators held in much esteem.

One must not neglect, however, a wide range of other drugs that may enhance cognition and memory indirectly. Psychostimulants and analeptics are examples (1), although their usefulness is debatable and they may even worsen the patient. Antidepressants are helpful in depressed, impaired elderly patients, and some psychogeriatricians advocate a trial of therapy with cautious doses of an antidepressant. Other symptomatic treatments include sedatives and hypnotics, of dubious risk-to-benefit ratios in the elderly.

New approaches encompass a wide range of drugs acting on many different neurotransmitter systems in the brain (2). The major ones are listed in Table 1. The number of compounds that has been suggested as therapeutic agents is becoming legion, but relatively few of these have been comprehensively evaluated.

DIVERSE INDICATIONS

Table 1 also shows some of the disorders that involve memory disturbances, although the list is not complete. In addition, there are a number of treatable dementias such as subdural hematomas, endocrine disorders, and nutritional deficiencies (3). The concatenation of many indications and many rather ineffective remedies has led to this field remaining inchoate. Progress is possible only by careful clinical dissection of syndromes and disorders and then the controlled administration of drugs.

The outcome of such diversity in both drug types and target symptoms, syndromes, and disorders is to make imperative careful focusing on drug actions at phase 1. No general rules can be laid down to cover all possibilities. Indeed, the overlap between the various categories of drugs is very small and relates to cognitive effects only. Nevertheless, other domains should be explored if only to exclude these actions.

OUTCOME MEASUREMENTS

What aspects of human behavior should be assessed? In typical phase 1 studies, prior animal investigations point to potential areas of interest. Unfortunately, preclinical studies have not been widely accepted as very helpful. For example, Hershenson and Moos (3) assert: *"unfortunately, appropriate animal models do not yet exist"* (authors' italics). The upshot is inevitable: screening programs of the type usually concentrated in preclinical testing have to be incorporated into phase 1 and phase 2 studies.

A wide range of body functions must be monitored to detect potential side-effects. However, side-effects (better termed unwanted effects) represent a value judgment on the part of both the patient and the physician. It is important, consequently, to scrutinize each drug effect to confirm that it is indeed unwanted in all cases. For example, mild drowsiness may be unacceptable in the inert individual but quite useful for the overalert insomniac.

EFFECTS ON MOOD

This should be a routine part of every phase 1 study. A wide range of instruments are available in different formats. Few, however, have been either validated or tested for sensitivity to drug effects. We developed a simple visual analogue scale (VAS) nearly 20 years ago and have used it routinely since (4). We know that it is sensitive to depressant drug effects but relatively few studies have been performed to establish its sensitivity to stimulant drug actions. It is important that mood scales are properly developed and used. The factor structure of such scales may not accord with the face validity of the items. Careful instructions are needed to prevent halo effects, scoring falsely at the extremes, and answering according to perceived social norms.

The two dimensions of most importance are stimulation/sedation and euphoria/depression. Such actions would be expected to occur in patients with memory disturbances if found in appropriate doses in phase 1 studies. In turn, these effects could have an indirect influence on cognitive and memory functions by affecting concentration, attention, and motivation. Therefore, effects on memory function should be co-varied against effects on general behavior and on mood changes. Only in this way can one begin to tease out important primary actions on memory from secondary general effects.

BIOCHEMICAL EFFECTS

We have seen that a wide range of different drugs have been used or suggested for use in patients with memory disorders. The mode of action of any of the existing compounds remains obscure. Others, however, such as the cholinergic compounds, have a biochemical rationale. In phase 1 studies it is useful to search for markers of such biochemical actions in both biochemical and physiologic terms. For example, a serotoninergic compound might be expected to alter serotonin turnover in a fairly gross way. A noradrenergic compound that releases norepinephrine will increase the amount of metabolites in the urine. Most of these measurements are fairly crude and can provide only gross indicators of whole-body actions. More focused measurements, such as the concentration of the serotonin metabolite 5-hydroxyindoleacetic acid (5-HIAA) in the cerebrospinal fluid, may be difficult to perform in phase 1 studies because of technical difficulties, cost and, above all, ethical considerations.

Indirect measurements of biochemical effects may be obtainable using the so-called "neuroendocrine window on the brain." Hormones such as prolactin, cortisol, and growth hormone are under the complex control of several neural pathways. However, providing appropriate care is taken, changes in the plasma concentration of these substances can throw light on the mode of action of the NCE and at the very least act as a marker for dose–effect and time–effect studies.

EEG EFFECTS

Some experts put strong emphasis on the use of quantitative electroencephalographic (EEG) techniques to predict the clinical properties of NCEs. Any drug effect can be used as an empirical marker to facilitate the construction of dose–effect and time–effect curves. It is more contentious to claim that each type of agent has its own characteristic EEG pattern both topographically and in terms of spectral composition (5). The argument can too easily become circular, with putative new classes of psychotropic action being invoked to explain each type of EEG change. However, some broad directions can be delineated. For example, if a new drug believed to enhance cognitive function were found to have an EEG profile resembling that of a psychostimulant, such as amphetamine, its development might differ from that of a compound with a "nootropic" or a totally novel profile.

Practical problems also obtrude. The technology is complex and fairly expensive, especially when multilead analyses and topographic imaging techniques are used. There is as yet no agreement on standardization of techniques. In summary, quantitative EEG techniques are not yet established as useful in phase 1 studies except as empirical indicators of dose and time effects of an unspecified drug action.

PSYCHOLOGICAL TESTS

A wide variety of assessments of cognitive and psychomotor functioning are potentially available for the evaluation of NCEs. The selection of appropriate tests to include in a battery requires carefully considered criteria. Minimal requirements are that the group of tests should be (a) sensitive to both increments and decrements in function, (b) available in equivalent forms for repeated testing to evaluate change, (c) appropriate for the study population, (d) of such a duration that they will not produce marked fatigue or decreased motivation; and (e) they should sample a specified and adequate range of functions (6). Major differences in the various approaches to the construction of a battery lie in the last criterion. Given time restrictions, one must balance the desire for breadth of assessment (sampling a wide range of functions) with that for depth (sampling specific functions in sufficient detail to allow clear interpretation of results).

In addition to these minimal requirements, certain further criteria are relevant to the assessment of psychotropic drugs. First, and most important, the battery should be capable of detecting not only changes in the main functions of interest (e.g., attention, memory) but also more global changes in alertness or arousal levels which might affect performance on cognitive tests as a byproduct. For example, an NCE may produce a generalized stimulant effect resulting in performance increments across a wide range of tests, and therefore the battery should be capable of distinguishing such across-the-board changes from a specific effect, such as enhancement of episodic memory.

Second, it may be appropriate to model the test battery on the clinical syndrome of interest. For example, if a drug is thought to have potential in the amelioration of early stage Alzheimer disease (AD), one would select tests that reflect the profile of both impairments and preserved functions of early stage AD.

Within this background of selecting appropriate criteria, how does one choose which tests to include in a battery? Three broad approaches are possible. The first aims for breadth of assessment using "off-the-peg" test batteries; the second, at the other extreme, is an in-depth theoretical approach from within experimental cognitive psychology; the third, and our own approach, is a multiphased assessment beginning with sufficient breadth and, where initial results seem appropriate, continuing in a structured way to increasing depth.

Early studies used an "off-the-peg" approach with clinical test batteries such as the Wechsler Adult Intelligence Scale (7), which had proved useful in the diagnosis of brain damage. However, in the detection of often subtle drug-induced changes in cognition, such batteries proved of limited usefulness. In being designed (for clinical reasons) to sample a wide range of psychologic functions, these tests usually provided only rough and superficial measures of each. Moreover, as our understanding of the complexities of cognition advanced, it became clear that these batteries were capable of assessing only limited aspects of human information processing.

Similar considerations apply to more recently developed batteries which aim primarily to assess global cognitive dysfunction for clinical purposes. Clearly, test batteries designed to detect global cognitive dysfunction in the elderly will tend to show ceiling effects when used in normal volunteer studies. For instance, CAMCOG is the cognitive assessment component of the Cambridge Diagnostic Evaluation for the Elderly (8). Although this may prove to be a useful screening tool in the detection and diagnosis of dementia, it has been criticized as being too nonspecific and insensitive to assess cognitive changes induced by NCEs (9).

Another approach is seen in the CANTAB tests (10,11). These were designed to relate to animal research and have taken advantage of computer technology and touch screens. The CANTAB tests provide sensitive measure of visuospatial aspects of memory, attention, and planning. In assessing a restricted range of cognitive functioning in greater detail, such tests used on their own are insufficient to provide a full evaluation of an NCE. As a minimum, additional verbal assessments would be required to form a reasonably comprehensive psychologic battery of tests.

Two recent batteries have aimed to augment the face validity of testing such that it resembles more the memory requirements of everyday life (12,13). For example, in both sets of tests the traditional digit span is presented as a telephone number recall task. However, in adapting traditional tests for computerized assessment, such batteries inevitably lose out on ecological validity: remembering a shopping list of groceries may be a real-life memory requirement but interacting with a computer for a five-trial recall of that shopping list is not. These batteries, therefore, lack the ecological validity seen in more behaviorally oriented assessments such as the Rivermead battery (14). The sensitivity of any of these batteries to nootropic effects, rather than to global clinical dysfunction, is doubtful.

Another variant in the "off-the-peg" approach merits little attention but will be mentioned because it unfortunately typifies many psychopharmacological assessments. This is the "I have-a-test-which-is-sensitive-to-drug-changes-so-let's-use-it" approach. Such studies litter the literature but are largely uninterpretable in terms of a drug's cognitive enhancing or impairing effects.

The in-depth theoretical approach is typified by an increasing number of studies that explore the effects of drugs from within an experimental cognitive framework. This research aims to produce detailed descriptions of changes in specified aspects of cognition, and studies often involve experimental manipulations as well as drugs. Although this approach has produced some excellent studies which are theoretically fruitful, it is not the appropriate *first* step for phase 1 studies of NCEs.

The third approach is to construct a battery on the basis of our knowledge of cognitive functions, clinical syndromes, and pharmacologic effects which, in the first instance, compromises between breadth and depth of assessment. Thus, to assess the memory effects of a drug, one would employ sufficient tests to sample a wide range of memory functions (working memory functions, episodic, semantic, and procedural memory) and sufficient additional tests to assess nonspecific (e.g., stimulant) effects of the drug (e.g., motor speed, simple reaction times, psychophysiologic indices). By careful selection and/or construction of tests, it is possible to assess all these aspects of performance and to collect data on subjective ratings of mood and body symptoms, in a battery taking just 50 min to complete. This not only avoids marked fatigue but allows for re-testing at different time points before and after drug administration.

Where results from this first-step battery show that an NCE may have some specific effects of enhancing particular aspects of functioning, the second step would be to replicate and explore this in greater depth by focusing on those aspects. In this way, one proceeds from breadth to depth of assessment in a structured, hypothesis-driven manner.

INDUCED DEFICITS

These tests can be used by themselves in normal subjects to establish the psychologic effects of an NCE, or they can be combined with an experimentally produced performance deficit. The most favored such approach is the induction of an impairment by giving the anticholinergic drug scopolamine.

As is well known, the rationale of the scopolamine "model" derives from the "cholinergic hypothesis" of AD. Memory impairments induced by scopolamine mimic some but not all of those observed in AD, and this in itself is one limitation of the scopolamine "model." A further main problem with this model, however, stems from the question of how specific are scopolamine's effects on memory (15). Although it is clear from a number of studies that scopolamine impairs the performance of normal subjects on tasks involving memory, it also impairs performance on tasks which have no obvious memory component—for example, finger tapping speeds (16) and simple reaction times (17). Indeed, many normal volunteer studies of scopolamine have used only tests of memory and have excluded assessments of nonspecific drug effects (e.g., on arousal). From our own work, we have found that scopolamine has a pronounced sedative effect, impairing performance across a wide range of psychomotor and memory tasks, and that both the level of sedation produced and the effects on those tasks are very similar to those of the benzodiazepine lorazepam (18). Our results suggest that scopolamine and lorazepam do not offer distinct models of explicit memory dysfunction.

Any novel drug that ameliorates scopolamine-induced impairments could therefore be acting nonspecifically, by attenuating or reversing scopolamine's sedative effects, specifically, by enhancing some aspect(s) of memory functioning, or a combination of both. Indeed, one could argue that lorazepam-induced impairments were an equally (in)appropriate model for memory dysfunction and would lead to similarly confounded interpretations.

Clearly, patients suffering from AD do not also suffer chronic drowsiness, and future research must aim toward models of cognitive dysfunction in which specific effects can be clearly distinguished from global sedative effects.

Another impairment model comprises performance in hypoxic conditions. In one such study, the oxygen tension was equivalent to an altitude of 5,300 meters. Piracetam in high dose counteracted the effects of hypoxia on a range of physiologic and psychologic tests (19). However, it is unclear which clinical syndromes hypoxia is modeling. In most forms of dementia, lower oxygen utilization is a result of neuron decay rather than neuron malfunction reflecting insufficient oxygen supply. Only in such conditions as carbon monoxide poisoning, with consequent dementia and other primary hypoxic conditions, is the model relevant. In other conditions such as multiinfarct dementia, further work is needed to establish the validity of the model.

SUMMARY

Phase 1 studies classically comprise the first introduction of a new chemical entity to humans, usually normal volunteers. Apart from toxicity and pharmacokinetic aspects, appropriate pharmacodynamic actions are sought. No drug for the treatment of memory disorders is sufficiently efficacious to act as a worthwhile comparator.

Biochemical and EEG tests are limited in scope. In addition to evaluating cognitive functions, mood and alertness should be assessed as part of a psychologic test battery. Both broad and in-depth approaches should be adopted, within a coherent theoretical framework. Induced deficits such as the scopolamine model may be too nonspecific to have predictive value in the clinical setting.

REFERENCES

1. Coper H, Herrmann WM. Psychostimulants, analeptics, nootropics: an attempt to differentiate and assess drugs designed for the treatment of impaired brain functions. *Pharmacopsychiatry* 1988;21:211–7.

2. Whalley LJ. Drug treatments of dementia. *Br J Psychiatry* 1989;155:595–611.
3. Hershenson FM, Moos WH. Drug development for senile cognitive decline. *J Med Chem* 1986;29:1125–30.
4. Bond A, Lader M. The use of analogue scales in rating subjective feelings. *Br J Med Psychol* 1974;47:211–8.
5. Saletu B, Grünberger J. Drug profiling by computed electroencephalography and brain maps, with special consideration of sertraline and its psychometric effects. *J Clin Psychiatry* 1988;49:8(suppl):59–71.
6. Ferris SH, Crook T. Cognitive assessment in mild to moderately severe dementia. In: Crook T, Ferris SH, Bartus R, eds. *Assessment in geriatric psychopharmacology*. New Canaan, CT: Mark Powley; 1983:36–51.
7. Wechsler S. *Manual for the Wechsler Adult Intelligence Scale*. New York: Psychological Corporation; 1985.
8. Roth M, Tym E, Mountjoy C, et al. CAMDEX: a standardised instrument for the diagnosis of mental disorder in the elderly with special reference to the early detection of dementia. *Br J Psychiatry* 1986;149:698–709.
9. Montaldi D, Brooks D, McColl J, et al. Measurement of regional cerebral blood flow and cognitive performance in Alzheimer's disease. *J Neurol Neurosurg Psychiatry* 1990;5:33–8.
10. Morris RG, Evenden JL, Sahakian BJ, Robbins TW. Computer aided assessment of dementia. In: Stahl S, Iversen S, Goodman E, eds. *Cognitive neurochemistry*. Oxford: Oxford University Press; 1987:21–36.
11. Sahakian BJ. Computerised assessment of neuropsychological function in Alzheimer's disease and Parkinson's disease. *Int J Geriatr Psychiatr* 1990;5:211–3.
12. Larrabee GJ, Crook T. A computerised everyday memory battery for assessing treatment effects. *Psychopharmacol Bull* 1988;24:695–7.
13. Ferris SH, Flicker C, Reisberg B. NYU computerized test battery for assessing cognition in aging and dementia. *Psychopharmacol Bull* 1988;24:699–702.
14. Wilson B, Cockburn J, Baddeley A. *The Rivermead behavioural memory test*. Reading: Thames Valley Test Company; 1985.
15. Curran HV. Benzodiazepines, memory and mood: a review. *Psychopharmacology* 1991; 105:1–8.
16. Nuotto E. Psychomotor, physiological and cognitive effects of scopolamine and ephedrine in healthy man. *Eur J Clin Pharmacol* 1983;24:603–9.
17. Callaway E. Human information processing: some effects of methylphenidate, age and scopolamine. *Biol Psychiatry* 1984;19:649–62.
18. Curran HV, Schifano F, Lader M. Models of memory dysfunction? A comparison of the effects of scopolamine and lorazepam on memory, psychomotor performance and mood. *Psychopharmacology* 1991;103:83–90.
19. Schaffler K, Klausnitzer W. Randomized placebo-controlled double-blind cross-over study on antihypoxidotic effects of piracetam using psychophysiological measures in healthy volunteers. *Arzneimittelforschung* 1988;38:288–91.

Guidelines for Drug Trials in Memory
Disorders, edited by N. Canal, et al.
Raven Press, Ltd., New York © 1993.

11

Discussion

Dr. Hachinski: Dr. Drachman, please clarify what you mean by "subset of responders."

Dr. Drachman: An example would be if you tested 20 outcome measures with variability, and five were found to be worse and five were "significantly" better. You could post hoc select the ones that were "significantly" better as the ones that you really wanted all along. This is roughly comparable to tossing a coin and picking those tosses that you regard as being the appropriate subset. All the heads belong to a subset. Of all the individuals you test, which ones benefit? If, of 100 people, 10 do better, and these are the ones selected, this could be considered a subset of responders.

Dr. McKhann: With regard to the problem of a heterogeneous population and about the issue of brain reserve and its fragility, is there a challenge test or a pharmacologic approach one could take that would allow you to determine a population at risk?

Dr. Drachman: Work that we have done makes it very clear that there is marked heterogeneity of cell loss and synapse loss among different brain structures in people with Alzheimer disease. Some individuals with clear familial Alzheimer disease lose few neurons in the entorhinal cortex and few synapses in the hippocampal gyrus. So there is variability. If you look at 10 structures, by the time someone is demented there is a total burden of loss that adds up to dementia. So patients with Alzheimer disease aren't all the same. If there were drugs that were known to help one or another of the replaceable brain areas that may be lost, then a stress-type test could be used. We could use scopolamine in Alzheimer disease and see whether we could treat those individuals who are borderline but become demented with a very tiny dose. But until we have enough replacement strategies this may not work. From the studies we've done, quantitative perikaryal and synaptic studies on 10 separate areas of brain, not everybody with Alzheimer disease and dementia loses neurons or synapses from the same place.

Dr. Ferris: Dr. Lader, I've often wondered why pharmaceutical companies, at least in the United States, perform only toxicity and tolerance tests as part of traditional phase 1 trials. Even though there are open studies with different doses and so forth, how much additional cost is there to find out if there are any behavioral or cognitive effects, particularly with a potentially cognitive activating agent?

Dr. Lader: I think you are absolutely right. What surprises me about pharmaceutical development is that a pharmaceutical company approaches you with normal subjects whom they recruited for quite expensive and elaborate pharmacokinetic studies. The subjects sometimes have to wait for hours on end for the studies to begin. If one suggests doing a few cognitive or performance studies on the subjects during that time, they say that's another group's responsibility. It seems to me, this is wasteful. With regard to memory enhancers' studies, I'm not sure that they are as valuable as studies with anxiolytics or hypnotics where quite a lot of data can be obtained early on in the study. However, I think it's worth doing even if it's negative, because at least you're using the subjects, and it's more ethical if you're compiling more data on them.

Dr. Drachman: Although I do not believe that scopolamine is an ideal model for Alzheimer disease or even normal aging, the issue is whether or not it is lethargy that contaminates its effect. I studied this issue a number of years ago when I gave scopolamine together with amphetamine to young controls. They were extremely alert, but indeed their cognitive and memory performance was worse than before they received the amphetamines. This was very interesting because, at the time, this was the exact combination of drugs that NASA was giving to the astronauts when they went into space. Subsequently, I believe that they have stopped using this combination.

Dr. Lader: We were very struck by the anxiogenic effects of scopolamine. People didn't like to take it. With amphetamine there was an extreme overarousal, causing the performance to fall because of overarousal rather than underarousal.

Dr. Saletu: I agree with the remarks of Dr. Ferris. A few years ago we had a very difficult time with the group that was designing the first phase 1 studies. There was a tremendous resistance with regard to what information could be gained by doing only quantitative EEG measurements in the initial trials. Now, of course, this is performed routinely because we have learned that information can be obtained about the CNS effect of the drug and its pharmacodynamics. So I think you pointed this out very well, for a pharmacodynamic purpose, specially in this group of substances where vigilance plays an important role. There is not one drug that would decrease vigilance, for instance, and which claims to be active. I personally found the hypoxia model of great interest.

Dr. Lader: We encountered a compound that had an interesting effect in animals. However, when we gave it to normal subjects, there was no effect whatsoever. Subsequently it was discovered that there is a metabolic pathway in animals not present in humans. Those types of mistakes can be avoided by early EEG studies.

Guidelines for Drug Trials in Memory Disorders, edited by N. Canal, et al.
Raven Press, Ltd., New York © 1993.

12

Statistical Issues in Designing Clinical Trials in Memory Disorders

Francesco Grigoletto

Department of Statistical Sciences, School of Medicine, University of Padua, 35121 Padua, Italy

Memory is difficult to measure with precision and reliability, and the methods employed suffer from low sensitivity to small changes. As a result, it becomes crucial to use an appropriate experimental design to reduce the sources of variability and bias that can affect such measurements. Only a well-designed trial enables one to tackle the difficulties inherent in carrying it out in an appropriate manner.

This chapter considers some basic clinical experimentation techniques and raises certain methodological questions on their use in drug trials on memory disorders. We will examine the need for a careful definition of the study population and for a knowledge of the characteristics of the outcomes or end points chosen to measure the effect of the drug. After considering certain aspects of sample size, the importance of random assignment, blinding, and stratification in study design will be discussed. To close, a number of considerations on statistical analysis will be made.

SELECTING THE STUDY POPULATION

The range of severity of the patients to be included in the study depends on many factors, including existing knowledge about the effectiveness of the study drug and the amount of resources available for the research. Only when pilot studies have shown the effectiveness of the drug in selected groups of patients is it advisable to consider a population that is more heterogeneous in terms of the level of severity. One consequence of the latter will be the need for a larger sample size, leading to higher costs. The statistical aspect of this problem is the variability of the drug effect measurement: the higher variability rises, the lower the power of the statistical test becomes, meaning, in other words, that there is less probability of showing that a given treatment difference is statistically significant.

On the other hand, a heterogeneous population facilitates the analysis of subgroups and a control on the consistency of the results of the treatment in different types of patients. In addition, the results of the treatment in a population that has not been highly selected can be more convincing than those in a very homogeneous population. In the specific case of memory disorders, however, heterogeneous populations do present a drawback: the scales generally available for measuring the outcome are not able to reflect changes in a wide range of degrees of severity. This is for two main reasons: First, the scales are not "ratio scales," meaning that changes of the same amount may assume a different meaning depending on the point in the scale concerned; and second, patients with measurements in the margins of the scale are not sufficiently able to express changes in either a positive or negative direction, so that there is a floor or ceiling effect. This makes it difficult to interpret the results. The problem could be overcome by using different measurement scales for different groups of patients. The statistical analysis could be performed separately on the different scales and the results of the different statistical tests then combined using a suitable method (1). This procedure could, however, present interpretation problems in cases where the individual results are inconsistent.

In conclusion, study population selection criteria have conflicting needs. A compromise can be reached by taking the following principle into account: the more homogeneous the population, the easier it becomes to identify suitable outcome measurements and analyze the results.

MEASURING OUTCOMES

Memory is typically measured using a quantitative score for a specific memory function. To produce a good outcome, a method of measurement should be a useful index of the severity of a pathology, easy to observe, reliable (meaning stable when repeated under identical conditions), and valid (an effective expression of the memory function it aims to measure) (2,3). Previous studies must provide an appropriate demonstration that the method of measurement is valid in groups of patients similar to those of the study population. It is also necessary for the tests to have a sufficient number of equivalent forms for the number of follow-ups in the study design.

Floor and Ceiling Effects

The effects of a drug are generally measured as a change in the outcome over time. Caution should be exercised in the choice of the appropriate outcome when very severely or slightly affected patients are included because

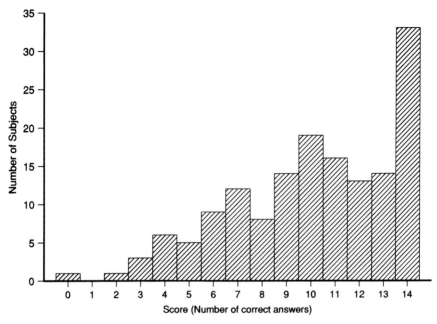

FIG. 1. Name–Face Association Test score of 154 patients with age-associated memory impairment: baseline evaluation (unpublished data).

it must be able to reflect changes in every category of patients considered in the study population. Potential floor and ceiling effects must be taken into account. For example, let us consider the score distribution for the Name–Face Association Test (4) on 154 subjects with age-associated memory impairment (AAMI) shown in Fig. 1. The subjects in this computerized test look at a video recording of 14 individuals, presented on the screen together with their names. These individuals are subsequently presented in a different order, and recall is evaluated by the number of correctly remembered names. The evaluation shown here is the baseline of patients considered for inclusion in a clinical trial. Forty-seven subjects (30.5%) had a score of 13 or 14. If the possibility of even a one-point improvement is envisaged, it is clear that there will be a ceiling effect, such that this test does not seem to represent a good outcome measurement for that particular AAMI population.

Multiple Outcomes

Measuring memory is typically a multidimensional problem, given the number of different memory functions that can be identified. One cannot think that a single elementary test would be able to evaluate this characteristic appropriately. It is, therefore, usually necessary to use multiple measurements, each for a specific memory function. The multiple results represent a difficult problem from a statistical point of view, above all where analysis of the clinical trial data is concerned, as discussed in the section on analysis. In all cases it is necessary to decide a hierarchy in advance for the relative importance of the outcomes concerned and to base the study design on what is considered the most important outcome from a clinical point of view and in relation to the properties of the test drug.

Outcome Variability

The variable described by the main outcome measurement should have a standard deviation known from pilot studies on the study population to be able to estimate the sample size. Its validity should also be optimal, so as to permit a reliable clinically significant minimal change in the outcome to be determined.

The undesirable variability of the outcome change variable can be reduced by acting on some of its sources. One such source, which we have already considered, is the heterogeneity of the study population. Another source is potential tester error. It is crucial to standardize the administration of the test because this reduces inter-tester variability. Tester training should continue through the follow-up stages to avoid the possibility of testers straying from their initial instructions. This will be facilitated if the tests are easy to transfer.

STUDY DESIGN

Pretherapeutic Evaluation

If the effect of the drug is measured in terms of change with respect to the baseline, as is usually the case, the study design should include a pretherapeutic evaluation. When cognitive tests are subsequently administered, it should be borne in mind that the response is affected by a certain degree of learning or practicing effect. For example, see Fig. 2, which shows the mean values of the Name–Face Association Test scores for 815 subjects divided into 10-year age groups. The data were collected for the Progetto Memoria, a study on reference values for memory in the Italian normal population (unpublished data). In Fig. 2, A, B, and C show three test trials which were administered consecutively, whereas the fourth (D) was delayed by approximately 40 min. The order of the faces whose names the subjects had to remember was changed at every trial. One can see a remarkable learning or practicing effect in the second and third trials, which is consistent across all the age groups. Which is the baseline evaluation? It could be argued that a

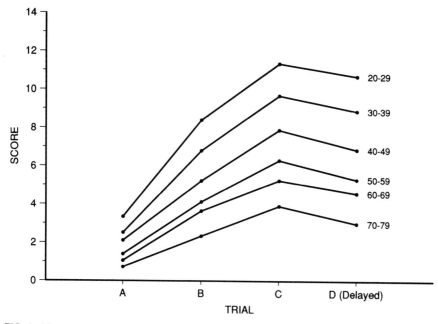

FIG. 2. Mean score of Name–Face Association Test on 815 subjects by age decade. Trials A, B, and C were consecutive, whereas trial D was administered approximately 40 min after trial C. (From Progetto Memoria, unpublished data.)

different characteristic is being measured in each of the different trials, but one ought to consider that this effect will be present in the evaluation of the subsequent follow-ups, which will, in their difference from the baseline, provide the change measurement. Because it seems that the learning effect tails off after the third administration, only the third trial can be considered as a measurement of the memory function both at the baseline and in the follow-ups, while the differences between the trials are able to provide information on the learning characteristic.

Observation Period

It takes time for the effects of a drug to alter the course of an illness in mental disorders. Certain authors are of the opinion that observation should continue for periods lasting from a minimum of 6 months to 1 or 2 years (5). This very long observation period imposes certain restrictions on study design. It becomes difficult to adopt crossover designs, for example, in which all the treatments under examination are administered to the patients in rotation. On the other hand, only a long period enables the emergence of a consistency effect sufficient to allow an acceptable sample size.

Control

Many factors, in addition to the drug being studied, can change the functional state of the patients in a treatment group, such as the natural evolution of the pathology or the administration of concomitant therapies. As a result, the net effect of the drug can be estimated only in relation to control patients. There can be two types of controls: external controls and internal controls (6).

External controls involve a group of patients who are in every respect similar to the patients treated with the drug apart from the treatment they receive. Usually they are observed in parallel with the group treated with the drug and are administered a placebo. All the patients involved in the clinical trial are assigned to the study drug or placebo group on a random basis. In addition, both groups of patients are kept unaware about what sort of treatment they are receiving. This is the preferred study design, known as the *double-blind, placebo-controlled, parallel-group design.*

Internal controls, on the other hand, involve the same subjects who receive the active treatment but are observed during a different period of time, as in the *crossover design* (7). In the simplest example of two treatments (A and B) and two time periods, the patients are assigned at random either to sequence AB, in which a patient receives treatment A during the first period and treatment B during the second, or sequence BA, in which B is administered first and A later. This design has the obvious advantage of ensuring that the treatment groups are comparable, avoiding between-subject variability in evaluating the effect of the drug. In addition, it is easier to obtain the patients' consent to take part in the clinical trial because they know they will all receive the active treatment. However, the crossover design is also subject to many potential problems, the most disturbing of which concerns pathologies connected with memory disorders, which are usually progressive. This rules out the necessary possibility of being able to consider patients' characteristics that are similar at the beginning of the second period to what they were at the beginning of the first period. This is made more difficult by the potential presence of the carryover effect. If, in addition to this, one considers the long periods required to observe the effect of the treatment, it becomes clear that the use of the crossover design is fairly problematic in clinical trials concerning the pathology in question.

Multiple Centers

A further characteristic of the study design of clinical trials on memory disorders results from the fact that the need for large sample groups, required to obtain definitive results on the effects of the drug, cannot be met by a single center. As a result, the study has to be organized on a multicenter basis. This makes it more important to standardize the test administration procedures to keep inter-center variability under control.

SAMPLE SIZE

Establishing the sample size requires prior experience with the pathology concerned and with the variables described by the outcome measurements. The calculation is based on the primary outcome of interest, for which one must establish the minimal change of clinical significance due to the action of the drug. The importance of this aspect must be stressed: the clinical trial will lead one to affirm the efficacy of the drug on the basis of the statistical significance of the minimum change. Consequently, any possible changes in the outcome that are a function of the action of the drug must have been investigated in preliminary studies and an estimate carried out for the standard deviation of the variable described by the changes.

In addition to the minimal change and the standard deviation of the change variable, the sample size is calculated using a predetermined α level of type I error (saying that there is a difference when there is none) and β level of type II error (saying that there is no difference when in fact there is one). The probability 1-β is the power of the test. A type I error level of 1–5% and a power level of 80–90% are usually adopted. The choice of α and β depends on the medical and practical consequences of the two kinds of errors.

Statistical testing sets out to test a null hypothesis of no treatment effect against a specified alternative hypothesis. The alternative can state that the drug effect is only beneficial (one-sided alternative) or that it is either beneficial or adverse (two-sided alternative). The choice between the two types of alternative essentially depends on the knowledge available about the drug effect. Here it is assumed that the clinical trial confirms a drug effect already shown by pilot studies. This would lead one to choose a one-sided alternative. When a drug is at an early stage of study, however, it can be advisable to use the two-sided alternative. The calculations of the sample size must take into account the type of alternative adopted, since the two-sided alternative demands a larger sample size than the one-sided alternative for the same α level.

Calculations

It goes beyond this scope of this chapter to illustrate the techniques for estimating the size of the sample group in relation to the types of variables described by the change (e.g., normal, binomial) and various different study designs (e.g., two treatments or more than two treatments). A good reference is the report by Dupont et al. (8), which also provides a computer program for the calculations. Our intention here is to consider an example of how one calculates the sample size by determining the minimal change, the period of observation, and standard deviation of the reference variable. Let us consider the mean values and standard deviation of the Buschke Selective Reminding Test score (9) shown in Table 1. These are for the 197 selected memory-impaired subjects who formed the placebo group in the GERMIS study (10) and were observed at 1, 3, and 6 months after the baseline evaluation. As one can see, the mean scores for each test function show an increase between the baseline and the third month, whereas they stabilize between the third and sixth month. Because the placebo group is concerned here, this progress must be due to a learning effect or practicing effect where the test is concerned, in addition to any potential "placebo effect." The clinically significant minimal change must be defined as over and above these effects.

Where the choice of the primary outcome of interest and the period required to observe the beneficial effects of the drug are concerned, one must be guided by information on the drug's potential effects on the various different memory functions. Let us suppose that the primary outcome of interest is the change in "total recall" 6 months after the baseline. The standard deviation to use in calculating the sample size is not that for 6 months (which is higher than previous valuations) nor that for the baseline (which is lower than those that follow), but is instead the variable for the *difference* between the evaluation for the sixth month and the baseline evaluation, which is equal to 6.9 for this group of subjects.

Following these assumptions, the calculation of the sample size leads to the results shown in Table 2, for a test comparing two placebo and drug groups with different minimum change values (two-tailed $\alpha = 0.05$, power $1-\beta = 0.90$). As one can see, assuming that every other condition remains constant, the smaller the minimal change the larger the sample size.

The population studied for memory disorders is usually elderly. It is highly likely that many patients will leave the studies during the long observation period because of death, transfer, or other reasons. The sample size should be calculated net of these *losses to follow-up* and should concern only those patients who can be analyzed for the main outcome.

TABLE 1. *Mean values (± SD) of Buschke Selective Reminding Test for 197 selected memory-impaired subjects (placebo group)[a]*

Memory function	Baseline	1 Month	3 Months	6 Months	Difference 6 month–baseline
Total recall	27.4 ± 7.8	28.2 ± 8.4	29.1 ± 8.0	29.2 ± 8.5	1.8 ± 6.9
Long-term storage	21.2 ± 11.6	21.6 ± 12.7	23.5 ± 12.2	23.4 ± 12.8	2.2 ± 11.4
Long-term retrieval	18.1 ± 10.9	18.8 ± 12.0	20.3 ± 11.7	20.4 ± 12.5	2.3 ± 10.4
Long-term retrieval consistent	11.1 ± 10.2	12.3 ± 11.5	13.1 ± 11.5	13.5 ± 12.7	2.4 ± 10.5

[a] From the GERMIS Study (10).

TABLE 2. *Sample size needed for achieving 90% power to establish some hypothesized treatment differences as significant (two-tailed* $\alpha = 0.05)^a$

True improvement			Sample size	
Placebo	Drug	Difference	Each sample	Total
1.8	2.8	1.0	1,000	2,000
1.8	3.8	2.0	250	500
1.8	4.8	3.0	111	222
1.8	5.8	4.0	63	126

[a] Based on change at 6 months from baseline of Buschke Selective Remaining Test (Recall) with standard deviation = 6.9.

It is essential for the drug effect estimate to be realistic. If the effect of the drug is only to cause small changes, then a large number of patients will be required. Although small numbers of subjects can produce clinically relevant differences, they cannot reach statistical significance. That is why establishing the sample size helps in designing a study, as it forces one to specify the primary outcome and discourages one from carrying out studies that would prove inconclusive because the sample group is too small.

TREATMENT-RELATED BIAS CONTROL: RANDOMIZATION AND BLINDING

The outcome of a study not only depends on the treatment but is also influenced by many prognostic factors which can only be partly foreseen and are sometimes not even suspected. These factors can influence the effect of treatments, making interpretation of the results difficult. The study consequently must be designed to ensure that the basal characteristics of the treatment groups are as similar as possible, thus ensuring there is a valid basis for comparison. This can be achieved using the *matching* technique. When two treatment groups are involved, this consists of identifying pairs of patients who are very similar to one another in all the important basal characteristics and assigning one member of the pair to the test treatment group and the other to the control treatment group. This method is not, however, a practical solution, partly because it demands the screening of large numbers of patients to identify the pairs required.

Randomization

Randomization is the procedure usually followed to avoid any systematic difference between treatment groups. This technique ensures that each individual has the same probability of being assigned to either of the two treatment groups. As a result, if there is a large number of subjects in the randomized study, it is unlikely that the groups will differ for any of the prognostic factors, whether or not every one of these factors is known to the investigators. Randomization can be carried out by tossing a coin, using a table of random numbers (e.g., for two treatment groups, assigning the patients with even numbers to one group and those with odd numbers to the other), or using computer-generated random numbers, with the latter offering the advantage of being easy to repeat and document.

Randomization based on a mathematical model adds a probabilistic model to the outcome differences between the groups and consequently makes it possible to carry out significance tests. If the design includes a pretreatment evaluation, the randomized assignment of the subjects to the treatment groups can be delayed until the treatment effectively begins, thus enabling the evaluation of the basal conditions on which it is based to be improved.

There are various different versions of the randomization technique, such as *adaptive randomization,* which satisfies particular requirements regarding the size or prognostic characteristics of the groups. Within this context it is important to mention the *blocking randomization* technique, a limited randomization method which is useful for ensuring balanced sample group numbers (3). A block is a limited number of patients consecutively recruited to the trial, whose size is a multiple of the number of treatment groups. The number of patients in a block assigned to each treatment is the same. If, for example, there are two treatments (A and B) which are planned to have the same number of patients, then if the size of a block is four patients, two will receive treatment A while the other two receive treatment B. Because the treatment groups are balanced on each occasion in this way, interim analyses are also facilitated when necessary.

Blinding

Randomization avoids selection biases resulting from investigators having a preference for a certain type of treatment for given subject characteristics. It is, however, always possible for an investigator to have a prejudicial attitude to one of the treatments, in some cases without even being aware of it. Such an investigator could therefore evaluate the eligibility conditions of a patient in a distorted manner, knowing the treatment that patient is to receive. For this reason, selection bias can be avoided more effectively if the randomization scheme is kept secret from the investigator. This will result in what is known as a *single-blind* trial. The same procedure can also protect against another form of treatment-related bias that can occur at the data collection stage. The bias in question particularly affects trials with outcome measurements that are subject to ascertainment errors, such as memory disorders.

If aware of the treatment, the patient, too, can lead to a bias in the evaluation, particularly when the patient's mood is able to influence the outcomes. Consequently, whenever possible, it is better for patients to be unaware of the treatment assigned to them. The term single-blind is used to describe trials in which the investigator or patient is unaware which treatment has been assigned, although it usually refers to the latter.

The results can be defended more effectively if the treatments have been administered with the highest possible level of blinding. Both the investigator and patient may be kept from knowing the treatment involved (*double-blind* trial), as can the statistician, analyzing the data without knowing the characteristics of the different treatments, and the review committees concerned (*triple-blind* trial). The principle is that every evaluation involving any degree of subjectivity is carried out by blinded personnel. In practice, the opposing needs of avoiding potential biases and keeping logistic difficulties under control lead one to find the double-blind design preferable for clinical trials on memory disorders. This notwithstanding, it is advisable for personnel who classify subjects in relation to compliance or drug safety characteristics to be kept unaware of the treatment.

OUTCOME VARIABILITY CONTROL: STRATIFICATION

Randomization tends to produce groups that are comparable in basal characteristics, but it is still possible for the resultant groups to differ regarding important factors able to influence the outcome. When these factors have been identified, the drawback can be dealt with by *stratification*. This technique involves separating those patients eligible for the trial into subgroups or *strata* that are homogeneous for the levels in which these factors occur. The comparison between the treatments can be carried out within the strata and will not be affected by outcome variability caused by stratification variables. This increases the power of the statistical tests, which is to say, the probability of showing a statistically significant difference between the treatments when one actually exists.

Typical factors that can influence the outcomes for measuring memory disorders are age and education, as one can see from the data in Table 3. The table shows the mean values and standard deviations of the Mini-Mental State Examination score (11) for "normal" subjects observed in the Progetto Memoria study. The mean values for the different age groups show a consistent pattern, decreasing as age advances and falling from 28.8 for the youngest age group to 24.8 for the oldest. It should be noted that the standard deviation increases with age, when the groups become less homogeneous owing to the action of new factors that change the cognitive state. The mean score also changes according to the subjects' education, with a value of 26.1 for the lowest level and 29.0 for the highest. If the sample is stratified for these factors and the randomized assignment of patients to the different

TABLE 3. *Mini-Mental State Examination score of 906 normal subjects from Italian population by age and education[a]*

Factor	No. of subjects	Mean	Standard deviation
All	906	27.7	2.6
Age (years)			
20–29	208	28.8	1.7
30–39	181	28.8	1.5
40–49	156	28.0	1.8
50–59	157	27.0	2.6
60–69	126	26.4	2.9
70–79	78	24.8	3.6
Education (years of schooling)			
Less than 5	371	26.1	2.7
6–8	194	28.2	1.9
More than 8	341	29.0	1.1

[a] From Progetto Memoria (unpublished data).

treatments is carried out *within the strata,* the groups being compared will be balanced for the stratification factors, and the variability concerning the comparison will only be that within and not between the strata. It is always advisable to use the blocking technique illustrated above when randomization is carried out within strata, to make it easier to balance the number of subjects assigned to the different treatments.

Other potential stratification factors in clinical trials on cognitive disorders are the severity and duration of the disease, the progress of cognitive decline before treatment, and depression (5). Furthermore, if the study involves more than one center it is always advisable to stratify by center, as centers may differ in characteristics that affect both the patients and investigators. However, it is difficult to take more than one or two stratification factors into account because the number of strata increases geometrically in relation to the number of factor levels (e.g., three age groups, two education groups, 10 centers equals 60 strata). An excessively large number of strata can cause the number of patients within the strata, which cannot be predicted, to become very small, making analysis of the data more complex, decreasing the power of the statistical tests, and making interpretation of the results more difficult. Indeed, because potential stratification variables are often highly dependent, only a few prognostic factors are of use in the design of a clinical trial.

DESIGN AND ANALYSIS

The statistical analysis of clinical trials is a vast and complex subject beyond the scope of this chapter. Therefore, this section will be limited to a number of comments on statistical analysis in connection with study design.

The study protocol for every clinical trial should include a complete analysis plan for both safety and efficacy. The analysis of the primary outcome on which the effectiveness of the drug will be judged must in all circumstances be decided before any data processing is carried out. Every patient exposed to the drug must be included in the safety analysis. Where the efficacy analysis is concerned, more convincing results will be obtained in a similar way by considering all the patients with an *intention-to-treat analysis*.

The protocol should include *interim data analyses* during the course of the trial for predetermined numbers of recruited patients, to monitor the effects of the treatment. These analyses could lead to a suspension of the trial should the drug group be affected by an unacceptably high number of adverse effects in comparison with the control group, or if there is a drastic difference in the effects of the treatments being compared.

Statistical Techniques

Where the statistical analysis technique is concerned, the positive results achieved by simple comparisons between treatment groups are usually the most convincing. In this way, when the patients have been evaluated both before and after the treatment, the comparison between the two treatments can be effected using Student's *t* test on the changes or, alternatively, the analysis of variance for repeated measurements (7).

In general, however, it is best to use statistical techniques that enable one to isolate the variability caused by the stratification factors, to increase the power in testing hypotheses. The statistical significance of the differences between the treatments will thus be tested by the analysis of variance, with the observations categorized by strata. If the study involves more than one center, the variable "Center" must be included in these factors. It should be noted that this technique is useful only when the stratification factors have a real prognostic value and the patient numbers are not distributed over the strata in an overly unbalanced manner.

Although randomization balances the basal characteristics of treatment groups, one cannot rule out the possibility of their imbalance for one or more variables. These variables can be balanced by carrying out a covariance analysis (12): this technique enables one to reduce the between-subject variance of the outcome through the use of covariates represented by baseline variables. Even though the covariates cost degrees of freedom, the statistical test will usually be more powerful. The role of covariate can also be usefully filled by the pretreatment evaluation of the primary outcome: in this case, the outcome can be either the posttreatment evaluation or the change.

Multivariate Analysis

The lack of appropriate testing when a multiple outcome study is analyzed can increase the probability of a type I error, finding a statistically significant difference when there is no real difference between the treatments. If separate comparisons are carried out for the different outcomes and the α level is 0.05 for each of them, on average one comparison out of 20 will emerge as significant simply by chance. The analysis is made more complex by the interdependence of outcomes. In theory, the best solution is to use multivariate analysis methods (13), which compare the treatments on all the outcomes simultaneously. Multivariate analysis can increase the power of testing: if the outcomes are not strongly correlated, it can reveal significant differences where no single test is significant.

However, the application of multivariate methods finds little support, in part because applying them correctly requires assumptions that are often not satisfied and in part because the results to which they lead are difficult to interpret. As a result, the usual approach involves carrying out individual comparisons and ignoring the problem of interdependence between outcomes. In such cases, however, one must reduce the α level in relation to the number of comparisons effected.

Subgroup Analysis

The analysis of the data can reveal a certain type of treatment-by-stratum interaction, such as a difference in favor of one treatment in all strata except one or two, where the difference is in the other direction. In cases such as this, the investigator must try and identify those patient subgroups for which the treatment can be noxious or, conversely, those that are able to benefit from the treatment. A significant effect within a segment of the entire group can provide a hypothesis for further study. However, it is necessary to proceed with great caution when proposing subgroup analyses, even if it is easy for the investigator to be led to do so by the presence of a number of outcomes. Subgroup analyses should under all circumstances be justified by baseline characteristics of the patients.

CONCLUSIONS

This chapter has considered several aspects of clinical trial design in relation to the statistical analysis of the data. Illustrations of the analysis techniques can be found in many publications, among which we can recommend Fleiss (7), Peto et al. (14,15), and Peace (16). The analysis can be carried out using the leading statistical software packages, which have different characteristics where comprehensiveness and ease of use are concerned. The SAS System is quite wide-ranging and is able to satisfy every aspect of data processing, whereas the BMDP Statistical Software supplies the most complete analysis of specific clinical trial designs such as, for example, crossover and repeated measurements.

Although much has been written about clinical trial methodology, it is not rare to find published studies that fail to satisfy certain fundamental methodological rules and which therefore present questionable results. The development of a consensus regarding important aspects of design can discourage inconclusive studies from being carried out. Furthermore, if a number of studies are similar regarding the characteristics of the pathology and basic design aspects, then it is easier to carry out data combining to perform a meta-analysis and to achieve more definitive results.

REFERENCES

1. Hedges LV, Olkin I. *Statistical methods for meta-analysis*. London: Academic Press; 1985.
2. Kelsey JL, Douglas Thompson W, Evans AS. *Methods in observational epidemiology*. New York: Oxford University Press; 1986.
3. Meinert CL. *Clinical trials: design, conduct, and analysis*. New York: Oxford University Press; 1986.
4. Larrabee GJ, Crook TH. A computerized everyday memory battery for assessing treatment effects. *Psychopharmacol Bull* 1988;24:695–7.
5. Jarvik LF, Berg L, Bartus R, et al. Clinical drug trials in Alzheimer disease: what are some of the issues? *Alzheimer Dis Assoc Disord* 1990;4:193–202.
6. Brouwers P, Mohr E. Design of clinical trials. In: Mohr E, Brouwers P, eds. *Handbook of clinical trials: the neurobehavioral approach*, Amsterdam: Swets & Zeitlinger; 1991: 45–66.
7. Fleiss JL. *The design and analysis of clinical experiments*. New York: Wiley; 1986.
8. Dupont DW, Plummer DW Jr. Power and sample size calculations: a review and computer program. *Controlled Clin Trials* 1990;11:116–28.
9. Buschke H. Selective reminding for analysis of memory and learning. *J Verbal Learn Verbal Behav* 1973;12:543–50.
10. Cenacchi T, Bertoldin T, Farina C, Fiori MG, Crepaldi G. Cognitive decline in the elderly: a double-blind, placebo-controlled multicenter study on efficacy of phosphatidylserine administration. *Aging Clin Exp Res* 1993;5:123–33.
11. Folstein MF, Folstein SE, McHugh PR. ''Mini-mental state'': a practical method for grading the cognitive state of patients for the clinician. *J Psychiatr Res* 1975;12:189–98.
12. Sokal RR, Rohlf FG. *Biometry*. 2nd ed. San Francisco: Freeman and Company; 1984.
13. Hand DJ, Taylor CC. *Multivariate analysis of variance and repeated measures: a practical approach for behavioural scientists*. London: Chapman and Hall; 1987.
14. Peto R, Pike MC, Armitage P, et al. Design and analysis of randomized clinical trials requiring prolonged observation of each patient: I. Introduction and design. *Br J Cancer* 1976;34:585–612.
15. Peto R, Pike MC, Armitage P, et al. Design and analysis of randomized clinical trials requiring prolonged observation of each patient: II. Analysis and examples. *Br J Cancer* 1977;35:1–39.
16. Peace KE, ed. *Statistical issues in drug research and development*. New York: Marcel Dekker; 1990.

Guidelines for Drug Trials in Memory Disorders, edited by N. Canal, et al.
Raven Press, Ltd., New York © 1993.

13

End Points, Duration, and Side Effects

G. K. Wilcock

Department of Care of the Elderly, Frenchay Hospital, Bristol BS16 1LE, England

Most of our knowledge about designing therapeutic studies for treating memory disorders is based on our experience of evaluating new treatments for the conditions that cause dementia. It is from this foundation that I will draw the points I shall be discussing; in general terms they will be applicable to designing studies for other conditions, such as age-associated memory impairment (AAMI).

Ideally, the design for a study evaluating a new compound for treating a memory disorder or a dementia should take into account the underlying hypothesis concerning the mode of action of the substance under investigation. Unfortunately, this is not always possible, as we are often uncertain about exactly how a new compound affects the brain, particularly the aging brain. Two examples of this, if one believes that they are in fact beneficial, are the nootropics and tetrahydroaminacridine (THA). Although the latter is considered to exert its effect through the cholinergic pathway, the evidence for this is beginning to look less convincing and alternative hypotheses are under investigation. In practice, therefore, we investigate as a treatment for dementia (using that term globally), substances that seem promising in restricted areas of cognition (e.g., cholinergic enhancing agents in relation to memory function), often hoping that they will improve a range of activities beyond those normally associated with cholinergic neurotransmission.

We must also bear in mind that what may be considered exciting by a scientist may not appear to be of much relevance to relatives caring for a person with dementia. We have to remember that we are treating patients who are people rather than scientific "objects." Our end points should therefore reflect the importance of this although, sadly, in the past this has not always been the case. Because we are dealing with people, not with simpler scientific concepts, we must remember that expectations and the way in which problems are appreciated may well differ in differing cultures. Our end points must therefore reflect the spectrum that ranges from scientific assessment of cognitive disturbance and its amelioration at one end to the more general issue of quality of life of both sufferer and caregiver at the other end.

We must also decide exactly to what we are referring if we use specialist terminology. This is an important area that requires general agreement. Surveys of the protocols for many studies over the last 20 years reveal that inadequately defined diagnostic criteria have often been employed, although happily this is now becoming more uniform because criteria such as those defined within DSM-III-R and ICD 10 are being more widely accepted. Nevertheless, until all centers that undertake research into the dementias, as well as the relevant pharmaceutical companies, can agree on common criteria, it will be very difficult to objectively compare the results of different studies, whether across centers or of different compounds. Even diagnosis based on the existing standardized approaches can be difficult to apply, as different investigators will interpret the gray areas in different ways. Similarly, when we try to be even more specific [e.g., making a diagnosis such as Alzheimer disease (AD)], the application of strict criteria such as those suggested by McKhann (1) becomes difficult because of the differing interpretation put on these and the heterogeneity of the presentation of AD.

TYPES OF END POINTS

It has been suggested by Kanowski and colleagues (2), although not necessarily generally accepted, that for at least one group of drugs, the nootropics, assessment for end point determination should be sought on different planes (e.g., the psychopathologic plane, a psychometric plane, a behavioral plane, and finally a neurophysiologic/functional dynamic plane). The psychopathologic plane includes measures such as clinical global impression, Reisberg's Brief Cognitive Rating Scale (3), and the Sandoz Clinical Assessment Geriatric Scale (4). The psychometric plane evaluates measures such as the SKT (5), trail-making tests (6), and the behavioral plane which concentrates on areas such as an assessment of the activities of daily living and behavioral assessment. The final plane (i.e., the neurophysiologic/functional dynamic plane) includes harder scientific objective assessments, including electroencephalograms (EEG), single-photon emission computed tomography (SPECT) scans, and measurements of cerebral blood flow. These authors consider that a relevant significant end point has been achieved if significant changes are demonstrated in one variable respectively from two of the first three planes. Although such an approach is attractive and may appear relevant to the assessment of other compounds, it is at present beset with practical difficulties. We have little knowledge about how these different tests relate to each other, either within a single plane or between planes, nor do we know how the individual assessment techniques used in most of these approaches perform when used for differing stages of dementia. Similarly, they probably all have different floor and ceiling effects.

WHAT END POINTS CAN WE USE?

We could choose one or more of the following end points: (i) improvement in cognitive ability (e.g., memory function, language use, apraxia); (ii) improvement in behavior; (iii) improvement in activities of daily life; (iv) quality of life for sufferer; (v) level of stress in caretaker; (vi) physiologic measurements (e.g., SPECT); and/or (vii) death.

Some of these measurements, such as stress levels and quality of life, may be applicable to the evaluation of any new antidementia drug, whereas others may be more specific for the presumed mechanism of action of the compound under evaluation (e.g., assessment of individual cognitive parameters and certain physiologic measurements).

Choosing the type of end point, as well as its magnitude, will to a certain extent also depend on the stage of the disorder at which the treatment is aimed. Although it is possible, it seems extremely unlikely that a single therapy will be worthwhile at all stages in a dementing illness, especially in conditions such as AD or multi-infarct dementia. In the earliest stages, for example, disorders of cognition may be the only significant symptoms. Further into the disease process, as already mentioned, the level of stress in caretakers and the quality of life for the patient may be of greater importance and easier to measure. This is a reflection of the fact that progressive neuro-degenerative conditions are probably associated with a similarly progressive pattern of neurotransmitter dysfunction, and that neurotransmitter-based therapies are likely to be maximally effective during a specific "window of opportunity." This will vary depending on the strategy, and a similar principle may operate in other potential therapeutic situations, such as the use of trophic factors.

Timing of death (i.e., duration of life) is a particularly important but infrequently considered end point. Its importance lies not so much in the effectiveness of the treatment in relation to specific symptoms but rather in the more general terms of quality and duration of life. We must ascertain whether or not life is prolonged by treatment and, if so, whether the increased lifespan occurs during the period when the treatment is helping or whether it merely prolongs the more undesirable vegetative state. In other words, is the benefit of therapy greater than any potential adverse effects of increased duration of life, if this occurs? This is of course a very different scenario from that in many other areas of medicine, in which effective therapy automatically confers benefit (e.g., the treatment of hypertension in postponing the occurrence of a cerebrovascular accident), and raises particular ethical and moral questions which are also a feature of other terminal illnesses.

HOW DO WE MEASURE END POINTS?

Measuring end points will be explored in detail elsewhere in this volume; therefore, this section will be limited to some general principles.

In general terms, it seems most sensible to start with the concept of improving the quality of life, first of the patient and then of the patient's caretakers. We have few validated and widely accepted measurements for assessing the quality of life of a dementia patient. More readily available are scales designed to assess the level of activities of daily living, which is at best an indirect measurement of quality of life. There are many of these, and although the instrumental activities of daily living (IADL) of Lawton and Brody (7) is frequently used we prefer the Functional Life Scale of Sarno (8). This provides greater scope for assessing the significance of improvement or lack thereof in individual items in relation to the severity of the patient's dementia. Whatever method is chosen, further studies of therapeutic agents for treatment of dementia should involve protocols that give considerable weight to changes in the patient's ability to undertake the important activities of daily life.

The quality of life of the caregiver is rarely included but is probably the second most important parameter as far as the patient, his caregivers, and the State are concerned. The caregiver who can no longer cope will have to come to terms with the emotional results of this, and the State will have to meet the not inconsiderable financial consequences. This area is badly served. There are few validated assessment schedules, and most are for conditions other than dementia (9–11). The behavior of patients may also be considered an indirect measure of their quality of life, and is certainly very important as far as the caregiver is concerned. This has been the subject of greater exploration in the last 5 years, and there are now several methods of assessing behavior or certain aspects of it (12–15).

It is important, when we consider protocols that measure different end points, to remember that the scores may not move in parallel (e.g., changes in cognitive parameters may occur at a different rate from those of improvement or deterioration in the ability to undertake activities of daily living). Early studies suggested that the extent of decline in cognitive ability, as tested neuropsychologically, does not necessarily reflect the level of functional capacity.

CHOOSING A METHOD FOR ASSESSING END POINTS

When an assessment technique is being chosen from the literature, it is usual to search for one that has been developed in an appropriate setting, that has been adequately validated, and whose inter-rater and test–retest reliability have been adequately established. This is usually all that is considered before a schedule is applied in, for instance, a multicenter study, forgetting that there are many other important issues that should be considered before assuming that the study is valid in one's own context as well as in that in which it was developed. Other important factors also must be considered, including, to take an example at a simple level, that the specialty of the investigator may well determine the characteristics of the subjects included in the study. For example, in the United Kingdom a geriatrician, a pychogeriatrician, and a neurologist will each attract referral of patients of a different type, even though each may be considered to have the same underlying condition (e.g., AD). Patients referred to a geriatrician are likely to be physically more frail and to have senile dementia of Alzheimer type; the neurologist is more likely to be referred younger patients with the more aggressive disease and a greater likelihood of a familial component; and the psychogeriatrician to be referred older people who are causing stress to their caregivers. Similarly, at a cross-cultural level involving different countries, there will again be differences in the way in which tests should be interpreted.

These issues are gradually being addressed, and it is encouraging to see that some of the commonly used assessment schedules [e.g., the Mini-Mental State Examination (MMSE)], now have data that can be interpreted in relation to age-specific norms (16), cross-cultural data (17), and education/socioeconomic status (18,19). This is at least a starting point, particularly as the correlation between the MMSE and other assessment schedules is also being explored (20,21). Any attempt to introduce a consensus with regard to international and cross-cultural use of assessment protocols to define and measure parameters that could be used as end points for assessing the efficacy of therapy must take such data into account.

Finally, it is important to remember that instruments developed for diagnosis of dementia are not necessarily appropriate for measuring change, particularly as they may be relatively insensitive and may also have pronounced floor and ceiling effects.

END POINTS: QUANTITATIVE ASPECTS

Most therapeutic studies in the field of dementia research appear to have been undertaken without prior consideration of what is an acceptable end point. Because assessment schedules usually represent one means of assessing efficacy, this leads to subsequent debate as to whether the changes reported are clinically relevant, irrespective of whether these are in the field of cognitive improvement, which is difficult to relate to quality of life, or in the area of change in the ability to undertake the activities of daily living.

Various factors could be considered in determining what is a meaningful or acceptable end point in this context. Recent studies with tetrahydroaminacridine (THA) have highlighted the need to relate the benefits obtained to the risk/side-effects profile of the substance involved. The more threatening the side effects, the greater the magnitude of benefit that must be obtained to offset them. Conversely, a drug with only modest claims for efficacy should be relatively nontoxic. It is important, however, to distinguish and differentiate between the severity of the potential morbidity in an individual and the frequency of a given unwanted effect within the population to which it has been exposed. A minor side effect in a majority of people may be viewed differently from a serious side effect in only a smaller proportion of those studied.

Magnitude of Change

The magnitude of any change on a given scale must also be interpreted in relation to factors such as the linearity of the scale and the severity of the disease process. A 2-point change, for instance, in an overall score for one individual may not necessarily be the equivalent of a 2-point change in another individual, even with the same degree of dementia. This is because it may result from an alteration in a different subscore component that may appear of equal value on paper but has a very different significance to the patient and the caregiver. Similarly, for an individual patient, a 2-point change at the bottom of the scale may not mean the same as a 2-point change at the top of the scale (e.g., a small improvement in a severely demented patient may be very important, whereas a change of similar magnitude in a patient with early dementia may not be so impressive). In other words, as implied elsewhere, end points may have to vary depending on the stage of the disease, and therefore the target population for any agent under evaluation must be considered carefully when the protocol is designed. Most of these points are, of course, already taken into account in the better-designed studies.

Minimum Acceptable Benefit

What should be considered as the minimal improvement constituting an acceptable end point? To a certain extent this is a philosophical question, but to put the answer in terms that most people could understand it might be easiest to relate it to the equivalent of the number of months or years of improved quality of life. This principle could be employed irrespective of whether a therapeutic agent is intended to improve quality of life or to prevent or retard further progression of the disease. Not only might this approach be useful in considering the benefit for a particular individual, but it might also be possible to transpose it as a measure of the benefit to a group of subjects under evaluation as a whole. Although it is important to have end

TABLE 1. *Mean change in Mini-Mental State Exam items per year*

	Mean	SD	Z
Orientation	1.298	2.820	0.460*
Registration	1.043	1.642	0.635*
Attention	0.499	1.284	0.389*
Recall	0.146	0.761	0.192
Language	1.203	1.631	0.738*
Total Score	4.180	4.798	0.871*

* $p < 0.05$.
Adapted from ref. 22.

points that can be applied to an individual, we also need to know how much benefit is accruing to the entire population being treated.

Data presenting rates of changes of common measures of impairment in AD, such as those reported by Yesavage and colleagues (22), could be used as a baseline. These authors present the rates of change for the Brief Cognitive Rating Scale, the Global Deterioration Scale (GDS), the MMSE, and the Alzheimer's Disease Assessment Scale (ADAS), as they considered that these measures of impairment were applicable during a significant part of the duration of illness. Others have adopted a similar approach.

It is apparent from Tables 1–3 that the rate of deterioration in different measurements over a 12-month period varies. If, however, we assume that the minimal benefit that should accrue to a subject taking a therapeutic agent for dementia was a saving of the equivalent of 6 months of deterioration, the figures shown in the tables provide a foundation for calculating potential numerical end points. However, the data provided must be interpreted in the context of the severity of the dementia and the number of subjects studied. For the Yesavage study this is represented by an initial mean score of 16.5 on the MMSE and 4.3 on the GDS. Such information can, however, be regarded only as a starting point, and much more data are urgently required to enable us to arrive at meaningful quantitative end points to complement

TABLE 2. *Brief Cognitive Rating Scale (BCRS) and Global Deterioration Scale (GDS), mean change per year**

	Mean	SD	Z
BCRS			
Concentration	0.634	0.985	0.644
Recent memory	0.549	0.830	0.661
Past memory	0.677	1.575	0.430
Orientation	0.683	1.337	0.511
Self-care	0.613	0.861	0.712
GDS	0.462	0.725	0.637

* $p < 0.05$.
Adapted from ref. 22.

TABLE 3. *Examples of Alzheimer Disease Assessment Scale change in items per year**

	Mean	SD	Z
Language comprehension	0.847	1.856	0.456
Object naming	0.548	0.937	0.585
Constructional praxis	1.021	1.265	0.807
Remembering instructions	0.623	1.679	0.371

* $p < 0.05$.
Adapted from ref. 22.

the many qualitative measures that can be employed. It is also clear from the data in the tables, where there is a wide variability of Z-scores reflecting the different rates at which different clinical phenomena progress (or differing sensitivities within the subscales for a similar degree of change in a given parameter). Yesavage and co-workers concluded that all four scales provided reliable data about the clinical and neuropsychological course of the illness, although of course each provides somewhat different information (e.g., the ADAS is the most comprehensive, whereas the MMSE has more limited cognitive testing and completely omits behavioral assessment).

Summary

In summary, despite originally being designed as a screening instrument, the MMSE is now so well validated in different contexts that one could argue that it would be a useful "common denominator" for different studies. This should be supplemented by similar information from the other scales, but inclusion of an MMSE-related end point in all studies would allow a degree of comparability of results across studies and would provide a "feel" for the data, as the MMSE is so well known to all workers in this field. Such an approach could also be adopted for other dementias, and perhaps a minimal improvement or halting of disease progression of at least the equivalent of 6 months of deterioration, as measured on validated scales, should be sought.

Further studies on larger cohorts would be helpful because there is some variability in the reports of annual rates of change in the rating scales. Salmon et al. (21) reported only a 2.8 point decline on the MMSE over a 12-month period, compared to the 4 points reported by Yesavage (22).

TRIAL DURATION AND SIDE-EFFECTS

Much of the above discussion has implications for both the duration of a trial and the importance of side effects in relation to risk/benefit ratios. In general, studies should be no longer than the reasonable length of time inferred from the drug's apparent mode of action. At the same time, however, there is a fluctuation in the course of most dementing disorders, even in many subjects with AD, and the study must be long enough to avoid misinterpretation of such random fluctuations if the study numbers are small. Although in certain circumstances 6 weeks could be considered appropriate, 12 weeks seems to be a more reasonable minimal period for assessment of drugs that are considered to improve a subject's status rather than merely to prevent deterioration. The latter is likely to need much longer periods of study, e.g., 6–12 months minimum. The overall study design (e.g., parallel group or crossover), and the need for washout periods must also be taken into account.

The side-effect profile, and particularly that of unwanted effects that should be subject to a special surveillance, will to some extent be determined by the drug's absorption, distribution, metabolism, and excretion characteristics, as well as by its intrinsic mode of action. The yield of potential unwanted effects will, of course, increase the longer the drug is given to each individual, and we must not forget that in AD and many of the other dementias it may have to be given for life. In addition, the greater the number of people studied, the greater the yield of side effects that will be observed. It is important, however, not to react emotionally to the presence of side effects, as has often been the case with some of the cholinergic agents such as THA, as the major disadvantage of side effects has been the withdrawal of therapy from many patients whose relatives felt they were benefiting, rather than any long-term morbidity and mortality.

A very strong case can also be made against using an uncontrolled cohort of subjects for long-term safety assessment when this stage in the drug's development is reached, particularly in the elderly, as they are an age group in which many symptoms and signs are likely to occur for other reasons. A new drug may be unfairly associated with such side effects in the absence of an adequate control group.

Finally, in addition to duration of study, we need information that will enable us to decide what the duration of treatment should be, i.e., not only when should we start treatment, but when should we stop it for reasons other than the development of adverse reactions. This is an issue which, for the dementias at least, has not yet been addressed.

The side-effect profile must be related to efficacy, not only in terms of harm versus benefit but also with regard to any link between benefit and side effects (e.g., is efficacy especially demonstrated in those subjects with unwanted drug-related symptoms?).

CONCLUSION

Study of these issues, i.e., end points, duration, and side effects, raises more questions than answers but it is apparent that we, as a scientific community, are beginning to recognize the questions and are beginning to attempt to provide some of the answers. The way ahead is likely to be both lengthy and challenging.

REFERENCES

1. McKhann G, Drachman D, Folstein M, et al. Clinical diagnosis of Alzheimer's disease: report of the NINCDS-ADRDA Work Group under the auspices of Department of Health and Human Services Task Force on Alzheimer's Disease. *Neurology* 1984;34:939–44.
2. Kanowski S. In: Maurer K, Riederer P, Beckman H, eds. *Alzheimer's disease—epidemiology, neuropathology, neurochemistry and clinics.* Berlin: Springer-Verlag; 1990:531–43.
3. Reisberg B, London E, Ferris SH, Borenstein J, Scheiei L, de Leon MJ. The brief cognitive rating scale: language motoric and mood concomitants in primary degenerative dementia. *Psychopharmacol Bull* 1983;19:702–8.
4. Venn RD. The Sandoz Clinical Assessment–Geriatric (SCAG) Scale. *Gerontology* 1983; 29:185–98.
5. Erzigkeit H. *Syndrom-Kurz-Test*, 2nd ed. Ebersberg: Vless-Verlag; 1986.
6. Oswald WD, Roth E. *Der Zahlen-Verbindungs-Test*, 2nd ed. Gottingen: Hogrefe; 1987.
7. Lawton MP, Brody EM. Assessment of older people: self-maintaining and instrumental activities of daily living. *Gerontologist* 1969;9:179–86.
8. Sarno JE, Sarno MT, Levita E. The functional life scale. *Arch Phys Med Rehabil* 1973;54: 214–20.
9. Robinson BC. Validation of a caregiver strain index. *J Gerontol* 1983;38:344–8.
10. Greene JG, Smith R, Gardiner M, Tinbury GC. Measuring behavioural disturbance of elderly demented patients in the community and its effect on relatives: a factor analytic study. *Age Ageing* 1982;11:121–6.
11. Zarit SH, Todd PA, Zarit JM. Subjective burden of husbands and wives as caregivers: a longitudinal study. *Gerontologist* 1986;26:260–6.
12. Yudofsky SC, Silver JM, Jackson W, Endicott J, Williams D. The overt aggression scale for objective rating of verbal and physical aggression. *Am J Psychiatry* 1986;143:35–9.
13. Baumgarten M, Becker R, Gauthier S. Validity and reliability of the dementia behaviour disturbance scale. *J Am Geriatr Soc* 1990;38:221–6.
14. Hope T, Fairburn CG. The development of an interview to measure current behavioural abnormalities—the present behavioural examination (PBE). *Psychol Med* 1992;22:223–30.
15. Patel V, Hope RA. A rating scale for aggressive behaviour in the elderly—the rage. *Psychol Med* 1992;22:211–21.
16. Bleecker ML, Bolla–Wilson K, Kawas C, Agnew J. Age-specific norms for the mini-mental state exam. *Neurology* 1988;38:1565–8.
17. Salmon DP, Riekkinen PJ, Katzman R, Zhang M, Jin H, Yu E. Cross-cultural studies of dementia: a comparison of mini-mental state examination performance in Finland and China. *Arch Neurol* 1989;46:769–72.
18. Brayne C, Calloway P. The association of education and socioeconomic status with the Mini Mental State Examination and the clinical diagnosis of dementia in elderly people. *Age Ageing* 1990;19:91–6.
19. Murden RA, McRae TD, Kaner S, Bucknam MR. Mini-mental state exam scores vary with education in blacks and whites. *J Am Geriatr Soc* 1991;39:149–55.
20. Thal LJ, Grundman M, Golden R. Alzheimer's disease: a correlational analysis of the Blessed Information-Memory-Concentration test and the Mini-Mental State Exam. *Neurology* 1986;36:262–4.
21. Salmon DP, Thal LJ, Butters N, Heindel WC. Longitudinal evaluation of dementia of the Alzheimer type: a comparison of three standardized mental status examinations. *Neurology* 1990;40:1225–30.
22. Yesavage JA, Poulsen SL, Sheikh J, Tanke E. Rates of change of common measures of impairment in senile dementia of the Alzheimer's type. *Psychopharmacol Bull* 1988;24: 531–4.

Guidelines for Drug Trials in Memory Disorders, edited by N. Canal, et al.
Raven Press, Ltd., New York © 1993.

14

Problems and Pitfalls of Some Clinical Trials in Memory Disorders

Andrea Lippi

Department of Neurology and Psychiatry, University of Florence, Florence, Italy

DEFINITION OF MEMORY DISORDERS IN OLD AGE

Cognitive evaluation in the elderly is often performed to determine whether the subject is likely to undergo significant cognitive impairments. Several empirical reports have established that memory processes decline during the later decades of life (1). Kral (2) labeled as "benign senescent forgetfulness" a mild type of memory dysfunction of later life characterized by the inability to promptly recall fragments of a remote experience that otherwise has been registered and retained. Such a memory impairment seemed to progress slowly during a 4-year follow-up period. More recently, Crook and Larrabee (3) isolated and defined the inclusion criteria for the age-associated memory impairment (AAMI) as a specific amnestic disorder observed in aging people that partially replicate Kral's findings. The disorder is characterized by: complaint of memory loss reflected in everyday problems; memory test performance at least one standard deviation below the mean established for young adults on a standardized test of recent memory; evidence of adequate intellectual function on the basis of performance at the vocabulary test of the Wechsler Adult Intelligence Scale (4); and absence of dementia as determined by a score of 24 or higher on the Mini-Mental State Examination (MMSE) (5).

AAMI is considered to exist when otherwise healthy individuals over the age of 50 years exhibit memory impairment that would be considered "normal" in later life (6). Whereas patients with senescent forgetfulness were compared with other elderly individuals, those with AAMI were compared with a young, normal control group (7). The question of whether these memory impairments represent isolated although progressive deficits or the first symptom of dementia is still unresolved.

In a clinical series of 71 outpatients referred during a 1-year period to our

Department of Neurology for cognitive problems, about 30% complained of memory impairment only. An extensive neuropsychological examination (8) enabled detection of benign forgetfulness in 13.5% of cases and early dementia in 41%, whereas in 45.5% no objective cognitive deficits were identified. On the other hand, memory impairment is often the first detectable symptom of dementia. Data obtained from a series of 64 consecutive Alzheimer disease (AD) patients referred to the Department of Neurology of Florence between 1982 and 1986 showed that memory impairment was the first reported symptom of dementia in 84.3% of cases, whereas apraxia was present as first symptom only in 7.8% of cases, disorientation in 5.7%, and aphasia in 3.1%. Patients with initial symptoms other than memory impairment at the onset of dementia always experienced memory disturbances 1 or 2 years later. Similar data were also obtained in an Italian population-based survey on dementia (9). In 20 cases of AD, memory impairment was reported to be present either alone or in combination with other symptoms during the early stages of the disorder in 16 patients. Finally, patients with memory impairment only, fulfilling the NINCDS-ADRDA diagnostic criteria for AD (10), investigated by positron emission tomography (PET) demonstrated metabolic reductions in the parietal association cortex, similar to those reported for patients with mild degrees of dementia (11). This study suggests that hypometabolism in the association neocortex is evident before associated patterns of neuropsychological deficits are demonstrable.

The so-called "benign forgetfulness" probably represents an early stage of AD in a high percentage of cases. Longitudinal studies are therefore needed to define the diagnostic criteria for "benign forgetfulness" and early dementia and to establish prognostic factors. A 2-year longitudinal study by Fliker and colleagues (12) demonstrated that verbal and visuospatial recall tests and language tasks can be used to discriminate between mildly impaired elderly subjects who will manifest progressive mental deterioration and those who will not progress to dementia.

CLINICAL TRIALS IN COGNITIVE DISORDERS AND DEMENTIA

In pharmacologic research, one of the main difficulties is to reproduce the experimental results in clinical practice. The clinical development of therapeutic agents for dementia is complicated by the poor correlation between animal models and human disease. In fact, advancing age alone does not represent a disease state, and animal models are either mechanically incomplete (e.g., lesions in the nucleus basalis of Meynert) or are primarily functional in nature. In no case do they represent the wide range of cognitive disorders observed in dementia. Furthermore, most of the studies conducted on lesioned animals have been based on simple conditioning procedures, such as the acquisition and retention of an avoidance response (13), but there is a poor analogy between human forgetfulness and the extinction of an avoidance response. Sahgal (14) showed that the acquisition and retention of various perceptual motor skills can be remarkably well preserved in amnesiac states, and Weiskrantz and Warrington (15) have demonstrated that conditioning can be normal in severely amnesiac patients. It will be necessary in the future to develop tests that are more analogous to those used to demonstrate the complex and global impairment that in humans is defined as dementia.

The evaluation of the true action of a given drug in human subjects requires numerous and extensive investigations. In particular, great care should be taken to confirm blindedness of investigators and patients, definition of objectives and characteristics of the studied population, identification of specific end points and outcomes, and methods of data collection and analysis. The possibility of obtaining valid results from clinical trials on dementia is strongly dependent on three principal factors.

1. Correct diagnosis of the disease underlying the dementia syndrome (e.g., AD) and definition of subgroups of patients with specific characteristics (e.g., early and late onset).
2. Detection of specific cognitive and behavioral disorders in demented patients by use of neuropsychological measurements that are minimally influenced by age, sex, and educational level, inter-rater variability, and repeated administration.
3. The identification of specific outcomes of the treatment.

In fact, the course of the disease is variable and the real impact of cognitive and behavioral disturbances on patients' performance in activities of daily living is not completely clarified. Indirect indicators of treatment outcome are also the rates of dropout and the shape of the dose–response curve.

High rates of dropout among patients sometimes invalidate treatment outcome studies. In fact, it is not possible to estimate or measure the potential benefit of any treatment when the patients who do not receive benefit from it later drop out. The results of studies with dropout rates that exceed 40% should be viewed with caution. On the other hand, low rates of dropout (below 20%) often identify good treatments.

As for the shape of the dose–response curve, a significant positive correlation between the dose of a specific drug and the amount of response indicates that some elements in the treatment have been beneficial in reducing the severity of the disease. Although the existence of a positive dose–response relationship does help to predict the outcome of treatment, its absence does not necessarily mean that beneficial effects are lacking.

The World Health Organization (16) has recently proposed some criteria for evaluating the effectiveness of treatment in organic mental disorders. The assessment should be broad in scope, including measurement not only of memory, thinking processes, and behavior but also of the reduction of disability in daily life and of improvement in quality of life as reported either by the patient or by the patient's caregivers. Even if the treatment leads to only a moderate reduction in symptoms, it may improve the quality of life of those who care for the patient, and therefore this effect should also be assessed.

The tests used for assessment of patients should be sensitive to change, their results should not depend on the number of times they are used, and they should be adapted to local cultural conditions. The effectiveness of treatment should be examined not only in the short term, but also for longer periods of several months or more. Finally, the only acceptable approach for the experimental trial design is a clinical trial that employs randomized, prospective, concurrent assignment of patients to the new drug and placebo under totally blinded conditions.

CLINICAL TRIALS IN AD

More than a hundred reports of drug trials in AD have been published over the last several years. A number of these apparently indicate positive results; some were carried out with control subjects, were single- or double-blind studies, and employed standard statistical methods to demonstrate efficacy. The drugs tried thus far have been used in an effort to improve memory and cognitive function, to alter the course of AD, or to modify behavioral disorders associated with AD, such as delusion, insomnia, and depression.

The majority of drugs under investigation for AD are proposed to improve memory and cognitive functions by enhancing neurotransmission. This group includes cholinomimetic and other neurotransmitter agonists, neuropeptides, and nootropic agents. Treatments to alter the course of AD have been proposed on the basis of the current etiologic hypothesis of the disease. They include chelating agents such as ethylenediaminetetraacetic acid (EDTA) and desferoxamine, hormone therapy, nerve growth factor, and neuronal transplantation. Finally, treatment designed to control behavioral disorders includes antipsychotic agents, minor tranquilizers, and antidepressant drugs.

Cholinomimetic Agents

It has been documented that intravenous physostigmine reverses the cognitive impairment caused by the anticholinergic drugs (17), and improvement of memory disturbances has been observed in several studies. Gustafson et al. (18) treated 10 AD patients with intravenous infusion of physostigmine for 2 h. The acute effects on cognitive functions, regional blood flow, and electroencephalograms (EEG) were compared with placebo using a double-blind crossover design. Physostigmine caused an improvement of cognitive performance and EEG and an increase in blood flow. The enhancing effect of low doses of physostigmine on memory has been confirmed by other authors (19), and it has been suggested that there is an inverted U-shaped curve, with decrements in memory above 50 ng/kg or 25% BuChE inhibition. Dosages of physostigmine should be assessed individually, as it is quite difficult to determine the useful dosage. One study (20) found that a low dosage of physostigmine improved memory in normal young adults but that higher dosages impaired memory and other cognitive functions. Furthermore, physostigmine has the additional disadvantage of a short half-life in plasma of approximately 30 min, necessitating frequent administration. On the other hand, a study carried out by Stern and co-workers (21) on 22 AD patients, using six different daily dosages of physostigmine, suggests that this drug had no pronounced effect on memory in AD. The lack of response to cholinesterase inhibitors could be due to poor absorption of orally administered drug or to the failure to achieve cholinergic enhancement because of extensive cell loss.

In addition to physostigmine, studies have been carried out with tetrahydroaminacridine (THA), a long-acting cholinesterase inhibitor. Some trials have shown encouraging initial results (22) and a remarkable clinical improvement with THA. On the other hand, other studies have failed to support these optimistic results and have pointed out problems with THA-induced liver toxicity (23). Several efforts are under way to synthesize compounds less toxic than THA but with the same effect on cognitive performance.

The possibility of increasing cholinergic transmission by administering additional precursor substances led to the performance of many clinical trials investigating the effects of choline and its dietary precursor phosphatylcholine (lecithin). Thus far, evidence on whether dietary choline can affect cognitive performance in human subjects is either inclusive or negative (24). A double-blind controlled trial of high-dose lecithin in 51 AD subjects with plasma choline levels monitored throughout the treatment period showed no difference between the lecithin group and the placebo group, but there was an improvement in a subgroup of relatively poor compliers, older and with intermediate levels of plasma choline. It has been suggested by the authors (25) that the effect of lecithin is complex and that there may be a therapeutic window for the effects of lecithin in this condition, more evident in older patients.

Randomized Controlled Clinical Trial with Phosphatidylserine

Phosphatidylserine (PS) is a phospholipid present in neuronal membranes. In the presence of cell damage, PS can act as an ''endocoid,'' an endogenous substance that, when necessary, can express pharmacologic activity (26). Membrane phospholipids can also influence neurotransmitter function. It has been shown that exogenous PS can increase dopamine release from the dopaminergic terminals of rat striatum (27) and can stimulate acetylcholine release from the cerebral cortex (28). Delwaide et al. (29) carried out an initial clinical trial on 42 patients affected by mild to moderate senile dementia of the Alzheimer type. One-half of the patients received 100 mg t.i.d. of the drug and the other half a placebo. After a washout period, the drug was continued for 6 weeks. Patients were evaluated basally and after 1, 6, and 9 weeks with two behavioral scales, the Crichton and the Peri scales, and with psychometric test, the Circle Crossing Test. The results indicated a trend towards improvement in PS-treated patients with a significant improvement of several Peri items, such as toileting, dressing, and relationship with the environment. After 3 weeks of washout, the effect was significantly reduced.

A study published by Palmieri et al. (30) also demonstrated positive results. Unfortunately, the patients included in this study were defined as generically affected by "organic dementia," and no more specific diagnostic definition is given. The study carried out by Villardita et al. (31) was also characterized by a large number of patients suffering from mild cognitive impairment and selected according to several exclusion criteria, even when no definite diagnosis had been made.

A multicenter study on a well-defined AD population was carried out by Amaducci et al. (32), in the Italian Multicentre Study on Dementia (SMID). In this study the subjects were selected according to rigorous inclusion and exclusion criteria and the clinical diagnosis of probable AD was based on a specific branching decision procedure (33). The blocks of randomization were set according to sex, age (above or below 65 years), and severity of dementia (score higher or lower than 14 on the Blessed Dementia Scale). The patients were evaluated basally, after 3 months of treatment with PS 200 mg/day or placebo, and after 3 subsequent months of washout. The assessment was based on a scale of daily living activities and on neuropsychological tests. After the first 3 months of treatment no significant difference between treated and placebo group was found. However, in the patient subgroup with severe impairment, 3 of 20 tests demonstrated better performance by the patients on PS than by those on placebo. Similar differences in favor of the treated group were observed 3 months after discontinuation of treatment. The daily living performance, as evaluated by the Blessed Dementia Scale, showed a progressive impairment in the placebo group, whereas a moderate, but statistically significant improvement was observed in the treated group. The same trend was noticed on the Information–Memory Concentration test and on the set test. The most evident effect of the drug was noted in seriously impaired AD patients. This effect may be due to the less variable course of the disease at this stage, which implies greater ease in detecting differences.

Randomized Controlled Clinical Trials with Oxiracetam

Preclinical research suggests that metabolic enhancers (nootropics) may improve cognitive functions such as vigilance, acquisition, and memory processes (34). The first studies were performed with piracetam. Oxiracetam is a more recently developed nootropic drug structurally related to piracetam (35). This drug has been found to be at least two to five times as active as piracetam in improving learning and memory in both normal and cerebrally impaired animals (36). At the neurochemical level, oxiracetam has been shown to activate protein synthesis and to stimulate the turnover of lecithin and phosphatidylethanolamine in the brain (37). Controlled clinical trials in elderly patients with organic brain syndrome indicated that oxiracetam is superior to both placebo (38) and provetam (39) in relieving symptomatology. Moreover, in comparison with piracetam, oxiracetam appears to induce a greater improvement in the memory factor (40). Unfortunately, the majority of clinical trials with oxiracetam have been carried out on patients with organic brain syndrome and no information has been given on the proportion of AD patients treated with the drug.

Randomized Controlled Clinical Trials with Acetyl-L-Carnitine

Acetyl-L-carnitine (ALC) is a naturally occurring molecule in the human body. Initial clinical observations of cardiopathic elderly subjects treated with ALC demonstrated psychotropic effects characterized by an improvement in mood, behavior, and cognition. This drug has been investigated for many years to elucidate its possible involvement in the cholinergic neurotransmission. Oral administration of ALC to human subjects produced modifications in brain bioelectric activity, brain metabolism, and modifications of hormone and peptide levels (41). Moreover, ALC was shown to improve performance in geriatric patients with degenerative or vascular disorders (42). Interesting results were obtained in two controlled trials on patients with senile dementia of the Alzheimer type (43). In these studies, a significant improvement at the MMSE (5) was observed in ALC-treated groups.

A large clinical trial with ALC has recently been carried out on 130 patients with AD (44). Patients were treated with a daily dosage of 2 g for 1 year. The efficacy of the drug was assessed with both behavioral and disability scales and neuropsychological tests. This study showed a slower rate of deterioration in the treated group for the majority of outcome measurements.

Taken together, the data obtained by these studies indicate a moderate although significant effect of several drugs on many neuropsychological functions and functional scales. The problem is to determine the clinical relevance of these to patients' performance of activities of daily living. It seems useful to define a priori, those changes in specific outcome measurements as related to the activities of daily living, that appear to be desirable in AD patients. As outcome indicators, we must rely on accurate records of daily living activities, neuropsychological evaluations, and the time elapsed before specific end points such as incapacity, incontinence, or death.

REFERENCES

1. Poon L. Differences in human memory with aging: nature, causes, and clinical implications. In: Birren J, Schaie K, eds. *Handbook of psychology of aging.* 2nd ed. New York: Van Nostrand Reinhold; 1985;427–62.
2. Kral V. Senescent forgetfulness: benign and malignant. *Can Med Assoc J* 1962;86:257 60.
3. Crook T, Larrabee G. Age-associated memory impairment: diagnostic criteria and treatment strategies. *Psychopharmacol Bull* 1988;24:509–14.
4. Wechsler D. *The measurement and appraisal of adult intelligence,* 4th ed. Baltimore: Williams & Wilkins; 1958.
5. Folstein M, Folstein S, McHugh P. Mini Mental State: a practical method for grading the cognitive state of patients for the clinician. *J Psychiatr Res* 1975;12:189–98.
6. Crook T, Bartus R, Ferris S, Whitehouse P, Cohen G, Gershon S. Age-associated memory impairment: proposed diagnostic criteria and measures of clinical change—report of a National Institute of Mental Health Work group. *Dev Neuropsychol* 1986;2:261–76.
7. Larrabee G, Crook R. Assessment of drug effects in age-related memory disorders: clinical, theoretical, and psychometric considerations. *Psychopharmacol Bull* 1988;24:515–22.
8. Bracco L, Amaducci L, Pedone D, et al. Italian multicentre study on dementia (SMID): a neuropsychological test battery for assessing Alzheimer's disease. *J Psychiatr Res* 1990; 24:213–26.
9. Rocca W, Bonaiuto S, Lippi A, et al. Prevalence of clinically diagnosed Alzheimer's disease and other dementing disorders: a door-to-door survey in Appignano, Macerata Province, Italy. *Neurology* 1990;40:626–31.
10. McKhann G, Drachmann D, Folstein M, Katzman R, Price D, Stadlan E. Clinical diagnosis of Alzheimer's disease; report of NINCDS-ADRDA Work Group under the auspices of Department of Health and Human Services Task Force on Alzheimer's Disease. *Neurology* 1984;34:939–44.
11. Haxby J, Grady C, Duara R, Schlageter N, Berg G, Rapoport S. Neocortical metabolic abnormalities precede nonmemory cognitive defects in early Alzheimer's type dementia. *Arch Neurol* 1986;43:882–5.
12. Flicker C, Ferris S, Reisberg F. Mild cognitive impairment in the elderly: predictors of dementia. *Neurology* 1991;41:1006–9.
13. Cohen NJ, Squire LR. Preserved learning and retention of pattern analysis skill in amnesia: dissociation of knowing out and knowing that. *Science* 1980;210:207–10.
14. Sahgal A. A critique of the vasopressin-memory hypothesis. *Psychopharmacology* 1984; 83:215–28.
15. Weiskrantz L, Warrington EK. Conditioning in amnestic patients. *Neuropsychology* 1979; 17:187–96.
16. World Health Organization. *Technical Report Series. Evaluation of methods for the treatment of mental disorders.* Geneva: WHO; 1991.
17. Drachmann DA. Memory and cognitive function in man. Does the cholinergic system have a specific role? *Neurology* 1977;27:783–90.
18. Gustafson L, Edvisson L, Dahlgreen N, et al. Intravenous physostigmine treatment of Alzheimer's disease evaluated by psychometric testing, regional cerebral blood flow (rCBF) measurement and EEG. *Psychopharmacology* 1987;93:31–5.
19. Ashford W, Kuwar V, Sherman K, Elble E, Giacobini E, Becker R. Physostigmine treatment of Alzheimer patients: memory vs. plasma cholinesterase. Presented at The Third Congress of the International Psychogeriatric Association. Chicago: August 28–31, 1987.
20. Davies P, Verth AD. Regional distribution of muscarinic acetylcholine receptor in normal and Alzheimer's type dementia brain. *Brain Res* 1978;138:285–392.

21. Stern Y, Sano M, Mayex R. Effects of oral physostigmine in Alzheimer's disease. *Ann Neurol* 1987;22:306–10.
22. Summers WK, Majowski LV, Marsh GM, Tachiki K, Kling A. Oral tetrahydroaminoacridine in long-term treatment of senile dementia Alzheimer type. *N Engl J Med* 1986;315: 1241–5.
23. Molloy DW, Guyatt GH, Wilson DB, Duke R, Rees L, Singer J. Effect of tetrahydroaminoacridine on cognition, function and behaviour in Alzheimer's disease. *J Can Med Assoc* 1991;144:29–34.
24. Bartus RT, Dean RL, Beer B. An evaluation of drugs for improving memory in aged monkeys: implication for clinical trials in humans. *Psychopharmacol Bull* 1983;19:168–84.
25. Little A, Levy R, Chuaqu–Kidd P, Hand D. A double-blind, placebo controlled trial of high dose lecithin in Alzheimer's disease. *J Neurol Neurosurg Psychiatr* 1985;48:736–42.
26. Toffano G, Bruni A. Pharmacological properties of phospholipid liposomes. *Pharmacol Res Commun* 1980;12:829–45.
27. Mazzari S, Battistella A. Phosphatidylserine effects on dopamine release from striatum synaptosomes. In: Di Benedetta C, Balazs R, Gombos G, Porcellai G, eds. *Multidisciplinary approach to brain development.* Amsterdam: Elsevier/North-Holland; 1980:569–70.
28. Casamenti F, Mantovani P, Amaducci L, Pepeu G. Effect of phosphatidylserine on acetylcholine output from the cerebral cortex of the rat. *J Neurochem* 1979;32:529–33.
29. Delwaide PJ, Gyselynck–Mamborg AM, Hurlet A, Ylieff M. Double-blind randomized controlled study of phosphatidylserine in senile demented patients. *Acta Neurol Scand* 1986; 73:136–40.
30. Palmieri G, Palmieri R, Inzoli MR, et al. Double-blind controlled trial of phosphotidylserine in patients with senile mental deterioration. *Clin Trials J* 1987;24:73–83.
31. Villardita G, Grioli S, Salmieri G, Nicoletti F, Pennisi G. Multicentre clinical trial of brain phosphatidylserine in elderly patients with intellectual deteriorations. *Clin Trials* 1987;24: 84–93.
32. Amaducci L, and the SMID group. Phosphatidylserine in the treatment of Alzheimer's disease: results of a multicenter study. *Psychopharmacol Bull* 1988;24:130–4.
33. Bracco L, Amaducci L. A clinical protocol for the assessment of senile dementia of the Alzheimer type. A progress report. In: Gispen WH, Traber J, eds. *Aging of the brain.* Amsterdam: Elsevier, 1982:275–282.
34. Saletu B, Grünberger J. Cerebral hypoxic hypoxidosis. Neurophysiological, psychometric and pharmacotherapeutic aspects. *Adv Biol Psychiatr* 1983;13:146–64.
35. Noël G, Jeanmart M, Reinhardt B. Treatment of the organic brain syndrome in the elderly. *Neuropsychobiology* 1983;10:90–3.
36. Banfi S, Dorigotti L. Experimental behavioural studies with oxiracetam on different type of chronic cerebral impairment. *Clin Neuropharmacol* 1984;7(suppl 1):768–9.
37. Trovarelli G, Gaiti A, De Medio G, Brunetti M, Porcellai F. Biochemical studies on the nootropic drug oxiracetam in brain. *Clin Neuropharmacol* 1984;7(suppl 1):776–7.
38. Saletu B, Linzmayer L, Grünberg J, Pietschmann H. Double-blind, placebo-controlled, clinical, psychometric and neurophysiological investigations with oxiracetam in the organic brain syndrome of late life. *Neuropsychobiology* 1985;13:44–52.
39. Ferrero E. Controlled clinical trial of oxiracetam in the treatment of chronic cerebrovascular diseases in the elderly. *Curr Ther Res* 1984;36:2,298–308.
40. Turan M, Mehon Gopi N, Bosak M, Songar A. The effects of oxiracetam (ISF 2522) in patients with organic brain syndrome (a double-blind controlled study with Piracetam). *Drug Dev Res* 1982;2:447–61.
41. Rossini PM, Di Stefano E, Febbo A, Gambi D, Collani M. Effects of intravenously administered L-acetylcarnitine on somatosensory-evoked potential. *Eur Neurol* 1985;24:262–71.
42. Hiersemenzel R, Dietrich B, Herrmann WH. Therapeutic and EEG effects of acetyl-L-carnitine in elderly outpatients with mild to moderate cognitive decline. Results of two double-blind placebo-controlled studies. In: Agnoli A, Cahn J, Lassen N, Mayeux R, eds. *Senile dementia. II International Symposium.* Paris: John Libbey Eurotext;1988:345–9.
43. Bassi S, Ferrarese C, Finoia MG, et al. L-acetyl-carnitine in Alzheimer disease and senile dementia Alzheimer type. In: Agnoli A, Cahn J, Lassen N, Mayeux R, eds. *Senile dementia. II International Symposium.* Paris: John Libbey Eurotext; 1988:461–6.
44. Spagnoli A, Comelli M, Lucca U, Menasce G. L-Acetylcarnitine and Alzheimer's disease: results of a controlled clinical trial. *Neurobiol Aging* 1990;11:342–3.

Guidelines for Drug Trials in Memory
Disorders, edited by N. Canal, et al.
Raven Press, Ltd., New York © 1993.

15

Placebos and Other Biases in Clinical Trials in Dementia

Amos D. Korczyn

*Department of Physiology and Pharmacology and Department of Neurology,
Sackler Faculty of Medicine, Tel-Aviv University, Ramat-Aviv 69978, Israel*

Biases exist in any drug study, and an effort must be made to prevent, eliminate, or at least recognize them. Extremely important among biases that limit the applicability of the results is the placebo factor. Surprisingly, many reviews of drug studies and potential therapies in dementia fail to mention the placebo factor altogether or do so only casually (1–4). This chapter discusses various issues that are relevant to the design of drug trials in dementia, with particular consideration given to placebo responses.

THE NATURE OF THE PLACEBO RESPONSE

Placebo responses are among the most interesting issues in medicine and should never be disregarded or taken lightly. They are common, frequently strong, and occasionally unexpected. Basically, they represent the mind–body problem. Under many conditions this is a self-fulfilling prophecy: the mere belief that a drug will have an effect (beneficial or otherwise) ensures that the effect will occur. A vast number of studies have attempted to characterize the placebo response and to define the conditions under which it is likely to occur. It is impossible to review these data here; however, it should be stressed that placebo responses, which inevitably occur in drug trials, attribute to the placebo the characteristics of the reference drug with which it is compared.

A commonly held assumption is that drug effect and the placebo response always add up algebraically in a straightforward manner. Obviously, placebo responses are not limited to inert substances. An active drug has two effects: the specific pharmacodynamic action and the nonspecific placebo response. If simple addition were the case, then performance of a drug study in which the experimental drug is compared with placebo in a parallel design could isolate the specific action of a drug by simple subtraction of the placebo response from the total effect of the drug. However, it is likely that in such a study a patient may detect the therapeutic action of an active drug (if the patient happens to be allocated to this treatment) and therefore will respond with a stronger placebo response than a patient who suspects, rightly or wrongly, that he or she is receiving placebo. Even a "side effect" may indicate to the subject that some biologic action is taking place and therefore suggests that a positive effect should be expected.

To evaluate accurately the efficacy of any drug in a clinical trial, the study should be conducted in a way that minimizes expectations on the part of the patient, the family, the treating physician, and the evaluator. This, however, is never the case for drug studies of dementia, in which patients join the experiment based on the hope that the medication they will be given will be effective, and the physician, whose interest is to recruit patients into the study, does not usually negate this possibility. Scientific considerations take priority over practical and ethical ones.

To circumvent this dilemma, it is important, in a drug study, to rely as far as possible on data that are as unambiguous as possible. For example, time elapsed until admission to a long-stay institution is a better indicator of the efficacy of a drug than subjective reports of wellbeing or activities of daily living, because the latter are highly dependent on patient motivation.

CLINICAL END POINTS

Drug trials should clearly define their end points, and this decision obviously depends on the expected effects of the drug. For example, in Alzheimer disease (AD), a drug likely to affect the progression of the disease should be studied with a protocol completely different from that which examines the acute memory-enhancing effects of drugs in patients with mild cognitive impairment.

The clinical end point in many drug studies is a test or a rating scale such as a short mental test (5,6). These instruments are very useful and important because of their relative objectivity and established reliability. Nevertheless, the main issue is not whether a demented patient improves or does not deteriorate according to such a test, but rather how the daily performance of the patient is affected in the home setting. This parameter should be evaluated independently by an observer unaware of the results of any test or rating scale.

PATIENT SELECTION

The selection of patients for inclusion in drug studies poses unique problems. Probably the most important is that in many neurologic diseases a definite diagnosis can be made only after death. In particular, when a study relies primarily on incident cases, a large proportion of these may eventually turn out to have alternate diagnoses. The problem of incorrect diagnosis is particularly relevant when studies include patients who have failed to respond to previous medication, as this group may be characterized by an even greater proportion of misdiagnoses. For example, elderly depressed patients who dropped out of a study of tricyclic drugs are more likely to have an underlying cognitive decline manifesting as ''pseudodepression.'' Similarly, it would be inappropriate to study the effect of a cholinesterase inhibitor such as tacrine on a mixed group of patients of whom some failed to respond to physostigmine, which is also a cholinesterase inhibitor. In addition, patients who did not respond to previous drugs are likely to have a negative attitude as well as fewer expectations, with a high potential for a negative placebo response to an active drug. For this and other reasons, it is probably methodologically incorrect to study a new drug on a mixed population of cases that comprises both patients who have been tested in previous therapeutic trials and de novo cases. In addition to the diagnostic difficulties, incident nontreated cases are relatively rare and may have a milder disease.

Each drug trial must define the population to be studied. By its very nature, this selection limits the conclusions that may be drawn. A study that demonstrates the efficacy and safety of a given drug in demented patients between the ages of 50 and 70 may not be applicable to older subjects. For example, dementia may have different etiologies in younger and older subjects. In addition, in patients of more advanced age there might be different or more marked side effects. Finally, the pharmacokinetics of a drug are frequently age-dependent.

Another relevant issue is that of the clinical characteristics of the recruited cases. In dementia, patients who are incapacitated primarily by aphasia may be quite different from those with impaired praxis, and their inclusion in a single study may mask an effect on one of those manifestations. Cholinergic agonists may be more effective in memory impairment than in other features of dementia. Many protocols dealing with AD exclude patients with aphasia or with affective changes, although both are well-known manifestations of the disease. There are good reasons for these exclusions, but obviously a clear definition of patients at the time of recruitment is important, as is a breakdown of responses according to clinical characteristics at presentation. Stratification may be a useful tool for analysis of the results obtained in a nonhomogenous population.

DIAGNOSTIC ISSUES

Many drug studies of dementia are designed for patients with either AD or multi-infarct dementia (MID). However, from the clinical standpoint the

TABLE 1. *Differential diagnosis of primary degenerative dementia*

Alzheimer disease	Frontobasal degeneration
Pick disease	Subcortical gliosis
Normotensive hydrocephalus	Alcoholic dementia
Subcortical infarctions	Age-associated memory impairment
Vascular dementia	Dementia associated with depression
Diffuse Lewy body disease	

differential diagnosis of dementia is far from simple (7) (Table 1). Drugs may be efficacious in one clinical entity and not in others.

Even rigid criteria for the diagnosis of AD (8) do not in actuality attempt to differentiate it from other primary degenerative dementias (PDD). A particular issue is the differentiation of PDD from other vascular dementias. Commonly used scales, such as the Hachinski Ischemic Scale (9), have been only partially validated (10).

Although the initial expectation was that PDD and vascular dementia could be completely separated on the basis of this clinical score, subsequent studies consistently identified a substantial intermediate group (11). This is an important problem because either inclusion or exclusion of patients belonging to this group may significantly bias the results. As discussed below, patients with vascular dementia may have not only a different pharmacologic response but also a different course, and therefore may differ from patients with AD.

RATING SCALES

To allow numerical analysis, drug studies must be quantitated in some manner, and it is therefore essential to use clinical rating scales. However, this is not always necessary. Data such as survival or time elapsed between diagnosis and loss of independence and hospitalization can be used to gauge the efficacy of drugs in slowing the progression of disease.

It is obvious that clinical rating scales must be reliable. It is therefore preferable for the same rater to examine the patient on repeated visits. Alternatively, an evaluation of interjudge reliability is required. Similarly, test–retest reliability applies to the degree that an investigator will grant the same rating if the patient is unchanged. In the study of drugs in dementia this can be evaluated, for example, by rating a videotape recording. Videotapes are very useful both for practicing and for adjusting different observers, as well as for actual recording, as rating can be done "blindly" after shuffling of the tapes so that the rater is unaware of whether the patient has or has not been treated, and for how long.

PLACEBO EFFECTS

In any trial, attention must be paid to placebo factors. Basically, patients respond to drugs not only because of the pharmacodynamic action but also because of their subjective expectations. As noted above, a frequently held assumption is that by use of a double-blind, controlled strategy the placebo response can be isolated and deducted from the total response, thus allowing an estimate of the true pharmacodynamic action. There are several reasons to suspect that this approach is an underestimation of the placebo problem. One reason is that when patients who are receiving an active drug feel its efficacy, they respond with greater placebo effect than those subjects who do not feel so (and who are more likely to be receiving inert dummies). This is particularly relevant for patients who have signed an informed consent and are therefore aware of the possibility that they may not receive an active drug. Patients who incorrectly suspect that they were assigned to the placebo group will be less likely to demonstrate the therapeutic effect of the drug. Thus, the pharmacodynamic and placebo effects are far from being simply additive, and a complicated and frequently unpredictable interaction exists between them.

Placebo responses may differ in different studies, reflecting the patients' conditions, their expectations, and the test drug against which the placebo is compared. It therefore follows that an ideal drug trial should consist of three groups: the treatment group, the placebo group, and a (concurrent) nontreatment group. The actual placebo response can, of course, be calculated by the difference between the last two groups.

What one measures as a "placebo response" in drug trials is not strictly the true placebo response and should be termed "apparent placebo response" (12). A frequent additional contribution to these apparent placebo responses is the expectations of the physician or rater. Obviously, the anticipations of the evaluator, the subject, and the caregiver are not independent of each other. In particular, the attitude of the treating physician affects the expectations of the patient and the caregiver. It is also reasonable to assume that when the tested drug is a potent agent, placebo responses will be stronger than when the comparison is made with a drug that the rater knows to have only borderline efficacy. Therefore, responses to placebos are stronger the more potent the reference drug against which placebo is being tested.

Evaluation of cognitive status through the use of rating scales depends, in many cases, on tests that are repeated on successive visits. Even demented patients may learn the correct responses to the Mini-Mental State Examination (MMSE) and, in fact, may practice and train at home, often with the support of the caregiver. The improved score will then be considered to be a placebo response if it occurs in the group that was not given active medication (obviously, antidementia drugs may improve the learning capacity).

Behavior problems are common in demented patients. Examples include agitation, restlessness, anxiety, paranoid ideation, delusions, and hallucinations. Many of these are classic targets for placebo responses. However, few pharmacologic agents are very specific, and even drugs with a unique action (e.g., cholinergic enhancers) can be expected to influence such behavior problems.

An important factor to consider is that of depression. Although patients with frank depression are usually excluded from drug studies of dementia, some affective manifestations may not be recognized or may be of a smaller magnitude than the cutoff point of the study. Depression is known to respond to placebos remarkably, and the improvement of the affective state may of course manifest itself as an improvement in activities of daily living and performance on the MMSE or similar instruments.

Included in the "apparent placebo responses" are random changes. When an active drug is examined against a placebo in demented patients, any improvement in cognitive function that is not directly related to the drug (e.g., when sleep is improved or anxieties relieved by medication or nonpharmacologic means), will be rated as due to a placebo response, as it would occur even in patients receiving the dummy medications. Any spontaneous fluctuation in the condition of the patient could also be ascribed to the drug or placebo. Spontaneous remissions are considered the hallmark of MID. Therefore, a larger response, which can be erroneously attributed to placebo, is expected in patients with vascular dementia as opposed to those with PPD.

A closely related issue is the problem of "regression towards the mean." This statistical term refers to the fact that when a biological parameter is measured once and again, the more extreme values often tend to approach the mean on repeated measurements. An example might be an improvement in scores on repeated MMSE of patients who initially had the lowest scores. Although the mean score of the entire group may not change or may even fall, a subset of "responders" (to an active drug or placebo) may be "identified."

The decision as to whether and when a patient is recruited into a drug study depends, of course, on study criteria. However, it is also dependent on decisions by the patient and the caregiver. This is more likely to be a factor when there has been a recent deterioration in mental state than when the patient has been stable for some time. If such a change were temporary (e.g., an acute delirium due to an infection) the improvement could be misinterpreted, and those patients who had been allocated to the placebo group would be described as representing a placebo response.

REFERENCES

1. Crook T. Clinical drug trials in Alzheimer's disease. *Ann NY Acad Sci* 1985;444:428–36.
2. Narang PK, Cutler NR. Pharmacotherapy in Alzheimer's disease: basis and rationale. *Prog Neuropsychopharmacol* 1986;10:519–31.
3. Orgogozo JM, Spiegel R. Critical review of clinical trials in senile dementia. *Postgrad Med J* 1987;63:237–40.

4. Cooper JK. Drug treatment of Alzheimer's disease. *Arch Intern Med* 1991;151:245–9.
5. Folstein MF, Folstein SE, McHugh PR. "Mini-Mental State." A practical method for grading the cognitive state of patients for the clinician. *J Psychiatr Res* 1975;12:189–98.
6. Treves TA, Ragolsky M, Gelernter I, Korczyn AD. Evaluation of a short mental test for the diagnosis of dementia. *Dementia* 1990;1:102–8.
7. Korczyn AD. The clinical differential diagnosis of dementia: concept and methodology. *Psychiatr Clin North Am* 1991;14:237–49.
8. McKhann G, Drachman D, Folstein M, Katzman R, Price D, Stadlan EM. Clinical diagnosis of Alzheimer's disease: report of the NINCDS-ADRDA Work Group under the auspices of Department of Health and Human Services Task Force on Alzheimer's Disease. *Neurology* 1984;34:939–44.
9. Hachinski VC, Iliff LD, Zilka E. Cerebral blood flow in dementia. *Arch Neurol* 1975;32:632–7.
10. Rosen WG, Mohs RC, Davis KL. A new rating scale for Alzheimer's disease. *Am J Psychiatry* 1986;141:1356–64.
11. Nussbaum M, Reider I, Korczyn AD. Vascular dementia and primary degenerative dementia: criteria for differential diagnosis In: Nagatsu T, Fisher A, Yoshida M, eds. *Basic, clinical and therapeutic aspects of Alzheimer's and Parkinson's diseases,* Vol 2. New York: Plenum Press; 1990:133–6.
12. Drory VE, Korczyn AD. Apparent placebo effect in epilepsy. *New Trends Clin Neuropharmacol* 1991;5:49–56.

Guidelines for Drug Trials in Memory Disorders, edited by N. Canal, et al.
Raven Press, Ltd., New York © 1993.

16

Special Considerations in the Design of Alzheimer Disease Trials

Leon J. Thal

University of California at San Diego Medical Center, Alzheimer Disease Center, San Diego, California 92103

In the United States, community surveys indicate that as much as 10% of the population over age 65 is afflicted with Alzheimer disease (AD) (1). With a population of 260 million, 15% of whom are over the age of 65, there were approximately 4 million individuals with AD in the United States in 1990. Prevalence figures from other countries, as reported in the Eurodem Study (2) and in studies from Shanghai (3), indicate similar although slightly lower figures, suggesting that prevalence does not markedly differ on at least three separate continents (North America, Europe, and Asia). Functionally, individuals with AD develop a syndrome of acquired intellectual deterioration which is severe enough to interfere with occupational or social performance or both. This syndrome manifests as memory loss accompanied by a variety of other cognitive impairments, including visuospatial dysfunction, dysphasia, and difficulty with abstraction, calculation, and concentration (4).

During the last decade, a combination of important discoveries and social factors have promoted dementia drug research. These include the knowledge that memory loss is not an inevitable consequence of aging, findings that the pathologic changes in AD and in senile dementia of the Alzheimer type are in fact identical, major advances regarding the neurochemistry of AD, and the increase in the elderly population in all developed countries.

PROBLEMS INHERENT IN THE CONDUCT OF CLINICAL TRIALS IN AD

A number of problems are associated with the development of drugs and the conduct of clinical drug trials in AD. At present, there is no biologic marker for this disease; therefore, clinicians are never 100% certain of the diagnosis. In a study by Ron et al. (5) of 51 patients diagnosed with dementia, misclassification of 31% was noted on careful follow-up 5–15 years later. More recent series indicate that diagnostic accuracy has improved considerably. A series of patients evaluated at the University of Western Ontario found that approximately 85% of individuals diagnosed with AD during life had that condition at autopsy (6). At the San Diego Alzheimer Disease Research Center (ADRC), diagnostic accuracy was evaluated on a cohort of 141 subjects examined pathologically. Diagnoses were made independently by two neurologists on the basis of a chart review comprising a focused history, neurologic and physical examination, neuropsychologic testing, laboratory data, and brain imaging. In this series, 90% of subjects clinically diagnosed as AD had that diagnosis at autopsy. In addition, approximately one third of AD patients met clinicopathologic criteria for the Lewy body variant of AD. Diagnostic accuracy was much lower for vascular dementia and mixed dementia (7).

In addition to the problem of diagnosis, subjects entering into clinical drug trials vary greatly. There is much heterogeneity in their innate abilities for memory function, language, and intelligence. Disease-related differences are also pronounced. Although all individuals enrolled in clinical trials have memory loss, many have additional disturbances of language, visuospatial relations, mood, and behavior.

A major question arises as to whether or not drugs designed to treat AD should enhance cognition alone, or whether these agents should be designed to improve noncognitive features as well. The original report of AD in 1907 described a 51-year-old woman with auditory hallucinations and delusions (8). A recent review of psychiatric symptoms in AD noted prevalence figures ranging from 10 to 73%, averaging about 30% (9). Based on the Diagnostic Inventory Schedule, 37 of 107 AD patients at the San Diego ADRC were found to have had delusions, hallucinations, or both. Patients with delusions were significantly more impaired than those without delusions on a wide variety of neuropsychological tests (10). In general, the prevalence of delusions was somewhat higher in patients in the middle stage of their dementing illness and declined with advancing disease state. Delusions may have disappeared in the later stages of the illness owing to progressing dementia or to the superimposition of expressive aphasia and an inability to verbalize the presence of delusions. Delusions occur so frequently in AD that they must be considered an integral part of the disease process. Whether or not drugs should be targeted to treat these behavioral features remains unanswered.

The issue of patient heterogeneity in AD is of great interest to the clinician and researcher. Many subclassifications have attempted to separate groups of patients on the basis of clinical features (11,12). Investigators have recently become increasingly aware of the Lewy body variant of AD. At the San Diego ADRC, approximately one-third of AD patients coming to autopsy had Lewy bodies as well as AD pathology (13). These patients usually present with memory impairment, and in the early stages are indistinguishable from other patients with classical AD. Later in the course of the disease, mild extrapyramidal features develop, including masked facies, bradykinesia, slowing of rapid alternating movements, and gait disturbance. These symptoms usually do not respond to levodopa therapy. Other classical signs of parkinsonism such as resting tremor do not occur. In addition, almost one half of these individuals in our series had an essential or action tremor (13). On neuropsychological testing, a severe impairment of attention is noted, as measured by total digit span score. A general deficit in verbal fluency that equally affects letter and category fluency tests is characteristic, as well as severe impairment on visuospatial performance. Pathologically, these patients meet the histopathological criteria of AD: all have sufficient senile plaques and many also have neurofibrillary tangles. In addition, Lewy bodies are regularly present in the substantia nigra and diffusely present throughout the neocortex. There are also spongiform changes in the temporal, entorhinal, and insular cortices, and in the amygdala. Lewy bodies in the cortex can readily be demonstrated by immunostaining against ubiquitin (13). This constellation of clinical symptomatology has become so familiar to us that we now regularly diagnose these individuals clinically. Whether or not patients with this syndrome should be included in conventional AD drug studies is unclear.

PRINCIPLES OF PHARMACOLOGICAL INTERVENTION

In conducting clinical trials in patients with AD, a number of key principles must be considered. First and foremost is the issue of the primary question. A clinical trial should contain a single primary question that can be answered with a single or a limited number of end points. Primary response variables must be defined before initiation of the study. The study population should be defined in advance and should have unambiguous inclusion and exclusion criteria. The design of drug-dosage schedules requires considerable attention. In psychopharmacologic studies of memory and cognition, many laboratory studies demonstrate inverted U-shaped dose–response curves with suboptimal performance at both low and high dosage. Therefore, dosage titration or exposure to a broad range of dosages is mandatory. The sample size should be sufficient that the clinical trial has the power to detect significant differences considered to be of clinical interest. Outcome measures should be objective, should sample a variety of cognitive functions, should be sensitive to the deficits characteristic of AD, should not be restricted by floor or ceiling effects, should be adaptable for repeated administration, should be relatively brief, and should correlate with changes in activities of daily living (ADL) (14).

The design of the trial for AD patients depends on the type of drug to be tested. At present, drugs are available to treat only secondary symptoms, such as agitation, anxiety, sleeplessness, and mood disorders. Such trials are reasonably brief and use behavioral end points as primary outcome measures. Most contemporary clinical trials are designed to treat the primary symptom of the disorder, memory impairment. Neurotransmitter-based replacement therapies are designed to produce short-term improvement in cognitive symptoms. Cognitive ADL and global improvement are the primary outcome measures. Several drug trials have now been implemented to prevent further decline in cognition or to slow progression. These trials are longer (6–24 months) and use outcome measurements similar to those for short-term cognitive trials. As our knowledge base increases and our ability to identify patients early in the disease course improves, drug studies designed to delay the onset of dementia will be attempted. Finally, as the mechanisms and the underlying pathophysiology of the disease unravel, trials will concentrate on the prevention of disease.

DESIGN CONSIDERATIONS

Many clinical drug trials that have been carried out have been poorly designed. Flaws in these studies have included lack of blinding, inappropriate design, small sample size, low power, or the use of multiple outcome measurements. It is virtually impossible to determine whether a drug has improved overall cognitive functioning when a study demonstrates improvement on one or two of 15 or 20 possible outcome variables. In addition, many outcome variables are based on psychometric testing and do not possess face validity. In contrast, the hallmarks of well-designed trials include adequate randomization, blinding, adequate sample size, few outcome measurements, and a meaningful correlation between the test variables and the clinical outcome.

For the evaluation of drugs designed to improve cognition in the short-term, three trial designs have been commonly used: crossover designs, randomized control parallel designs, and enrichment designs. The use of the crossover design is fraught with a number of difficulties. This design assumes that there are no carryover effects and that the treatment response is the same during both periods. The major advantage of this design is its economy. Randomized control parallel design studies, on the other hand, have two main advantages: the control population is uncontaminated by drug exposure and there are no period effects. The disadvantage of this design is that more subjects are required to answer the central question. A third approach recently used in the United States multicenter tacrine study employed an enrichment design combining features of both crossover and parallel design studies. In this design, all subjects meeting inclusion criteria underwent dosage titration in an attempt to determine their optimal dosage for response. Dosage titration was carried out because previous studies of cholinomimetic agents had demonstrated inverted U-shaped dose–response curves and a narrow therapeutic window (15). Subjects not responding to any dosage of drug were dropped from the study. Responding patients were subsequently randomized to treatment with either placebo or the optimal dosage of drug determined during the dosage titration phase, for evaluation in a double-blind, parallel, placebo-controlled study. Efficacy analysis was carried out on the double-blind parallel portion of the study. Although this design has many advantages, including individual dosage titration for each patient, its major disadvantage is that all subjects are exposed to drug at some point during the study, with the potential for carryover effects.

OUTCOME MEASUREMENTS

Each trial requires a series of outcome measurements that are objective, reliable, reproducible, and that measure meaningful change in the disease state. For a drug to be considered effective for the treatment of AD, it must improve cognitive performance. Many instruments are presently available that can be used to measure cognitive improvement. Instruments with well-defined anchor points, face validity, and known rates of change over time markedly enhance the ability of the clinician to calculate the amount of change the patient might be expected to undergo over time from psychometric test scores. In conjunction with cognitive improvement, enhancement of ADL or of other areas of overall functioning must be demonstrated to prevent the marketing of drugs that produce statistically significant improvements in cognition but trivial improvements in overall functioning.

RATE OF COGNITIVE DECLINE IN AD

Deterioration in cognition is a prominent feature of AD. However, it has been recognized that the rate of decline is quite variable, prompting interest in longitudinal studies designed to measure the rate of decline. Rates of decline have now been determined for a large number of neuropsychological screening instruments or composite tests. In a longitudinal study of rate of change in four cohorts that differed significantly from each other in regard to age, education, sex, and the degree of dementia, as measured by their initial Blessed Information–Memory–Concentration (BIMC) test score, the mean annual rate of decline was found to be 4.4 ± 3.6 points per year. This rate of decline was independent of residence, location of the study, patient sex, or education. Of particular importance was the finding that the rate of change in mental status test scores was independent of age (16). A number of other studies have now also found similar rates of decline on the BIMC (17–19). Rates of change have also been examined for the Mini-Mental State Examination (MMSE). Annual rate of decline was found to be approximately

2.8 ± 4.3 to 4.6 points per year in two studies (19,20). One single study examined the rate of decline on the Dementia Rating Scale of Mattis and found it to be 11.4 ± 11.1 points per year (19). Rates of decline have also been determined for the Alzheimer Disease Assessment Scale (ADAS), a composite instrument, and were found to be 8.3 (21) and 9.3 ± 9.8 points per year (22). An attempt to use the rate of decline during a 1-year period to predict future rate of decline during the following year revealed poor predictability (19). A number of important conclusions can be drawn from examination of these studies of rate of decline. First, the rate of decline for these common instruments appears to be similar for all degrees of dementia until a floor effect is reached. Second, the rate of decline is independent of residence, age, location, sex, or education. Third, whereas annual rate of decline is variable for individual patients, the rate of change is quite predictable for groups of patients. Fourth, for individual patients, the change in scores over 1 year does not predict the future rate of decline. Fifth, the standard deviation for the rate of decline for each test was approximately equal to the 1-year rate of decline. Finally, knowledge of the rate of decline allows the accurate computation of sample size for studies designed to slow the rate of decline in AD.

SURVIVAL ANALYSIS IN AD

Although many studies will examine whether or not rates of decline are altered in AD, the use of survival analysis techniques has not been widespread. There are a number of inherent advantages to survival analysis. First, end points can be real-life events rather than artificial constructs. Obvious real-life events include death and institutionalization. These require little interpretation and clearly possess face validity. Second, survival analysis can be carried out for multiple end points. Any patient who reaches one of several prespecified end points or who terminates the study provides useful data for analysis. Dropouts are not a problem, since every patient who drops out has clearly reached an end point and is available for statistical analysis. Third, for placebo-controlled trials the use of survival analysis allows patients to exit the study and seek treatment with other agents should significant worsening or attainment of an end point occur. This feature enhances recruitment for long-term placebo-controlled survival studies. Fourth, survival analysis allows comparison of the entire group despite various lengths of follow-up study. A potential disadvantage of survival analysis in AD is that the time to reach certain end points is likely to be more variable and to be affected by social support systems than is the rate of change on a cognitive measurement. In addition, if a large number of patients drop out of the study without reaching a prespecified end point, the validity of the primary end points may be open to question. Some examples of useful end points or milestones in AD include death, institutionalization, loss of ADL, loss of instrumental ADL, treatment with psychotrophic drugs, and decline in stage of disease.

HOW SHOULD RATE OF CHANGE BE INVESTIGATED IN THE FUTURE?

Several strategies merit consideration. One is to pool data from several types of measures such as mental status scores, ADL scores, neuropsychological testing, and possibly other variables. Certain items may change in a linear or otherwise predictable fashion for groups of patients in a manner analogous to the decline in measurements of muscle strength reported for amyotrophic lateral sclerosis. Selected items from different scales can then be combined into a composite scale sensitive enough to track short-term change over months or years. Alternatively, determining the time taken for patients to reach discrete outcomes, such as loss of complex ADL, can be utilized. Finally, the development of activity of daily living scales individually designed for the patient's particular level of severity might provide a sensitive and useful measurement for monitoring change. The overall challenge will be to validate a flexible and versatile set of assessment measurements which can be adapted to answering clinical questions about the natural history of AD, as well as in the evolving area of therapeutic drug trials.

REFERENCES

1. Evans DA, Funkenstein HH, Albert MS, et al. Prevalence of Alzheimer's disease in a community population of older persons. *JAMA* 1989;262:2551–6.
2. Rocca WA, Hofman A, Brayne C, et al. Frequency and distribution of Alzheimer's disease in Europe. A collaborative study of 1960–1990 prevalence findings. *Ann Neurol* 1991;30:381–90.
3. Zhang M, Katzman R, Salmon D, et al. The prevalence of dementia and Alzheimer's disease in Shanghai, China: impact of age, gender, and education. *Ann Neurol* 1990;27:428–37.
4. American Psychiatric Association. *Diagnostic and statistical manual of mental disorders,* 3rd edition. Washington, DC: American Psychiatric Association; 1980.
5. Ron MA, Toone BK, Garralda ME, et al. Diagnostic accuracy in presenile dementia. *Br J Psychiatry* 1979;134:161–8.
6. Wade J, Mirsen T, Hachinski V, Fishman M, Lau C, Merskey H. The clinical diagnosis of Alzheimer's disease. *Arch Neurol* 1987;44:24–9.
7. Thal L, Galasko D, Katzman R, et al. Patients clinically assessed at an Alzheimer's center generally have Alzheimer's pathology. *Neurology* 1991;41 (suppl 1):323.
8. Alzheimer A. Über eine eigenartige Erkrankung der Hirnrinde. *Allg Z Psychiatr Gerichtl Med* 1907;64:146–8.
9. Wragg RE, Jeste DV: Overview of depression and psychosis in Alzheimer's disease. *Am J Psychiatry* 1989;146:577–87.
10. Jeste DV, Wragg RE, Salmon DP, Harris MJ, Thal LJ. Cognitive deficits of Alzheimer disease patients with and without delusions. *Am J Psychiatry* 1992;149:184–9.
11. Chui HC, Tena EL, Henderson VW, Moy AC. Clinical subtypes of dementia of the Alzheimer type. *Neurology* 1985;35:1544–50.

12. Mayeux R, Stern Y, Spanton S. Heterogeneity of dementia of the Alzheimer type: evidence of subgroups. *Neurology* 1985;35:453–61.
13. Hansen L, Salmon D, Galasko D, et al. The Lewy body variant of Alzheimer's disease; a clinical and pathological entity. *Neurology* 1990;40:1–8.
14. Friedman LM, Furberg CD, DeMets DL. *Fundamentals of clinical trials*. Littleton, MA: PSG Publishing; 1985.
15. Mohs RC, Davis BM, Johns CA, et al. Oral physostigmine in treatment of patients with Alzheimer's disease. *Am J Psychiatry* 1985;142:28–33.
16. Katzman R, Brown T, Thal LJ, et al. Comparison of rate of annual change of mental status score in four independent studies of patients with Alzheimer's disease. *Ann Neurol* 1988; 34:384–9.
17. Thal LJ, Grundman M, Klauber M. Dementia: characteristics of a referral population and factors associated with progression. *Neurology* 1988;38:1083–90.
18. Ortof E, Crystal HA. Rate of progression of Alzheimer's disease. *J Am Geriatr Soc* 1989; 37:511–4.
19. Salmon DP, Thal LJ, Butters N, Heindel WC. Longitudinal evaluation of dementia of the Alzheimer type: a comparison of three standardized mental status examinations. *Neurology* 1990;40:1225–30.
20. Teri L, Hughes JP, Larson EB. Cognitive deterioration in Alzheimer's disease: behavioral and health factors. *J Gerontol* 1990;45:P58–63.
21. Yesavage JA, Poulsen SL, Sheikh J, Tanke E. Rates of change of common measures of impairment in senile dementia of the Alzheimer's type. *Psychopharmacol Bull* 1988;24: 531–4.
22. Kramer–Ginsberg E, Mohs RC, Aryan M, Lobel D, Silverman J, Davidson M, Davis KL. Clinical predictors of course for Alzheimer patients in a longitudinal study: a preliminary report. *Psychopharmacol Bull* 1988;24:458–62.

Guidelines for Drug Trials in Memory Disorders, edited by N. Canal, et al.
Raven Press, Ltd., New York © 1993.

17

Discussion

Dr. Baron: Dr. Grigoletto, the effects of age on the MMSE and the Face Recognition Test that you reported were surprising. Was the population studied screened for health? Did it strictly represent normal aged people? Were the results corrected for education?

Dr. Grigoletto: We believe that the series represents a sample of aged normal subjects free of any clear diseases. However, one should take into account that this was a cross-sectional study, not a longitudinal one. The findings presented were not corrected for education. There is a clear relationship between the MMSE score and education, and we are calculating factors to express the effects of education on the MMSE.

Dr. Levy: Were you advocating the use of repeated testing until you get a stable baseline, e.g., at 3 months? This makes a trial longer and more difficult. That was not really a placebo effect, it was a practice effect. It could also be related to the absence of parallel forms for the test. Using parallel forms, you might well be able to use the first baseline and shorten the whole procedure.

Dr. Grigoletto: I agree, it was the result of practicing or learning, which may be the result of many factors including the forms used and the test itself. If the people are feeling better only because they are considered for a therapy, this is a placebo effect.

Dr. Drachman: With the issue of multiple outcomes, one of the better ways of dealing with the statistical problems is to replicate the test. So if you want to cast a very wide net with 20 outcome measures, and you find three of them to be statistically significant, you can replicate these tests and you may validate the question. One other alternative is to divide your sample, do the statistical analysis on half of the subjects, and see whether the second half agrees with them. We have not used multivariate analysis.

Dr. Grigoletto: Correct. We have different ways of data management. Multivariate analysis is one, and dividing the population in half is another solution.

Dr. Hachinski: Dr. Wilcock, you have presented not only a nice theoretical framework but an approach tinged by experience and common sense. What would you consider to be a minimal duration for a study in Alzheimer disease? The minimal time to show both effects and side effects?

Dr. Wilcock: The minimum duration should be 6 months, in a study using a drug expected to improve the condition, rather than prevent the disease progression. In early stages the very minimum ought to be 6 months, preferable 12 months. In the midstages 6 months. If you get beyond that, I have no figures to support this, apart from the published data on rates of progression in different scales. I would not like to guess what is useful in the later stages, where the patient has reached the stage of being totally dependent.

Dr. Hachinski: You are probably familiar with the desferroxamine study published by McLachlin and his group from Toronto. They used a complex validated videotape assessment as a measure. The treatment group and the placebo group did not show differences at 1 year. But the groups began to diverge, and showed highly significant 50% improvement at 18 months. In view of this, do you not think that your estimates are a bit optimistic in terms of time span?

Dr. Wilcock: That particular study had a totally different concept for retarding the progression of the disease. I was talking about studies measuring the improvement in 6 to 12 months compared with the baseline, and not about studies preventing the disease progression in the next 12 months.

Dr. Reisberg: You wisely pointed out the issue of assumption of linearity of change, as well as the need to separate cognitive effects from behavioral ones. Our own data indicate that cognitive measures seem to proceed in a monotonic fashion with the functional progression of the disease. Behavioral changes, however, proceed in a very different fashion. In fact, all behavioral changes in the course of the disease peak at a certain point, before the final stage of the disease as defined cognitively or functionally. Consequently, scales that mix cognition and behavior are not entirely linear with the progression of the disease.

Dr. Gottfries: We have made both retrospective and prospective studies of the course of the disorder, both in Alzheimer disease and vascular dementia. They support what Dr. Hachinski said: If you separate the cases into early onset and late onset, the late onset of Alzheimer cases have higher variation and a faster course, whereas in early onset cases you need at least 1 year to catch any changes in a rating scale. However, using more sophisticated scales and psychological tests you can catch it earlier.

Dr. Korczyn: It was pointed out that depending on the sensitivity of the scales used, you may have to prolong the study. This is also related to the weakness of the drugs used. In Parkinson disease, for example, there is no need to extend the study for 3, 6, or 12 months. Three days or 3 weeks are probably enough to demonstrate efficacy. The problem is what we are going to study, what are the questions we are asking, and what is the basic mechanism we are talking about? If it is a replacement therapy we should expect an effect within a fairly short period of time. Whether the effect may or may not be maintained is a second question. Another goal is prevention of deterioration or progression of the disease. Obviously, replacement therapy is different from having a drug which will prevent further deterioration. Taking the example of Dr. Grigoletto, in which the placebo group showed improvement within 3 months and stabilized after that, showing training or learning effect, this in itself may be an important measurement between patients and controls; can the patients learn better under the effect of the drug? One should form a clear hypothesis first and then evaluate the appropriate length of the study.

Dr. Saletu: We have milder memory disorders as well, for example, alcoholic dementia. It has a different course of symptoms, and you may well see a difference from placebo within a shorter period of time. The same applies to the uremic syndrome in children.

Dr. Roth: Dr. Lippi, it is worth considering other objective long-term measures. Previously, Kay and I compared the life expectation of patients with dementia with the life expectation of comparable samples of the general population. Life expectation in the demented ones was only between 20 and 25% of the life expectancy of normals. Now there are new recent figures, but the life expectancy has not changed very much. This certainly provides a long-term criterion which should be examined. I do not know if drugs like THA improve life expectancy, and I don't know on what this could be based. Incidentally, another biologic point of interest came up: cause of death. It was extremely difficult to define post mortem the cause of death in patients with senile dementia. Their mortality was very high but post-mortem studies revealed very little in contrast to patients with depression whose mortality was low and the cause of which clearly evident in virtually every case, if it was specific. But the Alzheimer cases looked as if they had died of boredom. One other interesting feature of advanced dementia is the patients' loss of weight. They lose weight until they become cadaverous. What is happening in the metabolism of patients with Alzheimer disease is not known. Despite eating they lose weight. The weight loss can easily be ascertained during a drug trial.

Dr. Erkinjuntti: The duration of Alzheimer disease is now longer than 7 to 10 years, at least in Finland, the mean being 10 years. Measuring of life expectancy or survival time may be of use, but are we measuring the time of suffering instead of the time of good quality of life?

Dr. Roth: I do not think that recent data are strictly comparable, as the patients are now evaluated in a much earlier stage. When our studies were done, more than 25 to 30 years ago, we were measuring duration from the time of admission. Now, we are getting patients at a far earlier stage. Life expectancy would have no meaning without comparison with a control sample with the same demographic characteristics. Therefore, there is comparative, not absolute, expectancy.

Dr. Lippi: Our study on survival in Alzheimer disease shows that many variables that were supposed to influence survival are not important, e.g., age of onset, sex, or educational level. But a correlation between early aphasia and shorter survival was found.

Dr. Roth: These focal signs, aphasia or apraxia, are very likely related to the early-onset cases. If you compare them with the late-onset cases, the comparison is invalid. They may have the same life expectancy, but a life expectancy of 10 years at age 40 is different from that of 10 years at age 70. So you have to parcel out the effect of age of onset before you draw any conclusion.

Dr. Lippi: The aphasic patients were not those with early onset.

Dr. Joynt: While following patients with periodic neurologic examinations, the best information is usually provided by a relative: the patient is better or the patient is worse. None of you have mentioned how much you can use the relatives' information, which is becoming a very important measurement.

Dr. Lippi: I agree. In the clinic you cannot evaluate the functioning in activities of everyday life. The level of disability has to be evaluated in real life. Therefore, caregivers and relatives are a very important source of information.

Dr. Korczyn: It is rather important to know the level of functioning at home. This information can be given only by a close relative or another informant. However, we found that this is complicated by the fact that the patient is not always accompanied by the same caregiver, which creates great confusion and should be taken into account.

Dr. Lippi: For this reason, in our clinical protocol we try to identify a relative able to participate and to refer the patient's condition during the entire follow-up study.

Dr. Korczyn: We do the same. If the patient is not accompanied by the same person, we contact that person by phone to get information about activities of the patient's daily living.

Dr. Roth: Dr. Thal, I would like to comment first on the Lewy body problem. These are very important findings. Have you or others, clinically speaking, observed the very distinctive aspects of the clinical course? One group that I know well has described that the course was fluctuating, marked by periods of clouding of consciousness, a very rapid course, and early death, a far more rapid course than in Alzheimer disease. Therefore, it should be recognizable to some extent from its clinical course. The tangles are the most distinctive part of the Alzheimer pathology. If in the postmortem pathology two-thirds were lacking tangles, you cannot interpret this until you have done ultramicroscopy. Do they have paired helical filaments in dystrophic neurites? Are there intra- and extracellular tangles? Do they respond to amyloid antibodies, or to antibodies against fractions of the tau molecule? Nonspecific tangles occur in a whole range of other disorders, including dementia pugilistica. Therefore, the pathology needs to be examined in more detail, because it would tell us whether this is biologically different far more profoundly than what you have said. In relation to plaques, are there neuritic swollen neurites in the plaques or are they mere amorphous deposits of amyloid? We do not know these facts, and whether that is a quite distinctive pathology. The finding of the new mutation has caused everyone to search for the amyloid protein precursor molecule, spending thousands of hours looking for these mutations and, in most cases, not finding them. The fact that one kindred in a familial case is reported to have the Dutch hemorrhagic form of familial amyloidosis suggests that these may not have been cases of Alzheimer disease but something very remote from Alzheimer disease.

Dr. Thal: When we see these patients early in the course of the first 2 years they are indistinguishable from other patients with Alzheimer disease. A question would be whether or not they have a higher incidence of psychiatric findings. I do not know the answer, but I suspect that they do. In terms of course, it appears that they decline somewhat more rapidly. In terms of their fluctuating and showing disturbances in levels of consciousness, we have not observed that at all. If we see these patients very early on, they have a memory deficit and the neuropsychological testing looks like Alzheimer disease. Later they have some mild extrapyramidal findings and the neuropsychological profile has begun to shift. That is as far as we have come in characterizing the clinical features, but we won't be certain of that until we have more cases. The pathological features are really Dr. Robert Terry's concept, as you know. Obviously, we do not even always agree with our own colleagues on the other side of the country and the Atlantic. One issue is, what are the elderly patients, i.e. individuals over the age of 75, who have plaques only? Dr. Terry feels very strongly that individuals who have large numbers of senile plaques alone and are demented have Alzheimer disease. That is the precondition under which he looks at the brains of patients who also have Lewy bodies. It does not bother him that not all of these patients have neurofibrillary tangles, because he is perfectly willing to diagnose Alzheimer disease in the presence of plaques alone.

Dr. Roth: In terms of the Lewy body patients that we have looked at pathologically, they do have dystrophic neurites and they do have appropriate senile plaques with swollen nerve endings and amyloid cores. Biochemically, the plaques are indistinguishable and are stained with the same markers that a plaque stains in a patient with Alzheimer disease, and the neurofibrillary tangles are composed of paired helical filaments, but they are scanty on the cortex and, in my opinion, this is important.

Dr. Salazar: A slightly different design question. You implied that you would feel quite content doing studies in which you have two treatment arms.

Dr. Thal: No, that is unacceptable. In treatment versus placebo, one of those treatment arms has to be placebo.

Dr. Korczyn: To make a couple of points about today's diagnosis, we usually look at pathologists as having the "gold standard." Pathologists were blind to diffuse Lewy body disease until just recently. The same is true for

other entities such as frontal lobe dementia, which have clearly been identified recently as an important contribution to dementia in some areas, but
are not seen by other neuropathologists, who say these are local diseases.
This is unlikely. I think it is more likely that if you are looking for something
you are going to find it, and if you do not look for it you are likely to miss
it. Use ubiquitin and you see more Lewy body diseases, and once you find
an appropriate marker for the frontal lobe dementia you will see a larger
number than now. Dr. Thal, you said that you can clearly identify patients
with Alzheimer disease at the beginning, but a third of them will be diagnosed
later as having Lewy body disease or another entity. If you restrict your
diagnosis you may be right, but with vascular dementia the chances are
not as good. There is a contradiction, as most cases either have primary
degenerative dementia or vascular dementia. If you cannot diagnose vascular
dementia, which clearly has a misdiagnosis rate of 25%, obviously the rate
of misdiagnoses in Alzheimer disease will be influenced by that. If you restrict your diagnostic criteria for Alzheimer disease so that you exclude unknown, possible, mixed, or possible vascular dementia, you remain with a
selected group. This creates a problem in designing a drug study, as you
have to select cases from a very much larger population. Another problem
relates to patients with primary delusions. In many studies these patients
are excluded, either because of the delusions or because they are treated
with neuroleptic drugs. If about one-third of your patients have primary
delusions, there is a problem.

Dr. Thal: We do not have problems in diagnosing patients with pure Alzheimer disease. However, if we diagnose patients as having vascular disease
and pathology, they very often turn out to have Alzheimer changes as well.
This does not present a problem because we are an Alzheimer center and
therefore receive mostly patients with Alzheimer disease. We are not at-
tempting to study patients with vascular dementia. So that is not a great
problem in terms of coming up with patient numbers. The issue about paranoid delusions is important. In our drug studies we do not exclude patients
who have mild paranoid delusions. We clearly exclude patients who require
treatment with neuroleptic or other drugs for their paranoid delusions. A
good question is what to do with that cohort in the future.

Dr. Sano: We have found similarly that there is a steady rate of decline
with cognitive tests, not dependent on which mental status examination is
used. We do not find this with functional tests, and we even find some
variation with global impressions. We all agree that clinically the functional,
behavioral, and clinical impressions are of greater importance. What should
we do if we do not have a metric in which to measure them?

Dr. Thal: In reality, the cognitive tests do not decline linearly. They probably go down pretty linearly and then they flatten out. The problem with the
current ADL scales is that none of them was designed for Alzheimer patients,
and they do not have the appropriate psychometric properties. It would be

possible, with a lot of work, to design an appropriate ADL scale that would have at least a predictable rate of changes over time, possibly even linear.

Dr. Drachman: I do not agree that the pathology is the "gold standard." In a study that was published in 1986 in the *Journal of Epidemiology,* three of eight normal nondemented individuals over the age of 65 had many plaques, many tangles, or both. One subject in eight had both. If you do a calculation assuming a normal population of 100 individuals, seven of those over the age of 65 will have Alzheimer disease, and 35 of those who do not have Alzheimer disease will have many plaques, many tangles, or both. Thus, five times as many normal individuals as Alzheimer disease patients will have many plaques, many tangles, or both. However, we usually miss that. You had a total of four controls, two of whom showed many tangles. If you had 200 controls, you would have shown a very large proportion of individuals with plaques or tangles, or both. So the notion of the gold standard as being neuropathology is quite wrong. If you calculate the probability that a normal person with a temporal lobe biopsy or autopsy, single-punch biopsy or just a single section, will show many plaques or tangles, the chances that you will be wrong in calling what I refer to as Alzheimer's process, Alzheimer's dementia, will be very great.

As far as Lewy body disease is concerned, Lewy bodies are really mostly ubiquitin. Ubiquitin is found in very large amounts throughout the brain in Alzheimer disease. The fact that it comes together in particular locations may or may not define a separate entity. I wonder if it is simply another variant of people who have plaques but not tangles, tangles but not plaques, both of them but no amyloid, or amyloid but neither of the above.

Dr. Thal: Both your points are very well taken. Regarding the first, one raises the issue of what you would see in normal individuals. It may well be that these normal individuals are individuals who have subclinical Alzheimer disease, and if you had the luxury of following them for another year or two they would have indeed become demented. That is one possible explanation for these findings. To make a diagnosis of Alzheimer disease you need both the clinical picture and the pathologic picture, not just the pathology alone.

Dr. Erkinjuntti: As a conclusion to this discussion, I will outline three points of general agreement:

Rationale of the study. Define the main target and type of the treatment studied; intervention, substitution or facilitation. Duration of the study must be based on the assumed action of the therapy. The observation time should be long enough to reveal the effect and possible late responders should be taken into account.

Outcome variables. Select an outcome variable that is clinically meaningful, objective, and reflecting characteristic features of the disorder in question. Different planes (groups of domains) of end point should be considered, including not only the cognitive changes reflecting, e.g., learning and memory, but also those for activities of daily living, behavior changes, quality of life expectancy, and caregiver burden. These can also be divided as primary impairments and secondary ones. The outcome measures may be different for different subgroups, such as different degrees of severity. In addition, besides short-term end points, long-term ones also should be considered, which include delay in dependence in IADL or ADL, delay of institutionalization, or death. Only one major end point for each plane should be selected, and characteristics for the measure used should be previously known, including, e.g., standard deviations in equal study populations rate of change over time, effects of age, education, and ethnicity, as well as retest and interrater reliabilities. One should also be able to give the minimum change in the measure of clinically significance.

Study design, sample size. The sample size estimation is crucial, and a number of factors affect it. One is the number of end points; several end points require larger sample size. As stated, a given guideline is, have only one or most few clinical relevant end points, instead of tens of different measures. One other factor affecting the sample size is the homogeneity of the patient sample, including the diagnostic accuracy, possible subtypes of the disorder, degree of impairment, duration of disease, age, and, e.g., other associated disorders or clinical findings such as leukoaraiois (white matter changes) or, e.g., mood disorders such as depression. All these factors may affect patients cognitive abilities, modify the effect of the drug, and render the sample imbalanced. These factors should take into consideration in the sample size calculations, which still seem to be mostly neglected. They should also be considered in planning analysis of the study and use of possible strata.

We started with a list of obstacles, and conceivably we have made some progress in overcoming some of them. However, this area still looks for new discoveries, as well as more detailed basic guidelines for international use.

Guidelines for Drug Trials in Memory Disorders, edited by N. Canal, et al.
Raven Press, Ltd., New York © 1993.

18

Introduction

Drug Trials for Memory Disorders: The WHO Perspective

Jose M. Bertolote

Division of Mental Health, Organisation Mondiale de la Santè, Geneva 12, Switzerland

Complaints about memory malfunctioning constitute a frequent complaint and reason for health contacts in both general health care and in mental health care services. A closer look at the phenomenology of these complaints, however, reveals that they can be grouped into at least four distinct categories, with important implications for treatment:

1. Primary memory disorders: usually irreversible, these are found in patients with organic brain disorders, such as the dementias, of degenerative or vascular origin.
2. Secondary memory disorders: usually reversible, these can be (i) either secondary to or associated with other mental disorders (particularly depression and anxiety states); (ii) of iatrogenic origin (particularly associated with electroconvulsive therapy (ECT) and drug treatment, e.g., psychotropic medications); or (iii) toxic, caused by abuse of alcohol or other drugs.
3. Dissociative amnesia: a partial or selective loss of memory, usually of important recent traumatic events, such as accidents or unexpected bereavements, not due to organic mental disorder and too great to be explained by ordinary forgetfulness or fatigue.
4. "Hypochondriacal" dysmnesia: a persistent preoccupation with some degree of memory loss or malfunctioning that cannot be confirmed by objective examination.

WHO ACTIVITIES RELATED TO COGNITIVE IMPAIRMENT

Given the dimension and complexities of this problem, the World Health Organization (WHO) has oriented its actions in several directions.

Development of Instruments

A series of instruments with cross-cultural validity for both clinical and research purposes have been developed. These include the Composite International Diagnostic Interview (CIDI), the Schedules for Assessment in Neuropsychiatry (SCAN) and the International Personality Disorders Examination (IPDE), instruments for the assessment of dementia and for the differential diagnosis with depression. These instruments have now been tested in more than 20 countries and are presently available for use.

Standardization and Classification of Diseases

Since the preparation of the eighth edition of the International Classification of Diseases, a set of criteria and definitions has been proposed and has been undergoing continuous refinement. In the ICD-10 versions for both clinical (1) and research (2) use, internationally accepted operational definitions related to disorders of memory have been formulated. Both the psychiatric and the neurologic (3) adaptations of ICD-10 have now been finalized. The use of standardized operational definitions is fundamental for the cross-comparison of results obtained in different parts of the world and in different settings.

Epidemiological Studies of Cognitive Impairment and Dementia

WHO is engaged in large international multisite collaborative epidemiological studies aiming at obtaining more precise information on the dimension of cognitive impairments and dementia. Centers in six countries, using standardized protocols, have completed data collection in samples from general populations involving more than 10,000 subjects; another six centers started data collection in 1992. Initial results are available, and a first report is expected to be issued in 1993. WHO also has initiated a series of activities related to mild cognitive impairments; in these we also will be dealing with issues such as definitions and classifications, instruments and methods for identification, and prevention and treatment techniques.

Training and Fellowship Programs

WHO has been involved in a long-term program for the development of personnel. An international program of fellowships in the neurosciences has been operational for some years now and many fellows, particularly from developing countries, have benefited from it. Local training programs for both clinicians and researchers have also been implemented. Finally, the strengthening of a worldwide network of collaborating centers and institutions, for both provision of services and research, has been a constant preoccupation and has received a great deal of our attention and efforts.

Services for the Elderly

As part of the overall Mental Health Program, we have been enforcing activities for the improvement of both health and mental health care planning at a public health level, taking into due account local characteristics and needs and taking into consideration the realities of where the care takes place. An increasingly important part of these activities is related to the elderly, a group particularly at risk for developing different types of memory disorders.

GUIDELINES FOR CLINICAL TRIALS: SUGGESTIONS

Responses to many substances can be influenced by a variety of factors, among which we must include demographic and geographic factors, attitudes and beliefs related to health and disease, and service organization and prescribing practices. Therefore, one important principle to guide drug trials is that all clinical phases should be conducted in real-life situations, i.e., in places and settings where the drugs will probably be used and with populations to whom they will be administered. This principle can be translated into five main guidelines:

A. The trial should be conducted in a situation as close as possible to that in which practitioners find themselves. First, we have the important question of the population for whom the drug is expected to benefit. Researchers are eager to conduct studies in as "neutral" populations as possible, i.e., populations having only the target symptom they are studying. Those engaging in this type of activity frequently forget or overlook the fact that real clinical populations rarely have only one type of problem. Elderly people in particular usually have more than one type of physical, psychological, and social problem. They may, for example, have hypertension and sleep disorders, be smokers, and have suffered recent losses or bereavements.

It is essential to use the real situation in which the practitioner finds him or herself. In fact, it is not easy to find an ideal elderly person with only memory problems in clinical settings. It is even more difficult to find enough people in this situation to compose groups for adequate clinical trials. Our position in relation to this question is that we should not aim to find those ideal subjects, but rather to include in the trial people as they are to be found in real life, with the host of problems they normally have to face. There are enough methodological devices whereby we can take into due account these problems for achieving sounder conclusions.

B. An important consequence of this principle relates to the issue of drug interaction. Because the subjects with memory disorders will have other problems as well, they will also be receiving other medications. Therefore, it is also important to know the effect of the drug in subjects who must take other medications concomitantly. If a drug proves to be useful for memory problems but cannot be given to people receiving other medications commonly used for the elderly, its practical utility will be considerably diminished.

C. Nosologic diagnosis beyond the syndrome level should be obtained, preferably using standardized, internationally accepted diagnostic instruments. As we have seen earlier, memory problems can be found in different nosologic entities. Therefore, an attempt at reaching a nosologic diagnosis should be made when groups of patients with memory disorders are described in drug trials. Because the basic neurophysiopathology of memory disorders is not yet fully understood, we may identify drugs effective for some nosologic groups but not for others. There are now many internationally accepted standardized instruments for the diagnosis of mental and neurological disorders, and ICD-10 is available in both clinical and research versions.

D. Comparisons of the effects of the drug in trials should be made with the drug most effective for the same type of problem, whenever it exists. We should always compare any new drug with the most effective drug for the same type of problem, whenever such exists, instead of with placebo. This may not apply in the case of memory disorders because we do not have any drug with a proven efficacy for these disorders, but the principle nevertheless remains.

E. Costs, including side effects and eventual interactions with other drugs concomitantly taken, should also be taken into account to perform meaningful cost–benefit analyses. The consideration of costs should include not only economic costs but also personal discomfort and social costs. Much of the personal discomfort is usually taken care of under the analysis of side effects, which in some cases can even overcome potential benefits of a drug. It has become more and more relevant to include quality of life measurements in cost–benefit assessments of any drug, old or new.

Multisite collaborative work can set off many of the demographic (including race) and geographic (including climate) factors potentially interfering with drug effects. One useful and practical solution to the question of geographic factors interfering with clinical trials is the use of multisite collaborative work. The careful selection of centers in diverse places, from the very earliest stages in clinical trials, provides us with very useful information that can eventually redirect some inaccuracies or methodological flaws. Eliminating these problems at later stages when the study might be well advanced could be much more difficult.

Extensive past and present collaborative work in which WHO has been involved has proven this modality of research to be highly effective in many respects, but not without problems. One of these is related to the fact that in only a few countries can we find capable researchers and research teams. The development of new teams is always involved in the process of collaborative work, thus raising the global capability level for research. Collaborative work can be an invaluable method of learning from more experienced colleagues, and multisite collaborative clinical trials provide an excellent opportunity not only for learning but also for technical cooperation and technology transfer.

To set off some of the more frequently encountered problems in collaborative research, WHO's Division of Mental Health has proposed a "decalogue" addressing many of the ethical, legal, methodological, and economic issues involved in this type of work (4).

CONCLUSIONS

Memory disorders constitute important problems both in clinical practice and in the everyday life of many people. Measures to overcome this problem, including drug treatment, are needed and welcomed.

When trials are conducted to test the clinical usefulness of drugs potentially useful for memory disorders, special attention should be given to the characteristics of the population expected to use these drugs, the place and settings where they will be used, and the comprehensive cost–benefit analyses involving the drug's usage.

WHO will be pleased to participate in the development of guidelines and conduct of clinical trials of drugs for memory disorders, both by providing technical advice and by activating its network of more than 60 collaborating centers in biological psychiatry and psychotropic drugs, in mental health, in neurosciences, and in health, psychosocial, and psychobiological factors in more than 25 countries.

REFERENCES

1. World Health Organization. *Tenth Revision of the International Classification of Diseases Chapter V (F): mental and behavioural disorders. Clinical descriptions and diagnostic guidelines*. (Doc. WHO/MNH/MEP/87.1 Rev.4). Geneva: World Health Organization; 1990.
2. World Health Organization. *ICD-10 Chapter V Mental and Behavioural Disorders. Diagnostic criteria for research*. (Doc. MNH/MEP/89.2 Rev.2) Geneva: World Health Organization; 1990.
3. World Health Organization. *ICD-10 NA. The neurological adaptation of ICD-10*. (Doc. WHO/MNH/MND/91.2). Geneva: World Health Organization, 1991.
4. Sartorius N. Experience from the mental health programme of the World Health Organization. *Acta Psychiatr Scand* 1988;78(suppl 344):71–4.

Guidelines for Drug Trials in Memory
Disorders, edited by N. Canal, et al.
Raven Press, Ltd., New York © 1993.

19

Discussion

Dr. Levy: I detect a potential conflict in your attitude toward classification. On the one hand, you provide clear guidelines for diagnosis of Alzheimer disease and divide Alzheimer disease into type 1 and type 2. You also distinguish types of vascular dementia. On the other hand, your attitude toward drug trials in memory disorders seems to be to forget about the classifications because patients have more complicated presentations in the clinical arena.

Dr. Bertolote: My goal is to apply research instruments to patients for identification, in part because of the costs of identifying patients. In developed countries with established health care services that serve as filters, patients already are identified before entering trials. However, in the majority of countries without such filters, patient diagnosis is not always complete. Therefore, my suggestion is to include all patients with memory disorders in drug trials, irrespective of specific diagnosis, then consider diagnostic differences in the analysis of study results. Without such a system, patients with memory disorders would never be found in many countries in Latin America, Africa, and Asia because they present with memory disorders and a vast array of other problems. As an example, in one of our epidemiologic studies, standardized sampling procedures required finding subjects approximately 85 years of age, but we had to modify the procedure for Madras, India, because one does not find many people of that age in that area. The overall goal is to use standardized instruments or protocols of research to identify the most specific type of disorders, but it is best not to employ these protocols when initially collecting patients for the study because in most of the countries you will not find subjects.

Dr. Thal: I doubt that it is possible to move from the general to the specific with these trials. I don't think that the field will progress if one includes everyone with memory disorders in clinical drug trials, then later attempts to determine the specific diagnosis and decide where the drugs have worked. Unfortunately, we have to proceed in the opposite direction, even though that may be somewhat painful and slower, for two reasons. First, if a drug with a specific mechanism of action is tested in a group of patients with many different disease etiologies, it is perfectly plausible that the drug will not work in many of the disorders. Second, the degree of efficacy that we expect in the treatment of memory disorders is relatively small and, therefore, one initially wants to examine as homogeneous a population as possible.

The ideal procedure should be to find the most homogeneous population and the most specific agent, then ask whether findings can be generalized to larger populations, other populations with the same disease who have other concomitant conditions, or individuals who have other disorders of memory due to other etiologies.

Dr. Bertolote: If we knew the precise neuropathological bases of memory disorders, this would be the safer approach, but in fact, memory disorders are spread over a variety of conditions. As an analogy, if we had to develop an antibiotic without any knowledge of microbiology, it would be almost impossible to develop a drug. We do not really know if dementia of the Alzheimer type is a syndrome or clinical entity. The disagreement between clinicians and neuropathologists as to the gold standard is unresolved.

Dr. Thal: Your point is very well taken, but some differing etiologies of some memory disorders are known. Individuals who are depressed, for example, have a memory disorder associated with depression that probably would not be expected to respond to the same type of drugs that a patient with Alzheimer disease might. I think it would be inappropriate to consider all study entrants as having memory disorder or a particular etiology and then to expect them to respond to a single agent.

Dr. Bertolote: Then we should not talk about memory disorders per se, which is a clinical assessment. It is different if we are searching for a drug that can be effective in, to coin an imaginary entity, "pure Alzheimer disease type 1" memory disorders. I would suggest that we try to clarify the clinical entity we are addressing. If we are talking about memory disorders as such, then we have to specify the diagnosis. If we are talking about Alzheimer or cerebral vascular diseases with memory disorders, it is different. This controversy is exactly what justifies collaborative studies that encompass many different opinions and reach a consensus in the end.

Dr. Hachinski: Which of the instruments would you select if you had to choose only one or two?

Dr. Bertolote: The best instrument depends on the situation. Some instruments are excellent for use with clinical populations but not for general populations. Other instruments have been designed especially for general populations and cannot be applied in clinical situations. The *Source Book of Geriatric Assessment,* edited by Liliane Israel, Diorde Kozarevic, and Norman Sartorius (Karger, 1984) provides clear indications of proposed usage, such as general cognitive impairment, memory disorders, or attention disorders. However, these instruments have been designed for a particular use, and, in most cases, they are used for something different from what they have been designed to measure.

Dr. Reisberg: These volumes do contain many instruments, but many overlap. Additionally, certain categories of instruments that have been discussed in this conference, which are very important to the advancement of the field, will not be found in these volumes. Some examples include instruments to assess behavioral symptomatology in dementia patients, quality of life in dementia patients, and functioning that reflects the continuing cognitive decline.

Dr. Bertolote: Originally those were intended to be the first two volumes of a continuous publication, but the project appeared to be never-ending. However, the situation is different when talking about measuring such clinical aspects as quality of life. For some dimensions of the quality of life there are fully developed instruments and for some other dimensions there are no instruments.

Guidelines for Drug Trials in Memory Disorders, edited by N. Canal, et al.
Raven Press, Ltd., New York © 1993.

20

Introduction

Patient Selection Guidelines

Barry Reisberg

Aging and Dementia Research Center, Department of Psychiatry, New York University Medical Center, New York, New York 10016

The cognitive and behavioral disturbances associated with memory disorders represent important issues that must be addressed in the process of selecting patients to participate in drug trials. Determining the stage of the disorder in each patient is very important, particularly as it affects issues of diagnostic homogeneity. There also is a relationship between the stage of the disorder and a major confounding factor in pharmacologic trials of memory and dementia disorders, namely, behavioral disturbances. Behavioral disturbances are not simply a confounding factor, however; they also present an area of treatment opportunity. It will be necessary to conduct separate examinations of the cognitive and behavioral efficacy of drugs to treat these disorders. Finally, these factors must be examined interactively and individually to assess the risk–benefit ratio of treatment for either of these symptomatic domains.

USE OF STAGING

There are several reasons to use staging in the selection of patients for drug trials in memory disorders. The etiology of symptomatic changes, prognosis, symptomatology, and assessment all may vary, depending on the disease stage. Additionally, the range of utility of assessment measures and treatment side effects vary with stage. The Global Deterioration Scale (GDS) [1,2] (Table 1) and the Clinical Dementia Rating (CDR) [3,4] are two of the clinical staging instruments frequently employed. Elderly people with memory disorders, particularly Alzheimer disease (AD), can be assessed with either or both of these scales, which match specific clinical characteristics with general stages of cognitive decline.

TABLE 1. *Global Deterioration Scale (GDS) for age-associated cognitive decline and Alzheimer disease (AD)*

GDS stage	Clinical characteristics	Diagnosis
1 No cognitive decline	No subjective complaints of memory deficit. No memory deficit evident on clinical interview.	Normal
2 Very mild cognitive decline	Subjective complaints of memory deficit, most frequently in following areas: (a) forgetting where one has placed familiar objects; (b) forgetting names one formerly knew well. No objective evidence of memory deficit on clinical interview. No objective deficit in employment or social situations. Appropriate concern with respect to symptomatology.	Normal aging
3 Mild cognitive decline	Earliest clear-cut deficits. Manifestations in more than one of the following areas: (a) Patient may have become lost when traveling to an unfamiliar location. (b) Co-workers become aware of patient's relatively poor performance. (c) Word and name finding deficit become evident to intimates. (d) Patient may read a passage or book and retain relatively little material. (e) Patient may demonstrate decreased facility remembering names upon introduction to new people. (f) Patient may have lost or misplaced an object of value. (g) Concentration deficit may be evident on clinical testing. Objective evidence of memory deficit obtained only with an intensive interview. Decreased performance in demanding employment and social settings. Denial begins to become manifest in patient. Mild-to-moderate anxiety frequently accompanies symptoms.	Compatible with incipient AD
4 Moderate cognitive decline	Clear-cut deficit on careful clinical interview. Deficit manifest in following areas: (a) decreased knowledge of current and recent events; (b) may exhibit some deficit in memory of one's personal history; (c) concentration deficit elicited on serial subtractions;	Mild AD

TABLE 1. *Continued.*

GDS stage	Clinical characteristics	Diagnosis
	(d) decreased ability to travel, handle finances, etc. Frequently no deficit in following areas: (a) orientation to time and place; (b) recognition of familiar persons and faces; (c) ability to travel to familiar locations. Inability to perform complex tasks. Denial is dominant defense mechanism. Flattening of affect and withdrawal from challenging situations occur.	
5 Moderately severe decline	Patient can no longer survive without some assistance. Patient is unable during interview to recall a major relevant aspect of their current life, e.g.: (a) their address or telephone number of many years; (b) the names of close members of their family (such as grandchildren); (c) the name of the high school or college from which they graduated. Frequently some disorientation to time (date, day of the week, season, etc.) or to place. An educated person may have difficulty counting back from 40 by 4s or from 20 by 2s. Persons at this stage retain knowledge of many major facts regarding themselves and others. They invariably know their own names and generally know their spouse's and children's names. They require no assistance with toileting or eating, but may have difficulty choosing the proper clothing to wear.	Moderate AD
6 Severe cognitive decline	May occasionally forget the name of the spouse upon whom they are entirely dependent for survival. Will be largely unaware of all recent events and experiences in their lives. Retain some knowledge of their surroundings: the year, the season, etc. May have difficulty counting by 1s from 10, both backward and sometimes forward. Will require some assistance with activities of daily living: (a) May become incontinent. (b) Will require travel assistance but occasionally will be able to travel to familiar locations.	Moderately severe AD

continued

TABLE 1. *Continued.*

GDS stage	Clinical characteristics	Diagnosis
	Diurnal rhythm frequently disturbed. Almost always recall their own name. Frequently continue to be able to distinguish familiar from unfamiliar persons in their environment. Personality and emotional changes occur. These are quite variable and include: (a) delusional behavior, e.g., patients may accuse their spouses of being an imposter or may talk to imaginary figures in the environment or to their own reflection in the mirror; (b) obsessive symptoms, e.g., person may continually repeat simple cleaning activities; (c) anxiety symptoms, agitation, and even previously nonexistent violent behavior; (d) cognitive abulia, e.g., loss of willpower because an individual cannot carry a thought long enough to determine a purposeful course of action.	
7 Very severe cognitive decline	All verbal abilities are lost over the course of this stage. Early in the stage, words and phrases are spoken but speech is very circumscribed. Later there is no speech at all—only grunting. Incontinent of urine; requires assistance toileting and feeding. Basic psychomotor skills (e.g., ability to walk) are lost with the progression of this stage. The brain appears no longer to be able to tell the body what to do. Generalized and cortical neurologic signs and symptoms are frequently present.	Severe AD

Reprinted with permission from ref. 1.

GDS Stage 1

The first stage of memory capacity that can be distinguished is that in which elderly individuals have neither subjective complaints of cognitive impairment nor objective, clinically manifest impairments. These persons are considered at stage 1 of the GDS. The CDR does not distinguish this stage from the subsequent stage in which elderly persons exhibit only subjective decrements of memory, cognition, and cognition-related functioning. Consequently, on the CDR scale, persons at both this stage and the following GDS stage are classified as CDR stage 0.

A substantial, ever-increasing literature indicates that elderly persons as a group perform more poorly on certain cognitive assessment measures compared with younger cohorts. In general, cognitive test assessments that involve more levels of cognitive processing are more likely to evoke these deficits. By definition, the individuals at this earliest stage of memory capacity do not complain of memory problems.

The etiology of the deficits in complex cognitive processing tests that are frequently noted in many of these elderly persons who are free of subjective complaints of cognitive deficit or objective evidence of cognitive decline is not known at present. We can hypothesize that the test deficits, when manifested in persons at this stage, may be due to generalized pathophysiologic changes associated with aging, such as sensory or motor deficits. The prognosis for these individuals is excellent.

The treatment of these GDS stage 1 elderly persons poses special issues. Medications may be developed that purport to "restore former cognitive capacities," but the side effects of any possible treatments must be carefully sought, examined, and weighed in risk–benefit judgments.

The general ethical issue of improving cognitive capacity in these normal elderly individuals has been raised. These issues have not proven to be obstacles to physicians' and scientists' attempts to develop improved sensory, physiologic, and motor performance devices and treatments for age-related visual, auditory, cardiovascular, or musculoskeletal changes in the elderly. Analogies to these other age-related physiologic changes indicate that there would not appear to be ethical constraints on the development of pharmaceuticals for improved cognitive performance in the elderly, even in the absence of perceived deficits. The essential question for development of such therapies centers on the cost (primarily in terms of side effects) at which any observed gains are achieved.

GDS Stage 2

In the second stage of identifiable cognitive capacity, elderly individuals have subjective complaints of cognitive impairment without any clinically overt or manifest deficit (GDS stage 2). As noted previously, the CDR combines persons with these deficits with persons who are free of subjective deficits. These complaints are very common in the elderly and may, in fact, occur in as many as 80% of all elderly individuals. The terminology "age-associated memory impairment" has been suggested as a diagnostic rubric to describe this stage (5,6).

Therapeutic interventions at this stage may focus on the relief of perceived deficits or on improvements in psychometric performance. The prognosis for these individuals appears to be excellent (7). Recently, we have completed follow-up on a cohort consisting of more than 100 individuals in this stage and the two subsequent GDS stages. Individuals with diverse medical, psychiatric, neurologic, and neuroradiologic conditions that might have interfered with cognition at baseline or that might have progressed or recurred so as to interfere with cognition were excluded from the study. We followed 85% of these persons over a 9-year mean interval whose baseline mean age was approximately 70 years. There were no significant differences between the three GDS stage groups in terms of time to follow-up or loss during follow-up. Over the 9-year follow-up, 15% of uniformly healthy GDS stage 2 individuals died. Only approximately 8% of those still living exhibited clearly manifest dementia. Only 40% of all patients exhibited any type of negative outcome (death or a notable clinical worsening in cognition) during the follow-up interval. It should be noted that these elderly individuals initially came to the research center because of complaints of memory deficit and returned repeatedly because of the subjective complaints. Nevertheless, it would appear that the prognosis for individuals at GDS stage 2, given the limitations of this study sample size, is not notably different from what might be anticipated from a randomly selected group of healthy elderly individuals in the community. Assessments of treatment efficacy and the risk–benefit ratio of proposed pharmacologic interventions in this stage must be based on this relatively benign prognosis.

GDS Stage 3

At this stage of memory disorder, deficits are subtle, but manifest in the course of a detailed clinical interview. The CDR scale refers to persons at this stage as being at stage 0.5 (although this CDR stage may include persons in the subsequent GDS 4 stage as well). Individuals begin to show a deficit in their performance of complex occupational and social tasks. The precise functional equivalents of each of the GDS global stages can be described in the form of a separate scale known as the Functional Assessment Staging (FAST) scale (8,9). This scale, which is optionally concordant with the GDS, is shown in Table 2. The GDS stage 3 is one in which a professional, who formerly was quite capable of completing numerous reports on a regular basis, now, perhaps seemingly for the first time, cannot complete a single report. The same individual may begin to miss important appointments, seemingly for the first time.

The prognosis for individuals at this stage appears to be diverse (7). These people die at a greater rate compared with those in the GDS stage 2; approximately 35% of GDS stage 3 individuals were deceased at 9-year follow-up compared with only 15% of those in the GDS 2 stage. Additionally, 40% of GDS stage 3 patients who remained alive did not manifest any further cognitive deterioration at follow-up, but 60% did manifest overt dementia. These longitudinal data suggest that people at this stage are prognostically diverse.

TABLE 2. *Sequence of functional loss in normal aging and Alzheimer disease (AD)*
(Functional Assessment Staging with annotations)[a,b]

FAST stage	Characteristics	Clinical diagnosis
1	*No objective or subjective functional decrement.*	Normal adult
2	*Subjective deficit* in recalling names or other word finding and/or subjective deficit in recalling location of objects and/or subjectively decreased ability to recall appointments. No objectively manifest functional deficits.	Normal aged adult
3	*Deficits noted in demanding occupational and social settings* (e.g., the individual may begin to forget important appointments for the first time; work productivity may decline); problems may be noted in traveling to unfamiliar locations (e.g., may get lost traveling by automobile and/or public transportation to a "new" location or spot).	Compatible with incipient AD
4	*Deficits in performance of complex tasks of daily life* (e.g., paying bills and/or balancing checkbook; decreased capacity in planning and/or preparing an elaborate meal; decreased capacity in marketing, such as in the correct purchase of grocery items).	Mild AD
5	*Deficient performance in choosing proper attire, and assistance is required for independent community functioning*—the spouse or other caregiver frequently must help the individual choose the appropriate clothing for the occasion and/or season (e.g., the individual will wear incongruous clothing); over the course of this stage some patients may also begin to forget to bathe regularly (unless reminded) and automobile driving capability becomes compromised (e.g., carelessness in driving an automobile and violations of driving rules).	Moderate AD
6a	*Requires actual physical assistance in putting on clothing properly*—the caregiver must provide increasing assistance with the actual mechanics of helping the individual clothe himself properly (e.g., putting on clothing in the proper sequence, tying shoelaces, putting shoes on proper feet, buttoning and/or zipping clothing, putting on blouse, shirt, pants, skirt, etc., correctly).	Moderately severe AD
6b	*Requires assistance bathing properly*—the patient's ability to adjust bathwater temperature diminishes; the patient may have difficulty entering and leaving the bath; there may be problems with washing properly and completely drying oneself.	Moderately severe AD
6c	*Requires assistance with mechanics of toileting*—patients at this stage may forget to flush the toilet and may begin to wipe themselves improperly or less fastidiously when toileting.	Moderately severe AD
6d	*Urinary incontinence*—this occurs in the absence of infection or other genitourinary tract pathology; the patient has episodes of urinary incontinence. Frequency of toileting may mitigate the occurrence of incontinence somewhat.	Moderately severe AD

continued

TABLE 2. *Continued.*

FAST stage	Characteristics	Clinical diagnosis
6e	*Fecal incontinence*—in the absence of gastrointestinal pathology, the patient has episodes of fecal incontinence. Frequency of toileting may mitigate the occurrence somewhat.	Moderately severe AD
7a	*Speech limited to about 6 words in the course of an average day*—during the course of an average day the patient's speech is restricted to single words (e.g., "Yes," "No," "Please") or short phrases (e.g., "Please don't hurt me"; "Get away"; "Get out of here"; "I like you").	Severe AD
7b	*Intelligible vocabulary limited to generally a single word in the course of an average day*—as the illness progresses the ability to utter even short phrases on a regular basis is lost so that the spoken vocabulary becomes limited to generally 1 or 2 single words as an indicator for all things and needs (e.g., "Yes," "No," "O.K." for all verbalization-provoking phenomena).	Severe AD
7c	*Ambulatory ability lost*—patients gradually lose the ability to ambulate independently; in the early part of this substage they may require actual support (e.g., being physically supported by a caregiver) and physical assistance to walk, but as the substage progresses, the ability to ambulate even with assistance is lost; the onset is somewhat varied with some patients simply taking progressively smaller and slower steps—other patients begin to tilt forward, backward, or laterally when ambulating; twisted gaits have also been noted as antecedents of ambulatory loss.	Severe AD
7d	*Ability to sit up lost*—patients lose the ability to sit up without assistance (e.g., they need some form of physical brace—an arm rest, a belt, or other brace or other special devices to keep them from sliding down in the chair).	Severe AD
7e	*Ability to smile lost*—patients are no longer observed to smile, although they do manifest other facial movements and sometimes grimace.	Severe AD
7f	*Ability to hold head up lost*—patients can no longer hold up their head unless the head is supported.	Severe AD

[a] Adapted from ref. 8.
[b] The FAST stage is the highest ordinally enumerated score. Copyright © 1984 by Barry Reisberg, M.D.
These annotated descriptions can be found in ref. 15.

Independent data indicate that deficits at the GDS 3 stage also may be etiologically diverse. Therefore, any observed improvement in a cohort of patients at this stage may be related to an improvement in AD symptomatology, vascular disease symptomatology, or other factors.

It is very important to recognize that emotional changes occur even at this very early stage. A striking example of this is with "anxieties with respect to upcoming events," as illustrated by the patient who has an appointment with the doctor and continues to ask family members, "When are we going, when are we going, when are we going?" A recent study indicated that more than 40% of patients at GDS stage 3 had this specific emotional symptom (Table 3) (10,11). This and other related anxieties may be sufficiently disturbing to warrant treatment even at this early stage of cognitive and functional impairment. More than 45% of persons at GDS stage 3 also manifest other anxieties, and more than 20% engage in purposeless activity, nonverbal and nonphysical agitation (e.g., anger), tearfulness, and manifest symptoms of depressed mood (11).

GDS Stage 4

Stage 4 on the GDS and FAST scales is characterized by deficits that become clearly manifest in the course of a detailed clinical interview. Deficits occur in the ability to manage the complex activities of daily life. At this stage, for example, the ability to handle finances begins to be compromised in persons who previously managed their personal affairs. Complex meal preparation and marketing skills also begin to be compromised. Applying the McKhann et al. (12) criteria for probable Alzheimer disease permits a more specific diagnosis of early AD at this stage.

When we followed patients at GDS stage 4 prospectively for 9 years, 45% had died and more than 90% of all patients had a negative outcome (either death or clinical worsening of cognition). More than 90% of patients who remained alive manifested overt dementia at follow-up.

Dominant emotional features noted by family members at this stage include withdrawal, with the patient becoming quieter and showing decreased interest and slowed movement, which family members call depression. However, the clinician will note that patients do not exhibit pervasive dysphoria, feelings of guilt, or true suicidal ideation, although approximately one third of all patients at this stage will occasionally say, "I wish I were dead," or utter an equivalent statement in response to their condition (Table 3). However, those statements are not accompanied by suicidal intent. At this stage, there is also generally no weight loss.

Other emotional and behavioral changes frequently occur at this stage. At least 15% of patients manifest specific paranoid and delusional ideation, hallucinatory experiences, activity disturbances, aggressive symptoms, affective symptoms, and anxieties (Table 3) (11). However, these behavioral symptoms are generally less frequently manifest and/or less disturbing compared with subsequent stages.

Therapeutic intervention at this stage may focus on improved cognition or alternatively on the alleviation of behavioral symptoms. Treatment of the emotional symptoms may assist in alleviating the burden. The interrelationship of all symptoms in terms of any treatment is an important area

TABLE 3. Incidence of BEHAVE-AD[a] symptoms in aged and Alzheimer disease subjects at each Global Deterioration Stage (GDS) studied[b]

Symptom category	Specific symptom	Percentage of patients manifesting the symptom						
		GDS 2 (n = 15)	GDS 3 (n = 14)	GDS 4 (n = 24)	GDS 5 (n = 28)	GDS 6 (n = 22)	GDS 7 (n = 17)
(A) Paranoid and delusional ideation	"People are stealing things" delusion	0.0%	7.1%	16.7%	42.9%**	18.2%	0.0%
	"One's home is not one's home" delusion	0.0%	0.0%	12.5%	28.6%	22.7%	0.0%
	"Spouse (or other caregiver) is an imposter" delusion	0.0%	0.0%	4.2%	25.0%	22.7%	0.0%
	Delusion of abandonment (e.g., to an institution)	0.0%	0.0%	4.2%	17.9%	13.6%	5.9%
	Delusion of infidelity (social and/or sexual unfaithfulness)	0.0%	0.0%	4.5%	7.1%	9.1%	0.0%
	Suspiciousness and/or paranoia other than above	13.3%	0.0%	13.6%	57.1%**	36.4%	0.0%
	Delusion other than above	0.0%	0.0%	4.5%	32.1%*	36.4%*	0.0%
(B) Hallucinations	Visual hallucination	0.0%	0.0%	22.7%	10.7%	18.2%	5.9%
	Auditory hallucination	0.0%	0.0%	4.2%	7.1%	13.6%	0.0%
	Olfactory hallucination	0.0%	0.0%	0.0%	0.0%	0.0%	0.0%
	Haptic (sense of touch) hallucination	0.0%	0.0%	0.0%	0.0%	0.0%	0.0%
	Other hallucinations	0.0%	0.0%	0.0%	3.6%	4.5%	0.0%

(C) Activity disturbance						
Wandering (e.g., away from home or caregiver)	0.0%	0.0%	9.1%	35.7%*	50.0%**	17.6%
Purposeless activity (e.g., fidgeting, pacing)	0.0%	21.4%	31.8%*	60.7%***	68.2%***	17.6%
Inappropriate activity (e.g., storing and/or hiding objects in inappropriate places)	0.0%	0.0%	12.5%	39.3%**	59.1%***	17.6%
(D) Aggressiveness						
Verbal outbursts	6.7%	14.3%	22.7%	32.1%*	45.5%	17.6%
Physical threats and/or violence	0.0%	0.0%	9.1%	14.3%	27.3%	17.6%
Agitation other than above (e.g., nonverbal anger, negativity, panting)	6.7%	28.6%	22.7%	42.9%*	63.6%**	37.5%
(E) Diurnal rhythm disturbance						
Sleep (day/night) disturbance	6.7%	0.0%	9.1%	42.9%*	27.3%	17.6%
(F) Affective disturbance						
Tearfulness	33.3%	21.4%	25.0%	42.9%	59.1%	17.6%
Depressed mood other (e.g., statement such as "I wish I were dead")	6.7%	21.4%	36.4%	39.3%	18.2%	0.0%
(G) Anxieties and phobias						
Anxiety regarding upcoming events	7.1%	42.9%	22.7%	46.4%*	31.8%	0.0%
Other anxieties	26.7%	46.2%	27.3%	37.0%	18.2%	0.0%
Fear of being left alone	0.0%	0.0%	4.5%	42.9%**	45.5%***	0.0%
Other phobias	20.0%	7.1%	9.1%	17.9%	22.7%	0.0%

Incidence of symptom differs significantly from that observed in normal aged controls (GDS = 2 subjects). * $p < 0.05$; ** $p < 0.01$; *** $p < 0.001$; χ^2 test.
[a] From ref. 10.
[b] From ref. 11.

of concern, as is the risk–benefit ratio. Therapies directed toward increased socialization must be assessed in terms of their effects on cognition, behavioral changes, and overall functioning.

GDS Stage 5

This stage, also termed the early dementia phase, encompasses patients whose cognitive deficits are of sufficient magnitude that they no longer can survive on their own without assistance. On the GDS this is stage 5, and the CDR scale equivalent is CDR stage 1. Functionally, patients cannot handle such complex activities of daily life as the ability to choose the proper clothing for the season and for the occasion (Table 2). All of the cognitive and most of the emotional features referred to in the previous stage occur with increased magnitude and frequency in this stage.

Behavioral symptoms, which occur in more than 40% of patients in this stage, include the specific delusion that people are stealing things, miscellaneous suspiciousness, purposeless activity, agitation, frequent awakenings in the course of the night, tearfulness, anxieties regarding upcoming events, and a fear of being left alone (Table 3) (11). These emotional symptoms may cloud and color assessments of cognitive change and may themselves be worthy of therapeutic intervention.

Occasionally at this stage, patient embarrassment and the need to deny the loss of intellectual capacities combined with the emotional symptoms and cognitive deficits may render cognitive assessments unreliable and even preclude the ability to obtain some patient assessment. Consequently, judgments of cognitive efficacy should control for these factors. Additionally, effects on cognitive improvement together with effects on behavioral symptoms should be considered when assessing the overall benefit of putative treatments.

GDS Stage 6

At the next stage (GDS stage 6 and CDR stages 2 and 3), deficits are of sufficient magnitude to interfere with basic activities of daily life. A series of functional deficits occur over the course of this stage (Table 2). Early in this stage, in addition to not being able to pick out clothing properly, patients lose the ability to put on their clothing properly and to handle the mechanics of bathing. For example, patients no longer can adjust the hot and cold water temperature properly. With progression of this stage, patients lose the ability to handle the mechanics of toileting and subsequently develop incontinence. Generally, urinary incontinence precedes fecal incontinence. Traditional adult cognitive test measures yield uniformly "bottom scores," and mental status assessments also exhibit floor effects.

Family members or other caregivers no longer complain of withdrawal or of the patient being quieter at this stage. Rather, they complain of patient hyperactivity, agitation, sleeplessness, anxieties, and other behavioral symptoms.

Treatments directed toward making patients less withdrawn at an earlier stage of the disorder are likely to exacerbate the patient's behavioral, and very likely, cognitive deficits at this stage. Behavioral symptoms that are manifest in more than 40% of patients include wandering, purposeless activity, inappropriate activities, verbal outbursts, miscellaneous forms of agitation, tearfulness, and a specific fear of being left alone (Table 3) (11). Some behavioral symptoms peak in occurrence prior to the GDS 6 stage, while many peak during this stage. Behavioral symptoms may decrease in magnitude spontaneously as patients pass through the stage. This decrement in behavioral symptomatology clearly differs from the change in cognitive symptoms, which increase monotonically with the advance of AD.

Functionally, there is an overt decrease in ambulation, and patients characteristically begin to take very small steps. A major problem at this stage is falling, which is very relevant for pharmacologic drug trials at this and the subsequent stage. Approximately 50% of patients at this stage exhibit moderate-to-severe paratonic rigidity (13).

Therapeutic interventions may increase cognition or may improve behavioral symptoms, although assessment of cognition at this stage poses special problems because of floor effects and behavioral disturbances. Although treatment of behavioral disturbances can decrease the burden, side effects—including decreased ambulation, falling, and rigidity—require special consideration.

GDS Stage 7

In the final stage (GDS stage 7), individuals require continuous assistance with all basic activities of daily life. Although the CDR scale does not refer to patients at this stage, modifications of the scale have been proposed which would include patients at this stage as CDR stages 4 and 5. Even early in this stage, speech ability is severely compromised, essentially limited to only approximately six words (Table 2). Subsequently, there is a single-word substage in AD in which patients may say "yes," "no," or "ok" and repeat the final single word in response to all verbalization-provoking phenomena. Eventually, the ability to say even this final single word is lost. Ambulatory ability may be lost from the late GDS stage 6 onward, but at this point in the GDS 7 stage, after speech is lost, ambulatory ability invariably is lost. Those patients who survive then lose the ability to sit up, and the few patients who survive beyond this point lose the ability to smile. Finally, the rare patients who continue to survive lose the ability to hold up their heads.

Traditional psychometric assessments invariably result in bottom scores at this stage, as do mental status assessments. Recently developed tests based upon infant and childhood development models indicate continuing cognitive deterioration in association with continuing functional deterioration in these patients (14,15). Using the *Uzgiris* and *Hunt* ordinal scale of psychological development (OSPD) (16), a test battery developed from Piagetian ideas that was further modified for use in Alzheimer patients, we were able to obtain cognitive data on patients until the 7e stage on the FAST procedure (Table 2) (15). At this point, patients cannot walk, sit up independently, or smile. Nevertheless, using these procedures, we are still able to obtain cognitive data. These modified OSPD tests appear to bottom out only at the point when patients lose the ability to hold up their heads independently.

There is a strong correlation between continuing functional decline in AD and continuing cognitive deterioration. The magnitude of the relationship between continuing cognitive change measured using the OSPD and continuing functional deterioration is comparable to that observed earlier in the course of disease between, for example, Mini-Mental State Examination scores and functional decline (15).

Interestingly, behavioral changes seem to decrease in occurrence in this stage compared with the previous stage (Table 3) (11). No behavioral symptoms were noted to occur in more than 40% of the patients we have studied. Symptoms that occurred in more than 15% of patients included activity disturbances such as wandering, purposeless activities (such as fidgeting and pacing), and inappropriate activities (such as hiding objects). Aggressivity commonly occurs, including verbal outbursts and physical threats of violence, as do other forms of agitation, such as nonverbal anger, negativity, panting, and banging. Sleep disturbances, marked by frequent awakenings in the course of the evening, tearfulness, and screaming, also may be particularly burdensome behavioral symptoms in this stage. All patients in this stage manifest paratonic rigidity, at least to a mild or moderate degree (13).

Reflexes can provide clues about brain activity. A majority of patients at this stage have one or more at least moderately hyperactive deep tendon reflexes. A majority of patients also have at least an equivocally positive plantar reflex and at least a moderately positive prehensile release sign (i.e., a hand or foot grasp and sucking or rooting reflex).

Treatment at this stage may be directed toward decreasing functional disturbances. A decrease in incontinence, gait instability, or progressive motor losses all are worthy treatment goals. Treatment also may be directed toward improving behavioral disturbances, such as agitation, screaming, scratching, or refusal to bathe or to be dressed.

Treatment also may be directed toward improving cognition, although this becomes a relatively complex issue at this stage. Increased cognitive awareness should not be sought at the expense of increased suffering for the patient secondary to the increased awareness. The cognitive effects of behavioral treatments also must be examined. The philosophical meaning of continued existence as well as the validity of the goal of improved cognitive awareness can be questioned at this stage of the illness (17). One reasonable philosophical view is for optimization of cognition and consciousness to be the basic goals of medical therapy, with careful examination of possible negative effects of behavioral pharmacologic treatments, for example, on rigidity and other neurological symptoms.

DEMENTIA DIFFERENTIATION

The stage-specific cognitive, emotional, functional, and neurological aspects reviewed above apply to the dementia associated with AD. Dementias secondary to diverse other etiologies present and/or proceed differently. In some cases these presentations may be described homogeneously for the particular dementia diagnostic entity. In other cases, such as a head trauma or a stroke, the dementia diagnostic entity is diverse in its presentation.

The series of functional changes that occur characteristically with the progression of AD (Table 2) is characteristic of dementia of the Alzheimer type. These functional changes are not necessarily the same in other dementia disorders with which AD can be confused. For example, in normal pressure hydrocephalus, patients commonly present with gait disturbance as the earliest symptom, even antedating their cognitive or other functional disturbances, while the ambulatory disturbance occurs much later in AD and at a specific point in the evolution of the illness process. Similarly, in dementia associated with Creutzfeldt–Jakob disease, one-third of patients present with gait disturbance as the earliest symptom. In stroke, a gait disturbance is accompanied by varying degrees of cognitive and other functional disturbances. In normal pressure hydrocephalus, urinary incontinence commonly occurs after the gait disturbance and both the gait disturbance and the urinary incontinence commonly precede any manifest cognitive decline. In AD the urinary incontinence occurs long after cognitive disturbance is clearly manifest and at a specific point in the evolution of the dementia process. After a stroke, urinary incontinence may be present in the complete absence of dementia symptoms.

Characteristic behavioral symptoms also can be identified in the course of progressive dementia of the Alzheimer type. For example, the specific delusion that "people are stealing things" occurs in more than 40% of patients in the 5th GDS stage. Other specific delusions, such as that the patient's house is not his or her home, occur in 25% or more of all Alzheimer patients at specific stages. Generally, the occurrence of delusions peaks at GDS stage 5. Seven major categories of behavioral disturbances in Alzheimer patients have been identified: paranoid and delusional ideation, hallucinatory disturbances, activity disturbances, aggressivity, characteristic sleep disturbances marked by frequent awakenings in the course of the evening, affective disturbances, and anxieties and phobias. All of these behavioral symptoms peak in magnitude at a certain point in Alzheimer disease and subsequently

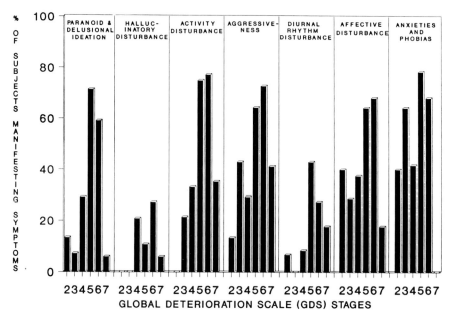

FIG. 1. Incidence of behavioral neuropsychiatric symptoms in normal aging and progressive Alzheimer disease. Adapted with permission from ref. 11.

are less frequently manifest (Fig. 1). They do not occur monotonically in relation to the cognitive and functional progression of AD. Clearly, these symptoms differ from cognitive symptoms that do deteriorate in a linear or monotonic fashion with the temporal evolution of AD.

CONCLUSION

Behavioral symptoms are a burden to caregivers that are likely to respond to pharmacologic intervention, and methodologies exist for systematic investigation of the treatment of these symptoms. Virtually all pharmacologic attempts to treat AD today have focused on treatment of the so-called cognitive symptoms, and studies of cognitive efficacy need to be conducted. However, such studies should examine cognitive changes in the context of behavioral changes, which can account for seeming cognitive effects. It is very important to avoid putative cognitive enhancers in AD which are, in actuality, only very weakly effective behavioral treatment modalities.

On the basis of the evidence presented here, the recommendation can be forwarded that future drug trials should differentiate the stages of central nervous system aging and progressive dementia of the Alzheimer type. Furthermore, we need optimal diagnostic homogeneity. We also must examine the behavioral and cognitive effects of interventions separately as well as salient side effects, for example, on ambulation and the rigidity that occur with the disease progression.

DISCUSSION

Dr. Hachinski: There is a strong parallel between Piaget's stages of mental development and your stages of mental breakdown. What percentage of patients go through these precise stages, and if there are some who do not conform to this pattern, what are the variants?

Dr. Reisberg: All patients with Alzheimer disease who survive progressively will lose the ability to handle a complex occupational task, handle finances, pick out clothing, dress, and bathe. These aspects of adult functioning are universally lost. All Alzheimer disease patients who survive also will lose continence. If they survive, they will all lose the ability to speak, to ambulate, and eventually to sit up, to smile, and to hold up their heads.

To determine the extent to which these deficits proceed ordinally, we have examined the ordinality of functional deterioration according to the FAST staging guidelines in 56 consecutive patients with probable Alzheimer disease, all of whom were at GDS stage 4 or greater (15). Fifty of the 56 patients manifested patterns of deficits entirely in accordance with the ordinal pattern described by the FAST staging procedures (Fig. 2) There were violations of ordinality in six patients. In two, deficits proceeded in the predicted manner, except that stage 6b deficit (loss of ability to bathe independently) was present whereas stage 6a deficit (loss of ability to put on clothing without assistance) was not. In two patients, deficits indicative of stages 6b and 6c were noted, but 6a deficit was not noted. In the remaining two not strictly ordinal cases, loss of ability to properly handle the mechanics of toileting (stage 6c) was noted in one patient who was still capable of independent bathing (stage 6b), and fecal incontinence (stage 6e) was noted in the absence of urinary incontinence (stage 6d) in one patient. A Guttman analysis (18) indicated that the FAST eminently fulfilled the Guttman criteria for an ordinal scale (15).

Developmental analogies also are relevant. The order of loss of the 16 FAST stages and substages in Alzheimer disease is a precise reversal of the order of acquisition of the same stages in the course of normal development (Table 4) (19). Interestingly, the temporal disparities between the reciprocal FAST stages is mirrored by the temporal disparities between the same stages and substages in normal development (albeit, in reverse ordinal sequence).

Dr. Drachman: How does the time frame relate to these stages? How do you explain that some people go through these stages in 3 years, and others go through them in 20 years?

Dr. Reisberg: Each of these functional stages is associated with an estimated mean time course (Table 5) (8). The third stage lasts a mean of 7 years, but it is difficult to discern the earliest point of the onset of this stage. However, from the fourth stage on, we can follow patients through each functional stage and substage. The fourth stage lasts a mean of 2 years, the fifth stage 1½ years, and the sixth stage 2½ years. Individuals in the seventh stage, of course, survive for varying periods, but for those who survive to the final substages, the mean time from the beginning of stage 7a to

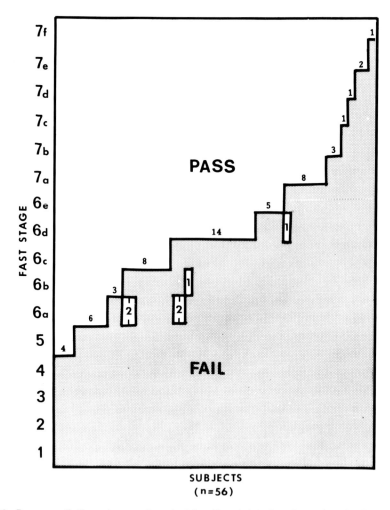

FIG. 2. Presence (fail) or absence (pass) of functional deterioration using the Functional Assessment Staging (FAST) procedure in patients with Alzheimer disease. Reprinted with permission from ref. 15.

the beginning of stage 7f is 6 years. Patients may survive for unknown time periods in stage 7f. The estimated time course is illustrated in Fig. 3, which also illustrates the range of utility of other tests measures and indicates the general bottoming out of other tests at some point in the sixth GDS and FAST stages (20).

We examined the actual temporal course systematically in a cohort of 103 patients (21). At baseline, all patients were at GDS and FAST stages 4 or greater, and the mean mini-mental state examination score at baseline was 15. At follow-up over approximately 5 years, 8% of patients were lost to follow-up and about 30% had died. Fewer than one third of the survivors were capable of returning to the clinic for follow-up. The majority of cases required residential home or nursing home visits,

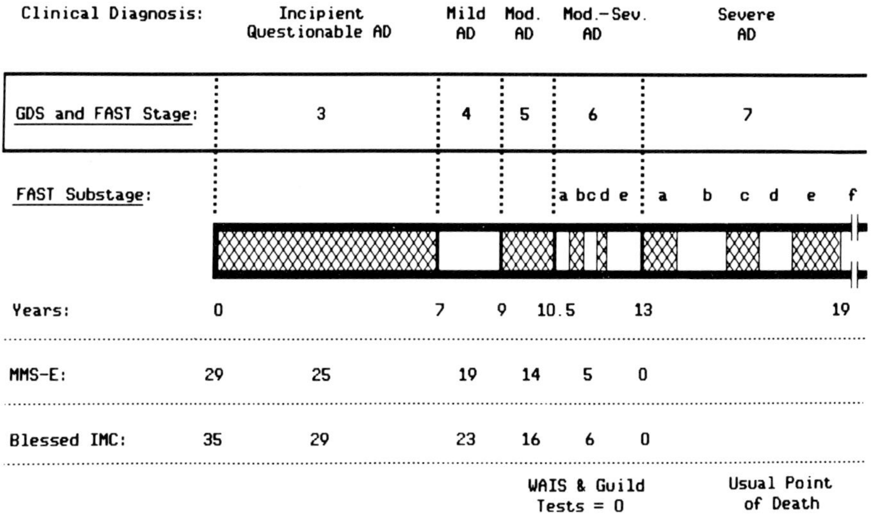

FIG. 3. Typical time course of Alzheimer disease (AD). GDS = Global Deterioration Scale; FAST = Functional Assessment Staging; MMS-E = Mini-Mental State Examination; Blessed IMC = Blessed Information, Memory, and Concentration test. Reprinted with permission from ref. 20.

TABLE 4. *Order of acquisition of the reciprocal Alzheimer disease FAST stages in normal human development**

FAST stage	Clinical characteristics	Age acquired
7f	Ability to hold head up	~4–12 weeks[a,b]
7e	Ability to smile	~8–16 weeks[a,b]
7d	Ability to sit up (without assistance)	~6–9 months[a,b]
7c	Ability to ambulate (without assistance)	~12 months[a,b]
7b	Speech ability limited to a single intelligible word	~12 months[a,b]
7a	Speech ability limited to about 6 intelligible words	~12 months[a,b]
6e	Fecal incontinence	~24–36 months[a,b,c]
6d	Urinary incontinence	~36–54 months[c]
6c	Requires assistance with mechanics of toileting	~48 months[b]
6b	Requires assistance bathing properly	~4 years[a]
6a	Requires assistance putting on clothing properly	~5 years[a]
5	Requires assistance choosing clothing properly for occasions	5–7 years
4	Requires assistance managing finances or with similarly complex activities of daily life	7 years to adolescence
3	Deficits in demanding occupational and social settings	Young adult

* Adapted from ref. 8 (copyright 1984 by Barry Reisberg).
[a] From ref. 23.
[b] From ref. 24.
[c] From ref. 25.

TABLE 5. *Sequence of functional loss in normal aging and Alzheimer disease (AD) (functional assessment staging)*[a,b]

FAST stage	Characteristics	Clinical Dx	Estimated duration in AD[c]
1	No decrement	Normal adult	
2	Subjective deficit in word finding or recalling location of objects	Normal aged adult	
3	Deficits noted in demanding employment settings	Compatible with incipient AD	7 years
4	Requires assistance in complex tasks, e.g., handling finances, planning dinner party	Mild AD	2 years
5	Requires assistance in choosing proper attire	Moderate AD	18 months
6a	Requires assistance dressing	Moderately severe AD	5 months
6b	Requires assistance bathing properly		5 months
6c	Requires assistance with mechanics of toileting (such as flushing, wiping)		5 months
6d	Urinary incontinence		4 months
6e	Fecal incontinence		10 months
7a	Speech ability limited to about 6 words	Severe AD	12 months
7b	Intelligible vocabulary limited to a single word		18 months
7c	Ambulatory ability lost		12 months
7d	Ability to sit up lost		12 months
7e	Ability to smile lost		18 months
7f	Ability to hold head up lost		12 months or longer

[a] Adapted from ref. 8.
[b] Copyright 1984 by Barry Reisberg.
[c] In subjects without other complicating illnesses who survive and progress to the subsequent deterioration stage.

and telephone follow-up was conducted in about 10% of cases. At follow-up, most of the patients were at GDS stages 6 or 7. Mini-Mental State Examination scores fell from a mean of 15 at baseline to a mean of 5 in survivors at follow-up. Blessed et al. (22) information, memory, and concentration test scores decreased from a mean score of 18 at baseline to a mean score of 5 at follow-up. A closer examination of mini-mental state scores at follow-up revealed that 50% of survivors had scores of zero, and 10% had scores of 1 or 2. The remainder of survivors had widely varying mini-mental state examination scores at follow-up.

We also examined the functional course of these patients over the 5-year interval. We worked with the assumption that every patient started in the middle of the respective FAST stage at baseline and ended in the middle of the respective follow-up FAST stage. We compared the estimated time projected for the 65 patients to travel from baseline to follow-up based on the typical time course of Alzheimer disease with the observed course. The observed and estimated times differed by less than

10%. Therefore, these time estimates for the duration of each of the FAST stages and substages appear to be very close to observed averages.

One third of the patients were within 1 year of the estimated course, and about two-thirds were within 2 years of the estimate. It should be noted that even if the FAST were a perfect measure, not every patient progresses from the middle of one stage or substage to the midpoint of another stage, so a certain degree of inherent variability remains in the analysis procedure utilized. The conclusion is that the mean durations of the FAST stages shown in Table 5 are very close approximations of the actual mean durations of these stages in patients with Alzheimer disease uncomplicated by additional brain or peripheral pathology, which can, of course, complicate the observed functional presentation.

ACKNOWLEDGMENT

This work was supported in part by U.S. DHHS grants AG03051, AG09127, AG08051, and MH43486.

REFERENCES

1. Reisberg B, Ferris SH, de Leon MJ, Crook T. The global deterioration scale for assessment of primary degenerative dementia. *Am J Psychiatry* 1982;139:1136–9.
2. Reisberg B, Ferris SH, de Leon MJ, Crook T. The global deterioration scale (GDS). *Psychopharmacol Bull* 1988;24:661–3.
3. Hughes CP, Berg L, Danziger WL, Coben LA, Martin RL. A new clinical scale for the staging of dementia. *Br J Psychiatry* 1982;140:566–72.
4. Berg L. Clinical dementia rating (CDR). *Psychopharmacol Bull* 1988;24:637–9.
5. Crook T, Bartus RT, Ferris SH, Whitehouse P, Cohen GD, Gershon S. Age-associated memory impairment: proposed diagnostic criteria and measures of clinical change—report of a NIMH Work Group. *Dev Neuropsychol* 1986;2:261–76.
6. Reisberg B, Ferris SH, Franssen E, Kluger A, Borenstein J. Age-associated memory impairment: the clinical syndrome. *Dev Neuropsychol* 1986;2:401–12.
7. Reisberg B, Ferris SH, Shulman E, et al. Longitudinal course of normal aging and progressive dementia of the Alzheimer's type: a prospective study of 106 subjects over a 3.6 year mean interval. *Prog Neuropsychopharmacol Biol Psychiatry* 1986;10:571–8.
8. Reisberg B. Dementia: a systematic approach to identifying reversible causes. *Geriatrics* 1986;41:30–46.
9. Reisberg G. Functional assessment staging (FAST). *Psychopharmacol Bull* 1988;24:653–9.
10. Reisberg B, Borenstein J, Salob SP, Ferris SH, Franssen E, Georgotas A. Behavioral symptoms in Alzheimer's disease: phenomenology and treatment. *J Clin Psychiatry* 1987; 48(suppl):9–15.
11. Reisberg B, Franssen E, Sclan SG, Kluger A, Ferris SH. Stage specific incidence of potentially remediable behavioral symptoms in aging and Alzheimer's disease: a study of 120 patients using the BEHAVE-AD. *Bull Clin Neurosci* 1989;54:95–112.
12. McKhann G, Drachman D, Folstein M, Katzman R, Price D, Stadlan EM. Clinical diagnosis of Alzheimer's disease: report of the NINCDS-ADRDA Work Group under the auspices of Department of Health and Human Services Task Force on Alzheimer's disease. *Neurology* 1984;34:939–44.
13. Franssen EH, Reisberg B, Kluger A, Sinaiko E, Boja C. Cognition-independent neurologic symptoms in normal aging and probable Alzheimer's disease. *Arch Neurol* 1991;48:148–54.
14. Sclan SG, Foster JR, Reisberg B, Franssen E, Welkowitz J. Application of Piagetian measure of cognition in severe Alzheimer's disease. *Psychiatric Journal of the University of Ottawa* 1990;15:221–226.

15. Sclan SG, Reisberg B. Functional assessment staging (FAST) in Alzheimer's disease: Reliability, validity and ordinality. *International Psychogeriatrics* 1992;4(suppl 1):55–69.
16. Uzgiris I, Hunt J McV. *Assessment in infancy: ordinal scales of psychological development.* Urbana, IL: Univ. of Illinois, 1975.
17. Reisberg B, Franssen E, Ferris SH, Bondoc EC. The final stage of Alzheimer's disease: Issues for the patient, family and professional community. In: Mayeux R, et al., eds. *Alzheimer's disease and related disorders.* Springfield, IL: Charles C Thomas; 1988;5–27.
18. Nie NH, Hull CH, Jenkins JG, Steinbrenner K, Bent DH. *Statistical package for the social sciences.* New York, NY: McGraw-Hill; 1975:531.
19. Reisberg B, Ferris SH, Franssen E. Functional degenerative stages in dementia of the Alzheimer's type appear to reverse normal human development. In: Shagass C, et al., eds. *Biological psychiatry 1985,* Vol 7. New York, NY: Elsevier Science Publishing Co.; 1986: 1319–21.
20. Reisberg B, Ferris SH, de Leon MJ, et al. The stage specific temporal course of Alzheimer's disease: functional and behavioral comcomitants based upon cross-sectional and longitudinal observation. In: Iqbal K, Wisniewski HM, Winblad B, eds. *Alzheimer disease and related disorders: progress in clinical and biological research,* Vol 317. New York, NY: Alan R Liss; 1989:23–41.
21. Reisberg B, Ferris SH, Franssen E, et al. Mortality and temporal course of Alzheimer's disease: a five-year prospective study (submitted for publication).
22. Blessed G, Tomlinson BE, Roth M. The association between quantitative measures of dementia and senile change in the cerebral gray matter of elderly subjects. *Br J Psychiatry* 1968;114:797–811.
23. Eisenberg L. Normal child development. In: Freedman AM, Kaplan HR, Sadock BJ, eds. *Comprehensive textbook of psychiatry/II.* Baltimore, MD: Williams & Wilkins; 1975: 2036–54.
24. Vaughn VC. Growth and development. In: Nelson WE, Vaughn VC, McKay RJ, eds. *Textbook of pediatrics.* Philadelphia, PA: W.B. Saunders; 1969:15–57.
25. Pierce CM. Enuresis and encopresis. In: Freedman AM, Kaplan HR, Sadock BJ, eds. *Comprehensive textbook of psychiatry/II.* Baltimore, MD: Williams & Wilkins; 1975: 2116–25.

Guidelines for Drug Trials in Memory Disorders, edited by N. Canal, et al. Raven Press, Ltd., New York © 1993.

21

Diagnostic Assessments and Criteria for Memory Disorders in Clinical Drug Trials

*†Timo Erkinjuntti, †Raimo Sulkava, and *Vladimir C. Hachinski

*Department of Clinical Neurological Sciences, University of Western Ontario and The John P. Robarts Research Institute, London, Ontario, N6A 5A5 Canada; and †The Memory Research Unit, Department of Neurology, University of Helsinki, Helsinki, Finland

Despite the growing awareness of and importance of memory disorders in clinical practice, there is unfortunate and often fundamental confusion about the conceptual bases and diagnostic criteria. Detailed multicultural, internationally agreed-on definitions are still required.

The main levels in clinical assessment of persons with subjective or objective memory problems include the symptom or syndrome diagnosis and the etiologic diagnosis. The most important symptom categories, especially with regard to clinical trials for memory disorders, include the age-associated memory disorder (AAMI), the amnestic syndrome, and especially the dementia syndrome. A number of factors that affect the brain cause the memory impairment, including transient, treatable, and progressive causes. Early diagnosis of the treatable causes and factors is particularly important.

In Alzheimer disease (AD), the initial and dominant symptom is memory impairment, which is also a feature of vascular dementia (VaDe). In these disorders an early diagnosis is becoming more vital as effective therapies are found. In clinical trials, accurate antemortem diagnosis is mandatory. However, in AD and VaDe the diagnostic accuracy and homogeneity of patient samples is still unsatisfactory.

This chapter reviews and comments on the clinically most important diagnostic assessments and criteria for memory disorders in clinical drug trials, especially those for the dementia syndromes, AD and VaDe.

SYMPTOMATIC DIAGNOSIS OF MEMORY DISORDERS

The main categories in the symptomatic diagnosis of patients presenting with memory problems are given in Table 1 (1–3). With regard to possible drug trials for memory disorders, the most important categories include AAMI, the amnestic syndrome, early dementia or diminished cognitive capacity, and the dementia syndrome or syndromes.

Mental retardation is usually a stable condition. Many retarded individuals can cope reasonably well and remain independent and unnoticed by health and social services until some additional handicap and social or physical decline due to aging overload their adaptive capacity (4). Elderly retarded persons may be believed to suffer from dementia if they are seen over a relatively short period of time and a proper history is not taken. Retarded individuals may also become demented, e.g., in Down's syndrome (5). Occasionally mild mental retardation restricted to some areas of cognition may have been missed in younger adults. If their occupational requirements increase considerably, the handicap may become evident and a progressive organic brain disorder may even be suspected.

Delirium, acute brain failure, is a medical condition that must always be considered in the diagnosis of memory disorders and dementia (1,6–8). The essential feature of delirium is reduced attention and disorganized thinking. In addition, reduced level of consciousness, disturbances in perception and in the sleep–wakefulness cycle, increase or decrease of psychomotor activity, disorientation, or memory impairment are present. The onset is relatively rapid and the course typically fluctuates.

Delirium is caused by a variety of disorders, including heart and lung diseases, infections, nutritional deficiencies, endocrine diseases, electrolyte disorders, head trauma, drugs, and intoxication (8,9). Predisposing factors include old age, chronic cardiovascular disease and other systemic disorders, and preexisting brain damage. Delirious patients should be examined and treated without delay, as most of the disorders that lead to delirium are treatable. Without proper treatment they may result in permanent brain damage and even death.

TABLE 1. *Differential diagnosis of suspected memory impairment*

Mental retardation
Delirium
Amnestic syndrome and other circumscribed neuropsychological disorders
Other organic brain disorder
Functional psychiatric disorder
Diminished cognitive capacity (early dementia)
Subjective change
Age-associated memory impairment (AAMI)
Dementia

Although demented patients, as well as other patients with organic brain disorders, are at a greater risk for delirium, one cannot diagnose dementia in the presence of delirium because its symptoms interfere with the proper assessment of dementia (1,10).

Circumscribed neuropsychological disorders to be considered in the differential diagnosis include circumscribed memory disorder, the amnestic syndrome (1,11–13), and aphasia, agnosia, and apraxia (4,14).

The clinical criteria for amnestic syndrome are impairment in both short- and long-term memory, not occurring exclusively during delirium and not meeting the criteria for dementia, and evidence of a specific organic factor judged to be etiologically related to the disturbance (1).

The amnestic syndrome may result from any pathologic process that causes damage, usually bilateral, to the limbic and paralimbic structures and the diencephalon (e.g., in the hippocampal complex or the medial dorsal nucleus of the thalamus and their connections) (15). Causes include head trauma, surgical intervention, hypoxia, infarction in the region of the posterior cerebral artery, and, for example, *Herpes simplex* encephalitis (13,15). The typical pure amnestic syndrome is that associated with thiamine deficiency, often related to chronic alcohol abuse.

In the course of both AD and VaDe, there may also exist a period when the symptoms resemble the amnestic syndrome. However, as the disease progresses other areas of cognition will be affected.

Other organic brain disorders, usually associated with psychiatric symptoms, include the organic delusional syndrome, organic hallucinosis, the organic mood syndrome, the organic anxiety syndrome, and the organic personality syndrome (1,11). This category also includes intoxication, withdrawal, and organic mental syndromes not otherwise specified.

Functional psychiatric disorders may be characterized by both subjective and objective changes in memory. Among these disorders are affective disorders, including depressive and manic syndromes; schizophrenic disorders; other psychotic disorders; anxiety disorders; somatoform disorders including conversion disorder; and dissociative disorders including psychogenic amnesia (1,4,6,16,17). The most common psychiatric disorders in which memory impairment may be seen are depression, anxiety, and the so-called "burnout" syndrome. Here the objective cognitive impairment is often mild, with alterations in such functions as attention, concentration, short-term memory, and speed of processing.

Attention has been paid in particular to the relationship between depression and dementia (17). Lists of clinical characteristics for distinguishing dementia from depression have been published (16–18), but the concept and criteria for depressive pseudodementia still show some variation (17,18). However, a dementia-like depressive syndrome appears to be rare.

One proposed scheme for coordinating work on affective illness and dementia divides the relationships between depression and dementia into four categories (18): depression presenting as dementia; depression with second-ary dementia; dementia presenting as depression; and dementia with second-ary depression.

Diminished Cognitive Capacity and Early Dementia

Regardless of what is being measured, human subjects are not readily separable into groups that are unequivocally normal or abnormal, and as the complexity of the capacity being measured increases, the range of uncertainty often widens (19), increasing the difficulty of determining a threshold level of morbidity. In addition to degenerative brain diseases many systemic disorders, such as cardio- and cerebrovascular diseases, affect the subject's intellectual abilities (20), therefore, it is only to be expected that a continuum exists which ranges from no change at all to mild or limited change in intellectual abilities and to global intellectual deterioration.

Differentiation of mild dementia from the less severe changes has been difficult (21). The borderline zone between normal age-related changes and dementia has been designated "limited cognitive disturbance," a state less severe than "pervasive dementia" (22), "very mild" in contrast to "mild" cognitive decline (23), "questionable" as opposed to "mild" dementia (24,25), or "diminished cognitive capacity" (26), which is used also here.

Dimished cognitive capacity is a category without agreed-on definition or criteria. It can be regarded as an organic brain syndrome between AAMI and mild dementia. Its symptoms, in addition to memory impairment, also include some impairment in either abstract thinking, judgment, or other major cognitive functions. These changes may interfere somewhat with the person's work, social activities, and relationships with others. However, the degree of change does not meet the criteria for mild dementia.

Subjective Change

The growing awareness of disorders leading to dementia, the increasing demands to retain learning capacity even in old age, and the necessity to live independently as long as possible, creates personal concerns about possible changes in memory. The same is true for families with members suffering from dementia. Therefore, even persons without clear objective evidence of memory impairment may be looking for advice. After appropriate assessment, some of them do not show any objective changes.

Normal age-related cognitive changes are defined as changes that occur in old age without any signs of overt disease affecting the central nervous system. Aging is accompanied by slow and sometimes continuous changes in specific functions (e.g., the speed of learning and central processing), but little or no change in certain other functions (e.g., crystallized intelligence)

(27). This mild alteration in cognitive abilities related to normal aging does not have serious effects on the individual's social functioning. It does not lead to inability to maintain an independent life style, nor does it shorten life expectancy (4). The changes seen in normal aging are clearly distinguishable from the changes in age-matched patients with mild dementia (28).

AAMI may be reversible pharmacologically. In addition, it is possible that drugs of potential use for treatment of dementias such as AD can be identified through research in healthy aged individuals. Drug development has not often focused on AAMI. One reason for this may be that regulatory authorities have argued that drugs should be targeted at clearly defined clinical entities. In view of such concerns and the broad clinical and therapeutic implications of issues pertaining to the diagnosis of AAMI, recommendations for the diagnostic criteria have been published (29). The criteria for AAMI include: age 50 years and over; subjective complaints of memory loss; memory test performance one standard deviation below the mean established for young adults on a standardized test of recent memory; evidence of adequate intellectual functioning; absence of dementia as determined by a score of 24 (or 27) and higher on the Mini-Mental State Examination (MMSE) (30); and exclusion of all organic and functional factors known to cause memory impairment (31).

"PROCESS CHARACTER" OF THE COMMON DEMENTING DISORDERS

The diseases that progress to dementia (e.g., AD and VaDe) may, in their course from normality to dementia, resemble AAMI, the cognitive changes in a functional psychiatric disorder, the amnestic syndrome, or diminished cognitive capacity. Because there is need to treat such patients *before* they meet the criteria for mild dementia (1), concepts and definitions of possible milder categories are needed. At present, there should be no rationale for waiting until the patient meets the DSM-III-R criteria for dementia before treatment is started. On the contrary, treatment should begin as soon as the diagnosis is suspected.

DEMENTIA SYNDROME

Dementia is usually regarded as an aquired syndrome of cognitive decline caused by some organic factor affecting the brain. The diagnostic criteria most widely used are those of DSM-III (32) and DSM-III-R (Table 2) (1). The diagnosis commonly requires a global cognitive impairment, including decline of memory and other cognitive functions such as abstract thinking, in comparison with the patient's previous level of function. This can be determined by a history of decline in performance and by abnormalities noted

TABLE 2. *Diagnostic criteria for dementia (DSM-III-R, APA 1987)*

A. Impairment in short- and long-term memory
B. At least one of the following:
    Impairment in abstract thinking
    Impaired judgment
    Other disturbances of higher cortical function (aphasia, apraxia, agnosia, "constructional difficulty")
    Personality change
C. A and B significantly interfere with work, or usual social activities, or relationships with others

from clinical history, clinical examination, mental status testing, and confirmed by neuropsychological tests (10).

The decline in cognitive functions must be of sufficient severity to interfere with social or occupational competence; therefore, dementia always includes a social dimension. The diagnosis and grading of dementia cannot be arrived at by standardized examination of the present mental state alone; this must be combined with data concerning the patient's social competence, the history and development of the condition, and the background of the individual (33). Dementia is a diagnosis based on behavior and cannot be determined by computed tomography (CT), magnetic resonance imaging (MRI), single photon emission computer tomography (SPECT), positron emission tomography (PET), electroencephalography (EEG), or other laboratory methods (10).

According to these criteria, an underlying organic cause is always assumed, and functional disorders such as depression causing a dementia-like syndrome are designated as pseudodementia (1,32). In addition, a diagnosis of dementia cannot be made when consciousness is impaired, e.g., by delirium or intoxication, or when other clinical abnormalities prevent adequate evaluation of mental status. The definition of dementia carries no connotation as to prognosis; thus, dementia can be progressive, static, or remitting (1,32).

SHORTCOMINGS OF THE DSM-III-R DEFINITION FOR DEMENTIA

Although there seems to be a wide acceptance of the clinical diagnostic criteria for dementia outlined in DSM-III-R, there are both conceptual and practical difficulties. In addition, the two editions, DSM-III and DSM-III-R, differ from each other to some extent (1,32).

Loss or Impairment

In the DSM-III definition, dementia was defined as "a loss of intellectual abilities," which refers to a decline from a previous level. In DSM-III-R, "impairment" of different cognitive funtions is required. A decline from previous level of function is not explicitly stated, which may create a problem, for example, in classifying cases with mental retardation.

Memory Impairment

In the DSM-III definition a memory impairment was required. In the revised edition both short-term memory (or recent long term-memory) and long-term memory (or remote long-term memory) impairment are required. This change may well limit inclusion of cases with early AD and VaDe.

Which Combination of Cognitive Impairments?

The DSM-III-R definition requires only some combination of short- and long-term memory impairment with one of the domains including abstract thinking, judgment, aphasia, apraxia, agnosia, constructional difficulty, or personality change. In a typical case of AD several of these domains are affected. However, in other disorders this may not be the rule. Therefore, the question of whether a person with only memory impairment and some personality change qualifies for the diagnosis of dementia may be justified. This is especially important in the differentiation between dementia and more circumscribed neuropsychological syndromes.

Social Axis

The DSM-III definition refers to "sufficient severity to interfere with social or occupational functioning." The revised one requires "significant interference with work or usual social activities or relationships with others." Which combination of these social factors is required? Does only significant interference with relationships with others qualify?

Measuring and Assessing Impairment

The DSM criteria neither include more detailed guidelines for measuring impairment in a given cognitive or social domain nor do they state what degree of impairment in each domain qualifies for the diagnosis (see below). Therefore, the widely accepted DSM-III-R criteria for dementia unfortunately have serious limitations. Because the conceptual base is unclear, the definition becomes imprecise. By observing these criteria, a rather nonhomogeneous group of patients with memory disorders may even be collected. In addition, these criteria exclude patients with early AD and VaDe, who do not show clear impairment in long-term memory.

SCREENING AND DIAGNOSIS OF DEMENTIA

In the assessment of cognitive functions in addition to the classic clinical methods (interview, examination, follow-up), short cognitive rating scales such as the MMSE (30) are used in the screening phase (34). In more detailed diagnosis, and especially in the differential diagnosis, neuropsychological tests and test batteries are required (10,28). In addition, assessment of social functions is an ongoing part of the diagnosis of dementia. To supplement the interview, different behavioral rating scales can be used (34). Evaluation of emotional functions, especially depression, should also be part of the examination.

The commonly used screening tests for dementia do not assess all the cognitive domains included in the definitions. In addition, they may have been validated according to different definitions of dementia. For example, the MMSE (30) gives estimates of attention, orientation, recent long-term memory, language skills, and contructional abilities. However, it assesses neither impairment in remote long-term memory, abstract thinking or judgment, nor apraxia or agnosia. If these screening tests are used for preliminary screening only, some of these limitations can be overcome by use of more detailed neuropsychological tests and test batteries. However, if the MMSE is the major cognitive test used in the diagnosis of dementia, the situation is less satisfactory, and may be even worse if the further trial includes only some measurements of efficacy, not covering the major cognitive domains. In addition, the MMSE is insensitive in screening for mild cognitive impairment, especially among persons with higher education (35). Therefore, the structure of these tests limits the ability to identify early cases.

Standardized assessments of social impairment, as well as of emotional and behavioral factors, also have limitations (34,36). With regard to the screening and diagnosis of dementia syndrome, a number of timely question can be raised. These include:

Which areas of cognitive (e.g., orientation, short- and long-term memory, language skills, praxis, attention, visual functions, problem-solving), social [e.g., activities of daily living (ADL), instrumental ADL, and complex ADL functions], and emotional functions (e.g., depression, anxiety, paranoid symptoms) should always be assessed?

Which tests should be used during the screening phase and which sets of more detailed neuropsychological tests should be used in further evaluation, including more detailed assessments of quantitative and qualitative factors related to memory?

What is the minimal degree of impairment in memory, other areas of cognition, and social capacity that justifies the diagnosis of a mild degree of dementia?

How should the test results be corrected according to age, education, socioeconomic, and cultural background of the person tested?

How can possible confounding factors (e.g., change in motivation, lowered expectations, fatigue, motor and sensory impairments, effects of drugs, or the time and place of testing) be avoided during the testing?

CONCEPTUAL BASES FOR DEMENTIA

Is dementia a syndrome or a disease? Even the conceptual bases of dementia is controversial. However, that dementia is a cognitive syndrome caused by organic brain changes, rather than a disease entity, is widely appreciated.

The question of whether there is one or a variety of dementia syndromes has already become a matter of controversy (37). Should we use different criteria for dementias arising from different etiologies, such as the AD dementia syndrome, the cortical vascular dementia syndrome, the subcortical vascular dementia syndrome, or the Parkinson dementia syndrome? Do different definitions of dementia exist for different treatment strategies?

Should we abandon the dementia concept? If these different etiologies are each associated with a different dementia, the dementia concept would no longer be needed, as these conditions may well be defined as cognitive symptoms related to the specific causes, e.g., cognitive symptoms related to AD or vascular factors.

Which cognitive symptoms seen in demented patients are of primary importance, features typical of the majority of cases, and which are merely secondary, has not been discussed or studied in detail. On the basis of our own clinical experience, we venture to suggest a hypothesis for further testing (Table 3). The primary changes in dementia syndrome include, in the early phase, impairment in learning, recent long-term memory, and processing. In a later stage impairment in remote long-term memory and some impairment in immediate memory (attention) are also seen. Therefore, impairment in learning (acquiring) of new information leading to impairment in retrieval and storage of recent long-term memory items represents an early change. This is followed by a defect in retrieval and storage of remote memory and also by a change in the attentional matrix.

TABLE 3. *Proposed concept and basic criteria for dementia*

Primary impairments
  Early
    Learning, recent long-term memory
    Processing
  Late
    Remote long-term memory
    Immediate memory; attention
Secondary impairments
  Other cognitive impairments
  Personality changes
  Behavior changes

TABLE 4. *Diagnosis of dementia: requirements for clinical trials*

Define the cognitive and social domains to be used
Define measuring selected domains and confounding factors
Define the degree of impairment considered as diagnostic

Changes in mental processing include impairments in sequencing, executive function, and self-awareness (38). These functions are related to the poorly defined symptoms: abstract thinking and judgment. Sequencing includes the ability to handle information in sequences and to combine bits of this with other material. Executive function includes anticipation, goal selection, preplanning, and monitoring. Self-awareness is "knowing about knowing," an organized and deliberate acquisition and use of knowledge, as well as the maintenance and generalization of facts and strategies (38).

The essential etiology for such alterations in brain response that produce these primary symptoms are suggested to be lesions in paralimbic and limbic cortical areas, diencephalon, basal forebrain, and surrounding white matter connections, especially in the frontal lobes. Secondary symptoms may or may not be present. These include other cognitive changes such as aphasias, apraxias, agnosias, and constructional difficulty. These symptoms are related to lesions in the unimodal and especially the heteromodal cortical areas (39). In addition, personality changes, mood changes (e.g., depression, anxiety), and other behavioral changes (e.g., paranoia, delusions, hallucinations, aggressiveness, and sleep changes) occur. These other cognitive symptoms, as well as personality and behavioral changes, contribute to the diversity of the clinical picture of dementia. However, dementia may be caused by deep lesions only (40,41), which give rise to the primary symptomatology.

DIAGNOSIS OF DEMENTIA: SUGGESTIONS FOR CLINICAL TRIALS

The main requirements in the diagnosis of dementia for clinical trials are shown in Table 4. On the basis of the conceptual base used, the different cognitive and social domains should be defined in detail. In addition, detailed descriptions of methods for measurement and evaluation of the selected domains should be given. The major confounding factors (e.g., mood and motivation) should also be evaluated. Finally, the norms for different measurements in different age and educational groups in defined populations should be given, so that the degree of impairment can be sufficiently evaluated to qualify a patient for the study in question.

ETIOLOGIC DIAGNOSIS OF MEMORY DISORDERS

Here we focus on the diagnosis and the differential diagnosis of the primary causes of dementia. Diagnosis of other causes of memory impairment, including other categories of organic brain syndrome, has been briefly reviewed above.

Causes of Dementia

Most of the diseases that afflict the brain directly or indirectly may present as dementia. In addition to the two most common causes, AD and VaDe, dementia can be caused by various degenerative brain diseases, deficiency states, drugs and toxins, endocrine disturbances, infections, intracranial conditions, and systemic illnesses. These have all been the subject of reviews (2,20,42,43).

The diagnosis and differential diagnosis of these conditions are based on the clinical interview and examination, chest x-ray, electrocardiography (ECG), screening laboratory tests, and brain imaging, including CT or MRI (44–46). In addition, EEG or quantitative EEG, as well as SPECT, can be used. The clinical chemical tests mostly used include erythrocyte sedimentation rate, hemoglobin, white blood cell count, vitamin B_{12}, glucose, potassium, sodium, calcium, and kidney, liver, and thyroid function tests. Often plasma lipids are tested and tests for syphilis and AIDS are done. In addition, analysis of the cerebrospinal fluid (CSF) may be needed.

The main strategies in the evaluation of underlying causes in patients with memory disorders include: diagnosis of the specific causes, especially of potentially treatable conditions; evaluation of secondary factors that can alter cognitive functioning; and diagnosis of other causes, including AD and VaDe.

Secondary Factors Contributing to Deterioration of Cognitive Functioning

An individual's cognitive capacity can be decreased by secondary factors. These include mood disorders and other behavior changes (e.g., depression, anxiety, paranoid symptoms), sleep disorders (e.g., insomnia, excessive daytime sleepiness, hypopneas, and apneas), medications (e.g., anticholinergic and sedative drugs, alcohol), a number of medical conditions (e.g., cardiopulmonary and metabolic abnormalities, deficiency states, infections), and environmental factors (sensory deprivation, excess of sensory input, social isolation) (6,20,44). Therefore, many somatic, psychological, and social factors, in addition to the organic brain disease itself, participate in the development, manifestation, and outcome of organic brain disorders. Many of these factors should be carefully recorded and monitored as possible confounding factors in drug trials for memory disorders.

Etiologic Diagnosis: Requirements for Clinical Criteria

The main requirements for the clinical criteria to be used include high antemortem accuracy of the clinical diagnosis, as verified postmortem, and homogeneity of the patient sample with regard to possible subtypes, age of onset, and degree of cognitive impairment. However, too restrictive exclusion criteria may cause the patient groups to be overselected. One question related to this is whether all patients should be excluded who have a condition known to potentially cause memory impairment (e.g., hypothyroidism) but who have been adequately treated before the onset of the cognitive symptoms.

ALZHEIMER DISEASE

AD, the most common cause of dementia in Western countries (47), is a slowly progressive, degenerative brain disease of unknown origin. There is no known biochemical or other antemortem marker specific enough for AD, and its etiology is still unknown (48–50). The diagnosis therefore rests on exclusion of other specific causes, including vascular dementia, and on careful evaluation of the clinical course and findings (10,51,52).

The most widely used clinical criteria for AD are those of DSM-III-R for primary degenerative dementia (PDD) of the Alzheimer type (1), and especially the NINCDS-ADRDA Work Group criteria for probable, possible, and definite AD (10). In the latter, the main criteria are dementia syndrome with deficits in two or more areas of cognition, insidious onset and generally progressive deteriorating course without any history, signs or symptoms of focal brain damage, and negative history and laboratory findings referable to any other etiology (10).

Limitations of the NINCDS-ADRDA Criteria for Probable AD

Exclusion of Early Cases

The criteria for AD are specifically criteria for an AD patient with dementia. However, AD actually begins several years before the process has developed to the point that the cognitive deficit fulfills the criteria for mild dementia. Exclusion of early cases of AD from clinical trials because of these criteria is a crucial point, as the disease process in AD should be treated before manifest dementia.

Inclusion of Other Degenerative Disorders

The criteria for probable AD have high inter-rater reliability (53) and they have an accuracy of over 80% during life (54,55). However, these criteria

TABLE 5. *Probable Alzheimer disease*

Features supporting the diagnosis
  Progressive slowing of background activity on EEG
  Early focal atrophy in the temporal lobes, especially hippocampus, on CT or MRI
  Bilateral relative hypoperfusion in temporoparietal lobes on SPECT or PET
  Clinical features such as early loss of insight, early visuospatial difficulties
Possible heterogeneity
  Early vs. late onset
  Familial vs. sporadic cases
  Leukoaraiosis positive vs. negative
  Early vs. late aphasia
  More vs. less cholinergic deficit

also include cases of other degenerative diseases, such as Pick disease and frontal lobe-type dementia (56), as well as, for example, diffuse Lewy body disease (57).

Diagnosis Based on Exclusion Only

The criteria for probable AD are based on exclusion only. Therefore, they lack specific or positive features that could support the diagnosis. Features supporting the diagnosis of probable AD include: progressive slowing of the background activity on EEG or quantitative EEG (58); early focal atrophy in the temporal lobes, especially in the hippocampus, seen on CT or MRI (59,60); bilateral relative hypoperfusion in temporoparietal lobes seen on SPECT or PET (61–63); or clinical features such as visuospatial difficulties or early loss of insight (64) (Table 5).

Heterogeneity of AD

There is also heterogeneity in groups of patients diagnosed as having probable AD (64) (see Table 5). These factors affect the clinical course of the disorder and may reflect differences in the underlying pathophysiology. Therefore, they should be taken into account in the planning of clinical trials. Features indicating heterogeneity in AD include early versus late onset of the disease, familial versus sporadic etiology, white matter changes [leukoaraiosis (LA)] versus lack of such changes, AD with early versus late aphasia, and less versus more pronounced cholinergic deficit (64–67).

Improving the Diagnosis of Alzheimer Disease

Despite the criticisms raised, the present criteria for diagnosis of AD could be improved by also including early cases, including positive and specific

TABLE 6. *Current problems related to vascular dementia*

Defining the syndrome
  The concept
  Factors causing, contributing, or only coexisting with dementia
  Subtypes
  Clinical criteria
Clinical diagnosis
  Possible noninfarct factors
  Clinically "silent" infarcts
  Radiologically undetected infarcts
  Coexisting infarcts only
  White matter changes
  Time and cause relationships

features in the diagnostic criteria, in addition to the well-known exclusion criteria, and by taking into account the possible heterogeneity in AD.

VASCULAR DEMENTIA

VaDe has commonly been considered a dementia syndrome evolving in connection with multiple ischemic lesions of the brain, without other changes known to cause dementia. This is based on the concept of multi-infarct dementia (MID) (3,68,69). However, there is growing confusion, and a number of questions related to VaDe have been raised (Table 6).

The Concept

VaDe is not a disease entity. Rather, it is a syndrome caused by different vascular factors. Although this statement is widely accepted, comparison of VaDe to AD as an entity has created confusion.

The role of ischemic brain infarcts as an etiology of VaDe has been accepted, but the possible role of so-called noninfarct mechanisms has created controversies. These include incomplete infarcts surrounding the infarcts (70), functional inactivity due to ischemia (71), vessel wall changes leading to blood–brain barrier or carrier dysfunction, and possible dysfunction of the oligodendrocytes leading to defective myelination (44,66,69,72).

Causative Factors

Different brain lesions, vascular mechanisms, and risk factors are involved in VaDe (69). To what extent these factors cause, contribute, or only coexist with the cognitive syndrome is not precisely known. Brain alterations associated with VaDe include location, side, number and volume of focal infarcts, as well as location, type, and extent of ischemic white matter changes (73–75). The vascular mechanisms include atherothrombotic stroke, cardiogenic embolic stroke, small-vessel arteriopathies leading to lacunar stroke or ischemic white matter changes, hemodynamic change, hemorrhage, and hematologic and hereditary factors (3,44,68,69,76,77). The risk factors of VaDe have been related to those of stroke; however, detailed data are lacking.

Subtypes

VaDe has usually been treated as a single group, although it is related to different brain changes, vascular mechanisms, and possible risk factors. However, a tendency to comfortable categorization has recently emerged (78,79). Unfortunately, this is not based on detailed clinical and neuropathologic data. This has even lead to fundamental conceptual confusion, as seen in the predominantly cortical MID related to lacunar infarcts in the proposal for the Tenth Revision of the International Classification of Diseases (79).

Clinical Criteria

The clinical criteria for MID widely used are those of the DSM-III-R, which are based on clinical descriptions only (1). These criteria include, in addition to dementia, features suggestive of focal ischemic brain lesions, such as stepwise deterioration, "patchy" distribution of deficits, focal neurologic symptoms and signs, and evidence of significant cerebrovascular disease that is judged to be etiologically related to the disturbance. However, these clinical features are not defined in detail, and brain imaging data are not used. Consequently, these criteria also cover a number of cases with AD with vascular changes, yielding a low accuracy of ante-mortem diagnosis as verified postmortem (for review see ref. 3).

To achieve a higher accuracy of antemortem diagnosis, Erkinjuntti (3,80) proposed more strict criteria for VaDe based on the infarct concept (Table 7). By use of these criteria the antemortem accuracy of the diagnosis of

TABLE 7. *Clinical diagnostic criteria for vascular dementia*

Dementia
Evidence of
  (a) clinical history and/or findings in clinical examination indicating stroke/strokes (i.e., event of focal cerebral dysfunction of vascular origin), and/or
  (b) findings on brain imaging (e.g., CT, MRI) compatible with vascular lesions of the brain (infarct/infarcts and/or moderate to severe degree of ischemic white matter change), indicating multiple cortical and/or vascular lesions of the brain which are judged to be timely and causally related to the disturbance
Absence of known specific causes of dementia revealed by clinical history and examination, laboratory investigations, and brain imaging

Adapted from refs. 3 and 80.

VaDe, as verified postmortem, has been near 90% (73). However, a number of vascular cases, including some of those who might benefit from treatment, may well be excluded.

Problems in the Clinical Diagnosis of Vascular Dementia

The use of clinical criteria for VaDe based on the multi-infarct concept and known to give sufficient antemortem accuracy raises a number of questions (Table 6).

Noninfarct Factors

As reviewed, in addition to ischemic infarcts other possible vascular factors may be important. These include, for example, areas of incomplete infarction, functional changes due to ischemia, or possible dysfunction of the oligodendrocytes. If these factors have a role in the genesis of VaDe, the problem lies in detecting and measuring their effects. In addition, detailed data concerning the extent to which they cause and contribute to the syndrome are needed.

Clinically "silent" infarcts may exist (81,82), and only the cumulative effect of these changes becomes clinically evident. However, often these are events that do not meet the criteria of focal ischemic stroke (83), such as the other cerebrovascular accidents and events characterized by diffuse cognitive symptoms without clear focal motor or sensory symptoms.

Radiologically undetected strokes include tiny focal cortical infarcts, cortical laminar necrosis, and infarcts in the limbic and paralimbic cortical areas. These areas are still less well-visualized on CT and MRI, not only because of concurrent atrophic changes.

Coexisting infarct is seen incidentally in patients with other causes of dementia (e.g., AD). In addition, an infarct may sometimes contribute to the clinical picture while not being the major causative factor.

Patchy and diffuse areas of white matter changes seen on brain images have been recently referred as LA (84). Some LA is seen in neurologically normal aged individuals (85). In nondemented subjects, LA is correlated with age and also with vascular risk factors and cognitive decline (86). LA is also seen in patients with AD, but these changes are mostly small, limited periventricular changes (45,73,74). By contrast, the VaDe patients typically show larger areas of LA, often extending to the deep white matter (41,73,74,87).

White matter has limited ways of reacting to different pathogenetic factors (45). Therefore different pathologic conditions can give rise to indistinguishable forms of LA. LA should not be used as a synonym for ischemic change. In addition, different types of LA (e.g., tiny paraventricular LA, spots of

LA in deep subcortical white matter, and dense LA extending to the deep white matter) may well have different profiles of causes and risk factors (69). This may be also true for LA in the vascular centrencephalon (89) and centrum semiovale.

Time and cause relationships of vascular events and the cognitive syndrome are critical. A time relation to clinically evident strokes may be clear, but "silent" infarcts and white matter changes represent a problem. Showing causative relations remains a difficult task, as stroke may only contribute to or coexist with the underlying ultimate cause of the cognitive decline.

Prospects

At present we are forced to recognize our limited knowledge with regard to VaDe (69,72). This can be overcome only by detailed prospective clinical, neuropsychological, neuroradiologic, and neuropathologic studies, which require international cooperation. In the meantime, however, agreement on clinical criteria as a starting point for further discoveries is needed. At present, a definition based on the multi-infarct concept is the solution, with some supporting evidence (Table 7).

The main issue in the diagnosis of VaDe is to show evidence of multiple cortical and/or deep vascular lesions of the brain that are in temporal association with the evolution of the cognitive syndrome and that are judged to be causally related to the disturbance. This can be based on a detailed clinical history and findings in clinical examination indicating stroke or other acute cerebrovascular episodes and/or on findings in brain images compatible with vascular lesions of the brain (e.g., infarcts and ischemic white matter changes) (44,45).

In cases where the core brain imaging evidence is based on white matter changes, other causes must be excluded. Among these potential causes are hypertensive encephalopathy, hydrocephalus, cerebral edema, brain irradiation, multiple sclerosis, systemic lupus erythematosus, and neurosarcoidosis (45,88). In addition, as the main evidence for the diagnosis of MID, these white matter changes should be rather extensive, present in two or more white matter areas and extending over one fourth of the total white matter area (41,45,74,90).

The limitation is that the strict criteria given for VaDe based on the multiinfarct concept exclude a number of patients in whom vascular factors may well have an adverse effect on cognitive function. These include patients with less obvious focal symptoms and signs, those with only minor changes on CT or MRI, and those in whom so-called "noninfarct" mechanisms affect their cognitive abilities, if in fact these cases have dementia on a vascular basis.

Detailed characterization of clinical findings is essential. These include the number, type, location, size, side, and timing of strokes and other cerebrovascular accidents, as well as the extent, type, and location of both focal infarcts and white matter changes. In addition, coexisting diseases and conditions, as well as possible risk factors, should be systematically noted. Detailed clinical neurologic examination and neuropsychological evaluation are also needed (44,91).

The specific causes of VaDe, such as the inflammatory and noninflammatory arteriopathies and the hereditary entities, should be treated in their own right in clinical trials. If typing is required, this could be done according to the known vascular mechanisms (e.g., atherothrombotic stroke, cardiogenic embolic stroke, lacunar stroke, and ischemic white matter change). In addition, although there are limitations, division into cortical and subcortical types is a possibility (37,41,92,93).

CONCLUSION

With a growing number of persons affected and the improving therapeutic possibilities, early diagnosis of AD and VaDe is most important. These cases should be identified when they have mild memory problems only, before they develop a full syndrome of dementia. Therefore, the clinical target should be memory disorders, not dementia.

Although there is heterogeneity in groups of patients with AD and VaDe, and although the primary cause may not be ascertained precisely, their antemortem diagnosis can be improved. However, this will require careful revision of clinical criteria for symptomatic diagnosis, such as those for dementia, and etiologic diagnosis, such as those for AD and VaDe. Many of the current obstacles can be overcome by international prospective, cooperative, clinical, neuropsychological, radiologic, and neuropathologic studies.

ACKNOWLEDGEMENT

Dr. Timo Erkinjuntti is supported by the Paavo Nurmi Foundation, Helsinki, Finland. Dr. Vladimir C. Hachinski is a career investigator with the Heart and Stroke Foundation of Ontario, Canada.

REFERENCES

1. APA, ed. *American Psychiatric Association Committee on Nomenclature and Statistics: Diagnostic and statistical manual of mental disorders (DSM-III-R)*, 3rd ed., revised. Washington, DC: American Psychiatric Association; 1987.
2. Katzman R. Differential diagnosis of dementing illnesses. *Neurol Clin* 1986;4:329–39.
3. Erkinjuntti T. Dementia. *Clinical diagnosis and differential diagnosis, with special reference to multi-infarct dementia*. Dissertation. Helsinki: Department of Neurology, University of Helsinki; 1988.

4. Gurland B, Toner J. Differentiating dementia from nondementing conditions. In: Mayeux R, Rosen WG, eds. *The dementias.* New York: Raven Press; 1983:1–17.
5. Oliver C, Holland J. Down's syndrome and Alzheimer's disease: a review. *Psychol Med* 1986;16:307–22.
6. Roth M. Diagnosis of senile and related forms of dementia. In: Katzman R, Terry RD, Bick KL, eds. *Alzheimer's disease: senile dementia and related disorders.* New York: Raven Press; 1978:71–85.
7. Blass JP, Plum F. Metabolic encephalopathies in older adults. In: Katzman R, Terry R, eds. *The neurology of aging.* Philadelphia: FA Davis; 1983:189–220.
8. Lipowski ZJ. Transient cognitive disorders (delirium, acute confusional states) in the elderly. *Am J Psychiatr* 1983;140:1426–36.
9. Lipowski ZJ, ed. *Delirium.* Springfield, IL: Charles C Thomas; 1980.
10. McKhann G, Drachman D, Folstein M, Katzman R, Price D, Stadlan EM. Clinical diagnosis of Alzheimer's disease: report of the NINCDS-ADRDA Work Group under the auspices of Department of Health and Human Services Task Force of Alzheimer's Disease. *Neurology* 1984;34:939–44.
11. McEvoy JP. Organic brain syndromes. *Ann Intern Med* 1981;95:212–20.
12. Kirshner HS, ed. *Behavioral neurology. A practical approach.* New York: Churchill Livingstone; 1986.
13. Benson DF, McDaniel KD. Memory disorders. In: Bradley WC, Daroff RB, Fenichel GM, Marsden CD, eds. *Neurology in clinical Practice.* Vol II. Stoneham, MA: Butterworth–Heinemann; 1991:1389–1406.
14. Walsh K, ed. *Neuropsychology. A clinical approach,* 2nd ed. London: Churchill Livingstone; 1987.
15. Signoret J-L. Memory and amnesias. In: Mesulam M-M, ed. *Contemporary neurology: principles of behavioral neurology,* 3rd ed. Philadelphia: FA Davis; 1987:169–92.
16. Wells CE. Pseudodementia. *Am J Psychiatry* 1979;136:895–900.
17. Bulbena A, Berrios GE. Pseudodementia: facts and figures. *Br J Psychiatry* 1986;148:87–94.
18. Feinberg T, Goodman B. Affective illness, dementia, and pseudodementia. *J Clin Psychiatry* 1984;45:99–103.
19. Wells CE, Buchanan DC. The clinical use of psychological testing in evaluation of dementia. In: Wells CE, ed. *Dementia.* Philadelphia: FA Davis; 1977:189–204.
20. NIA National Institute of Aging. Task Force Sponsored by the National Institute of Aging: senility reconsidered: treatment possibilities for mental impairment in the elderly. *JAMA* 1980;244:259–63.
21. Jorm AF, Henderson AS. Possible improvements to the diagnostic criteria for dementia in DSM III. *Br J Psychiatry* 1985;147:394–9.
22. Gurland BJ, Dean LL, Copeland J, Gurland R, Golden R. Criteria for the diagnosis of dementia in the community elderly. *Gerontologist* 1982;22:180–6.
23. Reisberg B, Ferris SH, DeLeon MJ, Crook T. The Global Deterioration Scale for assessment of primary degenerative dementia. *Am J Psychiatry* 1982;139:1136–9.
24. Hughes CP, Berg L, Danziger WL, Coben LA, Martin RL. A new clinical strategy for the staging of dementia. *Br J Psychiatry* 1982;140:566–72.
25. Berg L, Hughes CP, Coben LA, Danziger WL, Martin RL, Knesevich J. Mild senile dementia of Alzheimer type: research diagnostic criteria, recruitment, and description of a study population. *J Neurol Neurosurg Psychiatry* 1982;45:962–8.
26. Jacobs JW, Bernhard MR, Delgado A, Strain JJ. Screening for organic mental syndromes in the medically ill. *Ann Intern Med* 1977;86:40–6.
27. Katzman R, Terry R. Normal aging of the nervous system. In: Katzman R, Terry R, eds. *The neurology of aging.* Philadelphia: FA Davis; 1983:15–50.
28. Erkinjuntti T, Laaksonen R, Sulkava R, Syrjalainen R, Palo J. Neuropsychological differentiation between normal aging, Alzheimer's disease and vascular dementia. *Acta Neurol Scand* 1986;74:393–403.
29. Crook T, Barthus RT, Ferris SH, Whitehouse P, Cohen GD, Gershon S. Age-associated memory impairment: proposed diagnostic criteria and measures of clinical change. Report of a National Institute of Mental Health Work Group. *Dev Neuropsychol* 1986;2:261–76.
30. Folstein MF, Folstein SE, McHugh PR. "Mini-mental State": a practical method for grading the cognitive state of patients for the clinician. *J Psychiatr Res* 1975;12:189–98.

31. Crook T, Larrabee GJ. Age-associated memory impairment: diagnostic criteria and treatment strategies. *Psychopharmacol Bull* 1988;24:509–14.
32. APA, ed. *American Psychiatric Association Committee on Nomenclature and Statistics: Diagnostic and Statistical Manual of Mental Disorders (DSM-III)*, 3rd ed. Washington, DC: American Psychiatric Association; 1980.
33. Roth M, Tym E, Mountjoy CQ, Huppert FA, Hendrie H, Verma S, Goddard R. CAMDEX: a standardised instrument for the diagnosis of mental disorder in the elderly with special reference to the early detection of dementia. *Br J Psychiatry* 1986;149:698–709.
34. Israel L, Kozarevic D, Sartorius N, eds. *Source book of geriatric assessment*, Vols 1 and 2. Basel: Karger; 1984.
35. Ylikoski R, Erkinjuntti T, Sulkava R, Juva K, Tilvis R, Valvanne J. Correlation for age, education and other demographic variables in the use of mini-mental state examination in Finland. *Acta Neurol Scand* (in press).
36. Woods RT. Activities of daily living in dementia. In: Gottfries CG, Levy R, Clincke G, Tritsmans L, eds. *Diagnostic and therapeutic assessments in Alzheimer's disease.* Petersfield, UK: Wrighton Biomedical Publishing; 1991:71–80.
37. Cummings JL. Subcortical dementia. Neuropsychology, neuropsychiatry, and pathophysiology. *Br J Psychiatry* 1986;149:682–97.
38. Stuss DT, Benson DF. *The frontal lobes.* New York: Raven Press; 1986.
39. Mesulam M-M. Patterns in behavioral neuroanatomy: association areas, the limbic system, and the hemispheric specialization. In: Mesulam M-M, ed. *Contemporary neurology, principles of behavioral neurology*, 3rd ed. Philadelphia: FA Davis; 1987:1–70.
40. Ishii N, Nishihara Y, Imamura T. Why do frontal lobe symptoms predominate in vascular dementia with lacunes? *Neurology* 1986;36:340–5.
41. Roman GC. Senile dementia of the Binswanger type. A vascular form of dementia in the elderly. *JAMA* 1987;258:1782–8.
42. Cummings J, Benson DF, LoVerme S Jr. Reversible dementia. Illustrative cases, definition, and review. *JAMA* 1980;243:2434–9.
43. Rossor M. The dementias. In: Bradley WC, Daroff RB, Fenichel GM, Marsden CD, eds. *Neurology in clinical practice*, Vol II. Stoneham, MA: Butterworth–Heinemann; 1991: 1407–8.
44. Erkinjuntti T, Sulkava R. Diagnosis of multi-infarct dementia. *Alzheimer Dis Assoc Disord* 1991;5:112–21.
45. Erkinjuntti T, Sulkava R. Brain imaging and diagnosis of dementia. In: Gottfries CG, Levy R, Clinke G, Tritsmans L, eds. *Diagnostic and therapeutic assessments in Alzheimer's disease.* Guildford, UK: Wrighton Biomedical Publishing; 1991:17–31.
46. Erkinjuntti T. Differential diagnosis between Alzheimer's disease and vascular dementia: evaluation of common clinical methods. *Acta Neurol Scand* 1987;76:433–42.
47. Sulkava R, Wikström J, Aromaa A, et al. Prevalence of severe dementia in Finland. *Neurology* 1985;35:1025–9.
48. Hollander E, Mohs RC, Davis KL. Antemortem markers of Alzheimer's disease. *Neurobiol Aging* 1986;7:367–87.
49. Iqbal K. Prevalence and neurobiology of Alzheimer's disease: some highlights. In: Iqbal K, McLachlan DRC, Winblad B, Wisniewski HM, eds. *Alzheimer's disease: basic mechanisms, diagnosis and therapeutic strategies.* Chichester: John Wiley & Sons; 1991.
50. Rossor M. Primary degenerative dementia. In: Bradley WC, Daroff RB, Fenichel GM, Marsden CD, eds. *Neurology in clinical practice*, Vol II. Stoneham, MA: Butterworth–Heinemann; 1991:1409–22.
51. Roth M. The natural history of mental disorder in old age. *J Ment Sci* 1955;101:281–301.
52. Sulkava R. Alzheimer's disease and senile dementia of Alzheimer type. A comparative study. *Acta Neurol Scand* 1982;65:636–50.
53. Kukull WA, Larson EB, Reifler BV, Lampe TH, Yerby M, Hughes J. Interrater reliability of Alzheimer's disease diagnosis. *Neurology* 1990;40:257–60.
54. Sulkava R, Haltia M, Paetau A, Wikström J, Palo J. Accuracy of clinical diagnosis in primary degenerative dementia: correlation with neuropathological findings. *J Neurol Neurosurg Psychiatry* 1983;46:9–13.
55. Wade JPH, Mirsen TR, Hachinski VC, Fisman M, Lau C, Merskey H. The clinical diagnosis of Alzheimer's disease. *Arch Neurol* 1987;44:24–9.

56. Gustafson L. Frontal lobe degeneration of non-Alzheimer type. II. Clinical picture and differential diagnosis. *Arch Gerontol Geriatr* 1987;6:209–23.
57. Crystal HA, Dickson DW, Lizardi JE, Davies P, Wolfson LI. Antemortem diagnosis of diffuse Lewy body disease. *Neurology* 1990;40:1523–8.
58. Penttilä M, Partanen JV, Soininen H, Riekkinen PJ. Quantitative analysis of occipital EEG in different stages of Alzheimer's disease. *Electroenceph Clin Neurophysiol* 1985;60:1–6.
59. George AE, deLeon MJ, Stylopoulos LA, et al. CT diagnostic features of Alzheimer's disease: importance of the choroidal/hippocampal fissure complex. *AJNR* 1990;11:101–7.
60. Kesslak JP, Nalcioglu O, Cotman CW. Quantification of magnetic resonance scans for hippocampal and parahippocampal atrophy in Alzheimer's disease. *Neurology* 1991;41: 51–4.
61. Burns A, Philpot MP, Costa DC, Ell PJ, Levy R. The investigation of Alzheimer's disease with single photon emission tomography. *J Neurol Neurosurg Psychiatry* 1989;52:248–53.
62. Launes J, Sulkava R, Erkinjuntti T, et al. 99mTC-HM-PAO SPECT in suspected dementia. *Nucl Med Commun* 1991;12:757–65.
63. Fazekas F. Neuroimaging of dementia. *Curr Opinion Neurol Neurosurg* 1990;3:103–7.
64. Blennow K. *Heterogeneity of Alzheimer's disease [Dissertation]*. Gothenburg, Sweden: Department of Psychiatry and Neurochemistry, University of Gothenburg; 1990.
65. Erkinjuntti T, Sulkava R, Palo J, Ketonen L. White matter low attenuation on CT in Alzheimer's disease. *Arch Gerontol Geriatr* 1989;8:95–104.
66. Wallin A. *Vascular dementia—pathogenetic and clinical aspects [Dissertation]*. Gothenburg, Sweden: Department of Psychiatry and Neurochemistry, University of Gothenburg; 1989.
67. Rossor M. Alzheimer's disease: neurobiochemistry. In: Pitt B, ed. *Dementia*. London: Churchill Livingstone; 1987:140–53.
68. Hachinski VC, Lassen NA, Marshall J. Multi-infarct dementia. A cause of mental deterioration in the elderly. *Lancet* 1974;2:207–10.
69. Erkinjuntti T, Hachinski VC. Rethinking vascular dementia: escaping conceptual prisons. *Cerebrovasc Dis* (submitted).
70. Torvik A, Svindland A. Is there a transitional zone between brain infarcts and the surrounding brain? A histological study. *Acta Neurol Scand* 1986;74:365–70.
71. O'Brien MD. Vascular disease and dementia in the elderly. In: Lynn–Smith W, Kinsborne M, eds. *Aging and dementia*. New York: Spectrum Publications; 1977.
72. Hachinski VC. The decline and resurgence of vascular dementia. *Can Med Assoc J* 1990; 142:107–11.
73. Erkinjuntti T, Haltia M, Palo J, Sulkava R, Paetau A. Accuracy of the clinical diagnosis of vascular dementia: a prospective clinical and post-mortem neuropathological study. *J Neurol Neurosurg Psychiatry* 1988;51:1037–44.
74. Erkinjuntti T, Ketonen L, Sulkava R, Sipponen J, Vuorialho M, Iivanainen M. Do white matter changes on MRI and CT differentiate vascular dementia from Alzheimer's disease? *J Neurol Neurosurg Psychiatry* 1987;50:37–42.
75. DelSer T, Bermejo F, Portera A, Arredondo JM, Bouras C, Constantinidis J. Vascular dementia. A clinicopathological study. *J Neurol Neurosurg Psychiatr* 1990;96:1–17.
76. Loeb C. Vascular dementia. *Dementia* 1990;1:175–84.
77. Meyer JS, McClintic KL, Rogers RL, Sims P, Mortel KF. Aetiological considerations and risk factors for multi-infarct dementia. *J Neurol Neurosurg Psychiatry* 1988;51:1489–97.
78. Wallin A. A consensus on dementia diseases (I): classification and investigation. *Läkartidningen* 1990;87:3856–65.
79. WHO. *World Health Organization. The International Classification of Diseases 10th Revision (ICD-10)*. Chapter V: Mental, behavioural and developmental disorders. Geneva: WHO typescript document MNH/MEP/87.1; 1989;25–31.
80. Erkinjuntti T. Clinical diagnosis and differential diagnosis of multi-infarct dementia. *Rec Adv Cardiovasc Dis* 1990;11(suppl 1):35–47.
81. Fisher CM. Lacunes: small, deep cerebral infarcts. *Neurology* 1965;15:774–84.
82. Nelson RF, Pullicino P, Kendall BE, Marshall J. Computed tomography in patients presenting with lacunar syndromes. *Stroke* 1980;11:256–61.
83. NINCDS. National Institute of Neurological Communications Disorders and Stroke: a classification and outline of cerebrovascular diseases II. *Stroke* 1975;6:564–616.

84. Hachinski VC, Potter P, Merskey H. Leuko-araiosis. *Arch Neurol* 1987;44:21–3.
85. Inzitari D, Diaz F, Fox A, et al. Vascular risk factors and leuko-araiosis. *Arch Neurol* 1987; 44:42–7.
86. Steingart A, Hachinski VC, Lau C, et al. Cognitive and neurologic findings in subjects with diffuse white matter lucencies on computed tomographic scan (leuko-araiosis). *Arch Neurol* 1987;44:32–5.
87. Janota I, Mirsen TR, Hachinski VC, Lee DH, Merskey H. Neuropathologic correlates of leuko-araiosis. *Arch Neurol* 1989;46:1124–8.
88. Valentine AR, Moseley IF, Kendall BE. White matter abnormality in cerebral atrophy: clinicoradiological correlations. *J Neurol Neurosurg Psychiatry* 1980;43:139–42.
89. Hachinski VC, Norris JW, eds. *Acute stroke*. Philadelphia: FA Davis; 1985.
90. Erkinjuntti T, Ketonen L, Sulkava R, Vuorialho M, Palo J. CT in the differential diagnosis between Alzheimer's disease and vascular dementia. *Acta Neurol Scand* 1987;75:262–70.
91. Mahler ME, Cummings JL. The behavioural neurology of multi-infarct dementia. *Alzheimer Dis Assoc Disord* 1991;5:122–30.
92. Erkinjuntti T. Types of multi-infarct dementia. *Acta Neurol Scand* 1987;75:391–9.
93. Tatemichi TK. How acute brain failure becomes chronic. A view of the mechanisms and syndromes of dementia related to stroke. *Neurology* 1990;40:1652–9.

Guidelines for Drug Trials in Memory Disorders, edited by N. Canal, et al.
Raven Press, Ltd., New York © 1993.

22

Selection and Evaluation of Early Cases of Alzheimer Disease

Raymond Levy

Section of Old Age Psychiatry, Institute of Psychiatry, London SE5 8AF, England

This chapter deals with three main topics: how to obtain early cases of Alzheimer's disease (AD); how to select suitable cases for clinical trials; and how to evaluate them both initially and after medication. This chapter will inevitably overlap to a certain extent with other chapters in this volume. Such overlap may not necessarily be a disadvantage because it will serve to indicate similarities and differences of approach and thus stimulate the discussion necessary to reach a consensus in these matters. The material presented here is based more on direct personal experience than on literature review. Much of what is presented in each of the sections below is based on assumptions that may be and often have been questioned (1). When this is the case I will point to sources of disagreement that might form the focus for discussion and debate.

OBTAINING EARLY CASES

Before I deal with the problem of obtaining early cases, it should be pointed out that this aim is already a contentious one. The possible source of controversy sets a pattern for most of the disagreement with what I have to say. This runs roughly as follows: Why take such trouble to obtain access to early cases when the majority of cases seen in day-to-day life are late or advanced cases? I will not attempt to answer this in any detail except with the common-sense view, which may not necessarily be correct, that early cases are more likely to show predominantly functional changes in transmitter systems, whereas late or advanced cases are likely to be associated with structural damage and nerve cell loss. In addition, we are likely to learn more about the condition by studying its earlier manifestations. There are three main potential sources of cases for clinical trials: routine referrals, screening of "at risk" individuals in the community, and advertising for volunteers or other variants of this procedure.

Routine Referrals

Routine referrals to our old-age psychiatry service are numerous and readily accessible. However, despite the widely expressed need for early diagnosis, patients still come to light at a stage when they are usually too impaired to give valid consent or to cooperate fully in investigation. For example, in a cohort of 178 cases fitting the NINCDS-ADRDA criteria which is being followed-up systematically, the mean Mini-Mental State Examination (MMSE) was of the order of 8 (2), i.e., below the rough target minimum of 10 for entry into most trials.

Screening of Community Sample

Although screening of a community sample of subjects at risk appears attractive at first, practical experience has shown that this approach tends to be disappointing. For example in screening a sample of some 2,000 elderly subjects for a clinical trial (3), although we were able to identify 202 possible cases the majority either had to be excluded because they did not fulfill the entry criteria or refused to participate because they did not consider that they had a real problem.

Advertising for Volunteers

We therefore must resort to some form of appeal for cases through the media. In the United Kingdom the General Medical Council (GMC) does not allow direct advertisement by doctors, although this is generally understood to cover patients who are seen for private gain. (This has recently been modified to allow general practitioners to inform the public of the services they offer.) As far as I am aware, the GMC has not declared its intentions with regard to advertising for research purposes, particularly when no private gain is involved. Regulations are likely to vary in this regard in different countries.

To steer on the safe side, we have usually inserted information into previously planned articles and have sometimes given a name and address. Such statements in the press should be carefully worded, both for ethical and for practical reasons. They should make clear that treatment is experimental, that side effects may be involved, and also that the cases being sought must be mild or moderate in severity, live relatively near the trial center, and have a reliable caregiver who can ensure that the drug protocol is adhered to. It should also be borne in mind that the journalist writing the article may have no control over the headline, which is chosen by the subeditor. Therefore, an overenthusiastic account or headline can lead to literally thousands of often inappropriate letters from all over the world, whereas too discouraging a description will fail to attract any suitable volunteers.

SELECTING SUITABLE CASES

In the case of Alzheimer disease (AD) it is best to stay with well-known and explicit criteria such as the NINCDS-ADRDA or something similar. When these are applied rigidly, the diagnosis will be confirmed at autopsy in over 80% of cases (4). Other selection criteria have been mentioned above. As a guide to the severity of cases to be included, a lower cutoff score of 10 on the MMSE is a useful guide. Exclusions will emerge from the explicit criteria employed but must also include concomitant medication likely to interfere with the drug under investigation. Here, again, we came across two further assumptions that may be open to question: the attempt to select "pure" cases of AD and the exclusion of concomitant medication. Some will argue that most cases in real life are not "pure" and that because the patients under consideration are mostly elderly they are likely both to suffer from multiple pathology and to be receiving concomitant medication. Is it realistic to exclude such cases? I must state categorically that this is a view I reject absolutely and find at variance with customary scientific inquiry. It is surprising to me to see it espoused by people whose judgment I usually respect. I find it difficult to understand why the usual approach to a simple scientific problem which involves reducing the number of variables one deals with should be abandoned when dealing with the treatment of AD. It is surely more reasonable and heuristic to start with "pure" cases with a single pathology and no concomitant medication, however atypical these may be.

If one is able to demonstrate improvement in these cases, then we can proceed to widen the criteria. It has also been stated that exclusion of all but the simple "pure" cases is likely to be resisted by patients and their caregivers. The answer to that is surely that it is our duty as clinical scientists to educate the public rather than to pander to popular prejudice and to be pushed into inappropriate studies which will lead to results that will either be uninterpretable or wrongly interpreted as either positive or negative.

EVALUATION OF PATIENTS

In this context one should consider both the baseline evaluation and the measurements of change. Baseline evaluation should include the recording of demographic data together with important clinical information. A minimum will include age, age of onset, sex, family history, social class, and premorbid intellectual function, together with a standardized clinical profile of the cases involved. The latter may allow the isolation of important factors predicting response to medication. This baseline assessment should preferably use such schedules as the Cambridge Mental Disorders of the Elderly Examination (CAMDEX), the Geriatric Mental State schedule, or the Alzheimer Disease Assessment scale.

Measurements of change should distinguish key outcome measurements that will form part of the end points employed and additional measurements of change which are being employed either to confirm the main changes or for some other purpose. It is important to avoid "fishing expeditions" with the inevitable post hoc analyses that tend to follow. It is best to limit oneself to a simple measurement of cognitive function, such as the MMSE, which, although far from perfect, does have the advantage of wide use and some data regarding the expected rate of decline. Although one would ideally wish to have a measurement of activities of daily living (ADL), most measurements available are too insensitive, subject to ceiling effects, or are designed for more severely affected patients than those included in drug trials. Many also involve activities not usually carried out by men in the generation presently under study (e.g., housework). It is worth noting, for example, that in a recent study of tetrahydroaminacridine (THA) the Lawton and Brody ADL (5) showed no changes in either direction in either the placebo or the drug group at a time when clear changes in the MMSE were occurring. At first sight the GERRI scale (6) appears to have some advantage, but this is only an impression which must be tested in a real drug trial. The topic of ADL scales will be dealt with in greater detail elsewhere. This important area requires specific attention, since changes in test scores are less impressive than improvement in day-to-day life.

Finally, a measurement of noncognitive aspects of the disease is of some importance, although it should probably not be a key outcome measurement. Depression and other psychiatric symptoms are common in AD (2), and it is useful to know whether any change observed in patients arises indirectly from an alteration in mood or some other associated variable, as many so-called cognitive enhancers are weak antidepressants. A variety of other neuropsychological measures may be added provided that the purposes for which this is done are explicitly stated.

Once the key measures of changes have been selected and end points chosen on the basis of explicit statements about the minimal degree of improvement that is arrived at, the power of the trial should be calculated so that the number of subjects required to produce a statistically significant change can be determined. Too many trials report the results in studies involving as few as 10 patients or less in each group. In view of the heterogeneity of the condition, only a miraculously effective drug will produce significant changes in such a situation. Finally, it should be recognized that we are entering a new phase in the psychopharmacology of dementia and that, paradoxically, as effective drugs are developed and tested we will begin to have a better idea of the most appropriate measurements of change to select. This in itself will lead to wider consensus in this field. It is easy to disagree on what to measure when nothing changes but more difficult to do so in the face of unequivocal change.

REFERENCES

1. Jarvik LF, Berg L, Bartus R, et al. Clinical drug trials in Alzheimer's disease: what are some of the issues? *Alzheimer Dis Assoc Disord* 1990;4:193–202.
2. Burns A, Jacoby R, Levy R. Psychiatric phenomena in Alzheimer's disease. *Br J Psychiatr* 1990;157:72–94.
3. Little A, Levy R, Chuaqui–Kidd P, et al. A double-blind placebo controlled trial of high-dose lecithin in Alzheimer's disease. *J Neurol Neurosurg Psychiatry* 1985;47:736–42.
4. Burns A, Luthert P, Levy R, et al. Accuracy of clinical diagnosis of Alzheimer's disease. *Br Med J* 1990;301:1026.
5. Lawton MP, Brody EC. Assessment of old people: self-maintaining and instrumental activities of daily living. *Gerontologist* 1969;9:179–86.
6. Schwartz GE. Development and validation of the geriatric evaluation by relative's rating instrument (GERRI). *Psychol Rep* 1983;53:479–88.

Guidelines for Drug Trials in Memory Disorders, edited by N. Canal, et al.
Raven Press, Ltd., New York © 1993.

23

The Cambridge Mental Disorders of the Elderly Examination with Special Reference to Its Use in the Diagnosis of "Mild" or "Early" Dementia

Martin Roth

Addenbrooke's Hospital, Cambridge CB2 2QQ, England

The clinical diagnosis of persons suffering from mental deterioration in late and middle life and the accurate assessment of the decline in their cognitive ability and personality functioning entail eliciting information with regard to three different questions. These demand three interrelated but relatively distinct operations. The first is the formulation of a reliable categorical diagnosis with the aid of operational criteria such as those set down in DSM-III-R (1) or ICD-10 (2). A second operation involves the establishment of valid and reliable measures of the severity and extent of the wide range of cognitive impairment and also the changes in emotional life and volition experienced by the patients. These constitute the main features of proven cases of dementia. The third operation is to devise reliable and precise means for rating actual behavior and adaptation in everyday life. These require observations by independent persons able to explore and record patients' skills and failures in negotiating the problems of daily living, either at home or in hospital.

There are a number of scales for carrying out each of these forms of assessment. These have been reviewed in an earlier report (3). Difficulties and confusions have arisen, however, because of failure to differentiate clearly among the types of information that the three different approaches to assessment cited can be expected to provide. In consequence, cognitive tests such as the Kendrick Battery (4) and the Blessed–Roth Scales for measurement of the overall severity of dementia, from manifest behavior to the assessment of memory information and concentration (5,6), have been employed to establish a diagnosis. Alternatively, behavioral scales have been employed for measurement of dementia.

The Cambridge Mental Disorders of the Elderly Examination (CAMDEX) is an attempt to combine the three complementary approaches that are required to provide a comprehensive delineation of the status of individuals in whom the possibility of dementia or some kindred organic psychiatric disorder has arisen. It seeks to provide all of these elements within a single relatively compact and integrated instrument that has an acceptable measure of reliability and validity. It was also considered desirable that although possessing the advantages of a standardized instrument for scientific purposes it would replicate as closely as possible the main features of the clinical interview and examination. This has a degree of flexibility that gives it great advantages in clinical practice, and it also has a long record of achievement in the advancement of scientific knowledge.

There have been other attempts to develop comprehensive structured interviews and examination schedules of the kind described. The Geriatric Mental State Examination (GMS) of Copeland et al. (7) has been largely derived from the Present State Examination (PSE) of Wing et al. (8). The PSE was extensively employed in the International Pilot Study of schizophrenia developed by the World Health Organization and the United States–United Kingdom diagnostic project. In its original form it had certain limitations as an instrument for the diagnosis of other psychiatric disorders. The GMS did not provide information regarding the history and progression of neuropsychological deficits. As it had not been constructed or evaluated with the specific problems of the aged in mind, it was initially deficient in measurements of cognitive function.

The CAMDEX set out to rectify those defects in existing methods of assessment which focused attention mainly on standardizing the examination of the present mental state. Such information can lead to error if it is not set in the context of systematic inquiries regarding the evolution of the disorder, the individual's premorbid adaptation during different stages of life development, his basic personality, and observations of his behavior over a period of time adequate for determining competence in negotiating everyday tasks. To cite a simple example, the differential diagnosis between dementia and clouded/delirious states, as well as the disturbances in cognitive function that may complicate severe derangements of affect, may be difficult or impossible on the basis of a Mental State Examination alone. However, given a few reliable items of information concerning the history and development of the condition and the background of the individual, the diagnosis will rarely present difficulties.

A more extensive body of information is required for making a diagnosis and assessing the cognitive competence of the other common disorders that present in psychogeriatric practice. The objective in the development of the CAMDEX was to create a comprehensive instrument that would rectify the deficiencies in previously existing instruments described in this section.

THE CAMDEX SCHEDULE

In its present form the CAMDEX comprises the following sections. Basic demographic data are recorded on the first sheet. Thereafter the main components are as follows.

Section A

This covers items of inquiry regarding physical and mental state and, in particular, seeks evidence with regard to symptoms relating to organic disorders, depressive illness, and functional and paranoid psychoses. Inquiries regarding past history and family history are also made. If the patient fails to provide satisfactory answers to two of three questions in Section A, the interviewer abandons that section and moves on to Section B.

Section B

This consists of the cognitive examination. It incorporates the 19 items that comprise the Mini-Mental State Examination (MMSE) of Folstein et al. (9). There are many additional components. The section dealing with memory has been expanded by the addition of items that evaluate remote and recent memory and the recall and recognition of new information. This section also assesses orientation, language, memory, different aspects of praxis, attention, abstract thinking, perception, and calculation. Parts of each interview have been recorded so that the various aspects of spontaneous speech and the content of language can be systematically studied after interview. This section has come to be known as the Cambridge Cognitive Examination (CAMCAG).

Section C

The interviewer's observations of the patient's appearance, behavior, mood, speech, psychomotor retardation or agitation, insight, thought processes, and level of consciousness are written down. Bizarre behavior is also recorded. Additions are made to this section at the end of the interview, incorporating any other relevant observations made during subsequent stages.

Section D

This comprises a general physical examination, including a neurologic evaluation. Defects of hearing or sight, tremor, and other parkinsonian features are recorded. The purpose is to record all findings that have a bearing on the differentiation of "primary" and "secondary" dementias. Special attention is devoted to systems suggested by the interview as being of special relevance. The cardiovascular system would attract special attention in the presence of symptoms suggesting myocardial insufficiency and the central nervous system when there have been symptoms suggesting focal lesions, epilepsy, gait disturbance, or falls.

Section E

The results of laboratory and radiologic investigations are recorded in this section, including the blood count, vitamin B_{12} and folate, urea and electrolytes, liver function tests, and VDRL (veneral disease–related laboratory tests). Whenever possible, information from studies of brain imaging with magnetic resonance imaging or other methods are recorded.

Section F

A record is made of any medication currently prescribed for the patient and a note of the approximate period during which drugs have been taken. Information regarding all drugs in the possession of the patient should be set down. Random or excessive use of a variety of medications available in the homes of aged persons, particularly when they are defective in memory, is a common cause of clouded and delirious states.

Section G

This section provides for any additional items of information obtained in the course of the interview. The purpose is to amplify the picture already obtained with the aid of structured questions. A great deal of new and relevant information is spontaneously offered under this heading. It may prove especially valuable in atypical and difficult cases.

Section H

This section comprises a structured interview with a relative or caregiver who knows the patient well. Any personality change, difficulty in functioning in everyday life, or indications of cognitive difficulty observed by the caregiver is noted. Items needed to permit the Blessed–Roth Dementia Scale to be scored (6) are incorporated into this section. Questions relating to depressive and paranoid symptomatology are included, and also a family history and past history.

At the end of an interview the interviewer makes a psychiatric diagnosis based on all relevant and available information according to operational diagnostic criteria that are included in the schedule. Diagnoses are assigned to one of eleven categories: normal; four categories of dementia [senile dementia of Alzheimer type (SDAT), multi-infarct dementia (MID), mixed SDAT and MID, and dementia secondary to other causes (SD)]; two categories of clouding or delirium (clouded state, clouded state with dementia); depression; anxiety or phobic disorder; paranoid or paraphrenic illness; and other psychiatric disorders. Patients are also graded for severity of dementia and severity of depression, each on a 5-point scale.

DURATION OF ADMINISTRATION

The administration of the respondent's part of the interview can be completed in about 45–60 min. This takes between 70 and 80 min for demented patients. The Informant section takes 10–15 min to complete.

SUMMARY OF INITIAL INVESTIGATIONS OF RELIABILITY AND VALIDITY OF THE CAMDEX

Inter-rater Reliability

Sixty-one female and 31 male patients over the age of 65 years were interviewed to establish the reliability of the CAMDEX and to develop the main clinical diagnostic scales. There was good agreement with regard to diagnosis between pairs of psychiatrists who rated patients independently at the same time (Table 1). Complete agreement was reached in cases diagnosed by interviewers as normal or demented. One of five cases diagnosed by the interviewer as clouded was classed as demented by the observer. There was less agreement in the relatively small number of four cases of depression, but subsequent investigations in a larger material of patients in the period that has intervened have established satisfactory measurements of interobserver reliability in the diagnosis of depression.

TABLE 1. *Inter-rater reliability of CAMDEX for major diagnostic groups*

Interviewer's diagnosis	Observer's diagnosis			
	Normals	Dementia	Clouding	Depression
Normals	9			
Dementia		22		
Clouding		1	4	
Depression	1		1	2

Subsections of the Scales

The phi (ɸ) coefficients were calculated for each item in Sections A, B, C, and H of the CAMDEX. The medians and ranges of the values are shown in Table 2. It will be seen that the median coefficients for all the sections are high. The lowest value was derived for record of observed behavior, but at 0.83 this section can be judged as satisfactory. Reference has already been made to a probable source of disagreement concerning this section. Psychomotor retardation may be severe in elderly depressives, and indecision may contribute to poor performance. It has been recognized that scoring instructions and also the items devoted to the evaluation of psychomotor retardation (a depressive characteristic of central importance) must be made more explicit and perhaps need other modifications to increase reliability.

Cognitive Performance

The cognitive section yields two overall measures of cognitive function: total score on the MMSE, and total score on the Cambridge Cognitive Examination (CAMCOG), which includes 14 of the 19 MMSE items plus 43 items covering additional aspects of memory and other aspects of higher cerebral functional activity. Maximum scores are 30 on the MMSE and 106 on the CAMCOG.

Table 3 shows the cognitive scores in the four major groups. The normal and depressed groups did not differ significantly from each other on either test but performed significantly better than either demented or clouded groups ($p < 0.001$). These groups did not differ significantly from each other.

In calculating sensitivity and specificity of the MMSE, the recommended cut-off value of 21/22 for those aged 60 or over was used. This yielded 96% sensitivity and 80% specificity for our population, meaning that 96% of those with a MMSE score of 21 or less earned a clinical diagnosis of organic mental

TABLE 2. *Inter-rater reliability of sections of CAMDEX*

Section	ɸ Coefficients (2 × 2 agreement/disagreement on individual items)		Pearson correlations of total scores for each section	
	Median	Range	r	p
A, Interview with patient	0.94	1.0–0.28	0.99	0.000
B, Cognitive examination	0.90	1.0–0.30	0.97	0.000
C, Observations	0.83	1.0–0.30	0.81	0.000
H, Interview with informant	0.91	1.0–0.56	0.90	0.000

TABLE 3. *Total scores for the Cambridge Cognitive Examination (CAMCOG) and the Mini-Mental State Examination (MMSE) in the major diagnostic groups*

		Mean and range of CAMCOG scores (maximum = 106)		Mean and range of MMSE scores (maximum = 30)	
Normal	(n = 17)	90.0	(72–101)	26.7	(22–29)
Demented	(n = 49)	44.2	(8–82)	13.4	(1–25)
Clouded	(n = 14)	52.3	(38–79)	15.3	(9–27)
Depressed	(n = 12)	83.9	(68–98)	24.8	(14–30)

disorder (dementia or clouded state) while 80% of those with an MMSE score of 22 + had been diagnosed as normal or depressed. Conversely, 20% of those scoring 22 + had a clinical diagnosis of organic syndrome and were consequently misclassified on this cutoff.

In the case of the CAMCOG examination, the distribution of scores showed the optimal cut-off to be 79/80. This yielded a 92% sensitivity and 96% specificity. Only one organically impaired patient was misclassified by this instrument, compared with four who were misclassified by the MMSE.

Several patients obtained near-maximal scores on the MMSE. Sixteen scored 27 + (including five depressed and one clouded patient). Five patients scored 29 + (three normals, two depressed), the highest score [30] being obtained by a depressed patient. In contrast, only two patients (both normals) obtained a CAMCOG score of 100 +, while an additional two (one normal and one depressed) scored within 10 points of the maximum and a further five (two normal, three depressed) scored within 20 points of the maximum. It appears that the CAMCOG part of the CAMDEX can discriminate between individuals even at the high end of the ability range.

Relationship Between Subjective and Informant's Assessments and the Measurements of Cognitive Function

The patient's self-assessments of cognitive function did not correlate significantly, for the group as a whole, with performance on different aspects of cognitive performance. In contrast, the responses of informants to a wide range of cognitive items, including memory, concentration, language, praxis, and abstract thinking, showed a highly significant correlation with the relevant subscales on the CAMCOG. There were some exceptions with regard to a few items. It was concluded that whereas a patient's self-report of cognitive function bears no relation to cognitive performance, the informant's assessment provides a reliable guide.

Depressed Mood and Cognitive Function

The severity of depression can be assessed in a number of ways in the CAMDEX for all patients. For the group as a whole, scores on the depression severity scale were significantly related to orientation and memory scores ($p < 0.01$) but not to any other measurements of cognitive performance. The informant's assessment of depressed mood correlated significantly with scores on the depression severity scale but not, in this group, with any measure of cognitive function. Responses to a key item in the depression severity scale ("Do you feel sad, depressed or miserable?") were found not to be related to cognitive performance but correlated 0.64 ($p < 0.001$) with the informant's assessment. It appears that the presence of the signs and symptoms of depression is related to impaired memory functioning but that complaints about depressed mood are not.

DEVELOPMENT OF CLINICAL DIAGNOSTIC SCALES

The number of patients in the three main groups (SDAT, MID, and Depressive Disorder) of depression was sufficiently large to consider the development of diagnostic scales from items in the CAMDEX. Items likely to prove of value in differential diagnosis were selected and their frequency distribution was estimated for all diagnostic groups identified with the aid of the CAMDEX. Items that differed in frequency between the diagnostic groups were selected for development of the diagnostic scales. The result was an organicity scale (18 items), a scale for depression (14 items), and a scale for MID (12 items).

The detailed data concerning the development of these scales are to be found in the original publication (3). The plot of cumulative frequency curves of the scores in each scale for SDAT, depressive illness, and MID made it possible to determine optimal cutoff points for diagnostic purposes. The proportion of patients correctly classified using these optimal cutoff points is shown in Table 4.

The diagnostic discrimination achieved by the tests with the aid of these cutoff points was investigated. Using χ^2 tests and Fisher's exact test and applying a cutoff point of 4, the organicity scale differentiated between SDAT patients and normals ($p < 0.0001$) and depressed patients ($p < 0.005$) but did not differentiate between SDAT and MID. The cutoff point of 2 on

TABLE 4. *Classification of diagnoses by clinical diagnostic scales using approximate cutoff points*

	Cutoff score	% Correctly classified			
		Normal	SDAT	MID	Depression
Organicity scale	4/5	100	85	85	92
MID scale	2/3	95	85	85	83
Depression scale	10/11	100	100	85	75

the MID scale yielded significant differences between MID cases and normals ($p < 0.01$), SDAT ($p < 0.0001$), and depression ($p < 0.001$). The cut-off point of 10 on the depression diagnostic scales produced significant differences between the depressive groups and the normals ($p < 0.0001$) and SDAT ($p < 0.0001$).

Table 4 shows the percentage of patients correctly classified using the cut-off points cited. It is plain that none of the scales in isolation achieves complete discrimination. However, a combination of the results obtained with the aid of two or all three measurements yields results that agree closely with clinical diagnosis. For example only 85% of patients with Alzheimer disease (SDAT) are correctly classified by the organicity scale, but the depression scale achieves 100% success in discriminating between them. Conversely, only 75% of patients with depression (DD) are correctly classified with the depression scale. However, the organicity scale classifies 92% correctly.

In the algorithms for arriving at a final diagnosis published at the end of the CAMDEX for each entity clinical, diagnosis is on the basis of operational criteria. The scores on the "Depression," "Organicity," and MID scales and CAMCOG score taken separately are combined to arrive at "definite," "probable," and "possible" diagnoses for each category.

The independence of these scales when tested by their intercorrelations was high, as reflected by very low correlations between the depression scale and the other two scales, and showed low and insignificant correlations between them. Discrimination can be considerably improved by using the scores obtained on each of the scales ($r = 0.15$ and 0.18 for the O and MID scales, respectively). As was expected, there was a significant positive correlation between the organicity and MID scales.

The reliability of the scales, as tested by an odd–even split-half method, showed high levels of reliability for the organicity scale (0.95) and the depression scale (0.90). That for the MID scale (0.77) was acceptable in the present state of knowledge, considering the fact that a substantial proportion of those diagnosed as MID by any method during life prove to have been of mixed pathology post mortem. This is true for a smaller proportion of cases diagnosed as Alzheimer disease.

An acceptable test of validity must await the results of follow-up investigations and post-mortem studies of the brain. These are in progress. A certain measure of validation was provided by a principal component analysis of items from the cognitive section. The scores of the first three components proved to be correlated with the three scale scores. The pattern results on component 1, a general component, were strikingly similar to those obtained for the total score on CAMCOG as a whole. Both correlated highly with the organicity scale, providing substantial support for its validity (Table 5).

TABLE 5. *Correlations between clinical diagnostic scales and factors derived from cognitive items*

	Factor 1 (66.5%)	Factor 2 (9.5%)	Factor 3 (6.7%)	Total score on CAMCOG
Organicity	−0.61***	0.19	0.13	−0.63***
Multi-infarct dementia	−0.27**	−0.10	−0.01	−0.25*
Depression	0.21*	−0.12	0.02	0.22*

Figures in brackets are variance explained by each factor.
* $p < 0.05$; ** $p < 0.01$; *** $p < 0.001$.

The last part of the CAMDEX contains the following sections:

1. Items for arriving at various measures of severity.
2. Items relevant for selected DSM-III-R diagnoses and also those relevant for selected diagnoses using ICD-10 diagnostic criteria for research.
3. Items relevant for the ischemia score of Hachinski et al. (10).
4. Items required for reaching diagnoses according to operational criteria set out in the CAMDEX.
5. A range of algorithms to provide methods for combining selected subscales of the CAMDEX for arriving at clinical diagnoses in nine groups of mental disorder in late life at different levels of confidence ("definite," "probable," and "possible").

THE FOLLOW-UP STUDY OF DEMENTIA IN A COMMUNITY SAMPLE USED IN THE CAMDEX

A full account of this investigation has been published (11). This account will be limited to a summary of the findings relevant for the main theme of this chapter.

The first stage of the inquiry consisted of the screening of 2,311 patients aged 75 years and older using the MMSE. Respondents who scored 23 or less on the MMSE (out of a maximum of 30) were selected for a full CAMDEX assessment together with a one in three sample of those who scored 24 or 25 points. Response rates were 91% in the screening phase and 82% in the diagnostic phase.

In the first year, 44 elderly persons were judged to be minimally demented and 208 to be demented (94 mild, 85 moderate, 29 severe). The CAMDEX was administered for a second time to surviving minimally demented and demented subjects as close as possible to 12 months after the first assessment.

The CAMDEX category of "minimal dementia," which was tentative and hypothetical, was defined as "a limited and variable impairment of recall, minor and variable errors in orientation, blunted capacity to follow arguments and solve problems and occasional errors in everyday tasks." These patients were therefore judged not to be demented. The term "dementia" was employed to denote mild, moderate, and severe degrees of cognitive, emotional, and personality deterioration.

The follow-up of respondents who had been found to be cognitively intact was confined to the following subsamples in one of the general practices that was invited to repeat the MMSE 12 months after the screening interview. The groups investigated were: (i) Those who had scored 26 or more on the MMSE in the first year. (ii) Those who scored 24 or 25 but were not part of the one in three sample of patients who had been selected for full CAMDEX assessment. (iii) Those who had been assessed using CAMDEX but were found to be neither demented nor depressed.

In the remaining five practices, investigations were limited to review of a random one in ten sample of patients who fulfilled the criteria described. Four hundred seventy-eight normal subjects were selected for review from a pool of 2,059.

One part of the study consisted of a comparison of the changes in the MMSE scores of normal, minimally demented, and demented subjects over the course of the year. In the second part, the results of the initial examination with the CAMDEX were compared with the gradation of the severity of dementia recorded in the first examination.

The mean interval between initial and review CAMDEX interview for minimally demented and demented subjects was 13.4 months and for normal subjects 14.5 months. It proved possible to review 80% of the normals who were alive at 1 year, 88% of the "minimal" subjects, and 95% of surviving demented subjects. This confirmed the previous impression formed: that the demented elderly are less likely to refuse to participate in community surveys than nondemented persons.

The CAMDEX evaluation in the second year confirmed the diagnosis of dementia in 133 of the 137 cases of mild to severe impairment (97%) (Table 6). Two of the elderly originally judged to be mildly demented were reclassified as minimally demented, a grading which, as will be seen later, signifies nonprogressive disorders in the majority of those so graded in the final examinations. In fact, both these patients were diabetics whose physical health and mental state had improved after closer supervision of insulin medication and diet.

The most important findings, and those that are at the focus of interest in

TABLE 6. *Comparison of CAMDEX severity ratings in first and second years of study*

		Year 2					
		Normal	Minimal	Mild	Moderate	Severe	Total
Year 1	Minimal	13	10	5	1	—	29
	Mild	2	2	38	23	2	67
	Moderate	—	—	3	37	16	56
	Severe	—	—	—	1	13	14

this chapter, were the observations concerning those patients described as having "mild" dementia on first examination. Of these patients, two were rated as being normal and not demented on review. In each case there had been sound reasons for the initial diagnosis. However, only in the case of the second patient was there an explanation available for his improved performance, in the form of an abatement of anxiety manifest in the earlier test.

Of the 29 "minimals," six showed some progressive impairment, but five of these were only "mildly" demented. Thirteen were judged to be normal. In the light of additional information provided by the patients, three of these were thought to have been depressed at the time of the first investigation. Two patients were revealed as having labored under the influence of paranoid symptoms in the first examination and, in the case of one man who had made a good recovery from stroke, the impairment noted in the initial examination may have been due to mild and transient clouding of awareness. The remaining seven were thought to be indubitably normal. The follow-up study thus far shows the "minimal" group to be made up mainly of patients with nonprogressive disorders.

Perhaps the most significant changes were those observed in patients originally classed as suffering from "mild" dementia (Table 6). This grade of dementia has in the past been thought in many epidemiological inquiries to be an ambiguous and unsafe diagnosis. In this study, however, the diagnosis of dementia was sustained in the great majority of cases. Of the 67 patients who were observed, the diagnosis of mild dementia was confirmed in 38 patients, and 23 patients had advanced to a "moderate" and therefore indubitable dementia.

Only in four cases was improvement registered. Because two of these were judged as "minimal," a question as to the correctness of diagnosis remained. The other two were judged to be normal. In the "moderate" group the diagnosis of dementia was confirmed in 53 of the 56 cases. The largest group comprised cases again as "moderate" dementia (37 cases), and 16 had advanced to the grade of "severe" dementia. The remaining three were regarded as "mild" dementia. In the light of the outcome of the main group graded as "mild" in the first interview, it appears that these patients are, at least, at considerable risk for further deterioration at a later stage.

Among "severe" cases, only one patient out of 14 seemingly improved in rating, albeit to a "moderate" grade. The other 13 were judged, as in the first instance, to be "severe" cases. Hence, in 94% of patients rated as mildly, moderately, or severely demented, 129 of 137 were thought to be unchanged in their clinical state or to be worse.

Table 7 compares changes in MMSE average scores of the normal subjects in the course of a year with the changes in CAMDEX–MMSE scores of those minimally demented or demented. The scores of 71 subjects who had been unable to participate because of physical infirmity or noncompliance in one or both examinations had to be excluded. Normal subjects had shown

TABLE 7. *Changes in mean MMSE scores of normal, minimally demented, and demented subjects over 1 year*

Year 1 severity ratings	Year 1 MMSE scores	Year 2 MMSE scores	Mean change (SD)	Cases	Missing cases[a]	Significance values**
Normal	26.3	25.4	−0.9 (2.5)	297	64	NS
Minimal	20.7	18.1	−2.6 (6.0)	29	1	NS
Mild	17.7	15.0	−2.7 (5.4)	67	2	$p < 0.05$
Moderate	10.7	7.6	−3.1 (6.0)	56	4	$p < 0.001$
Severe	1.2	0.5	−0.7 (1.5)	14	—	NS

[a] Cases excluded if any MMSE1 or MMSE2 items missing.
** Mann–Whitney significance values, demented versus normal.

an average decline of less than 1 point. In contrast, the CAMDEX–MMSE scores showed a sharper decline except for the severely demented, most of whom registered very low or zero scores. Of the 361 normal subjects, only 20 (6%) showed a drop in MMSE scores of 5 or more points (two standard deviations). Four seemed to have undergone considerable decline. On review they were disoriented, and were described by the screening interviewers as being vague, rambling, and forgetful. Their MMSE scores of 28, 27, 24, and 25 in the first year of the study declined to 20, 22, 15, and 17, respectively. The two initial scores of 24 or 25 could not have been "false negatives"; neither had been part of the one in three sample in this score range who had been selected for full assessment with the CAMDEX schedule. The remaining subjects who had shown a marked decline were found to be alert and active, and some recalled their initial interview. Another two were extremely deaf, making testing impossible, and one man died of cancer within a few weeks of being seen. Schedules of the 23 subjects whose scores had been dropped by 4 points were examined but none showed clear evidence of dementia. It was concluded that only four of 361 subjects in whom the MMSE score had declined by 5 or more points were suffering from a severe form of mental disorder. However, the possibility that they had been demented at the first examination could not be excluded.

The subjects who had scored 23 or less (i.e., at threshold or below) on the MMSE in the first examination but were assessed as normal on the basis of the CAMDEX were of particular interest. The possibility that they may have been false negatives was examined. Two hundred ninety-five subjects who registered high scores at the initial interview (MMSE ≥24) showed a larger mean decline (and a significant one) in the course of the year than the 66 low scorers. This had been due to a small number of high scorers who had refused all or most MMSE items. However, even when seven subjects who missed one or more MMSE items in either examination were excluded from analysis, the original low scorers showed a mean decline of zero points compared with 0.9 points among the original high scorers.

DISCUSSION

The diagnosis of dementia made with the aid of the CAMDEX in a large general practice sample of elderly subjects was reviewed after an interval of approximately 12 months. The diagnosis of dementia was confirmed in 133 of 137 surviving cases (97%). Subjects classed as normal in the first year were reviewed with the aid of the MMSE. The number who are developing dementia is uncertain or the strength of their examination is uncertain. However, MMSE scores proved stable in the population of normal elderly people studied in this inquiry. Only a small proportion of subjects showed a decline of 5 or more points on the MMSE, and only 4 of 361 appeared to have developed probable dementia, judging from their cognitive performance and the observations of screening interviewers. These findings should be interpreted with caution; further cases may materialize at a later stage. However, on the basis of a detailed analysis of all individual cases who had shown a significant decline in MMSE scores, only a small number of negative diagnoses could be made within the first year.

The success achieved by the schedule in the diagnosis of dementia can probably be attributed in large part to the fact that it eliminates a number of the sources of error inherent in cross-sectional methods of assessment with the aid of psychiatric examination confined to the presenting mental state and/or measurement tests limited to current cognitive performance alone. Detailed history-taking from an independent observer as well as the patient helps to eliminate erroneous diagnoses of dementia that may be made in cases of severe depression and of severe clouding and delirium. Observations made on patients' behavior and performance in everyday tasks in a domestic or hospital environment further help to minimize diagnostic errors. Some patients may score poorly in cognitive tests but perform adequately or with skill in a whole range of tasks requiring accurate perception, memory, and coordination that would defeat some subjects in the relatively early stages of dementia. Those with clouding or delirium may perform poorly in everyday tasks as well as in tests. However, the history will usually be of no more than a few weeks' duration and their mental state, including their cognitive competence, will show marked fluctuations. Further errors arise from the tendency of some persons of relatively low intelligence, poor education, and low social class to perform poorly in cognitive tests (11,13).

The sections devoted to history, previous adjustment, a range of scales and a neuropsychological battery, independent observers' testimony, operational criteria for diagnosis, and algorithms for making diagnostic decisions and grading the level of confidence in diagnosis provide for comprehensive evaluation of all relevant sources of evidence required for diagnosis. All sections of the CAMDEX have been shown to have high interobserver reliability and there is preliminary evidence testifying to its validity. Further evidence in this last respect is being sought from follow-up studies and postmortem findings.

There are certain lessons to be learned from failure to attach sufficient importance to some of the observations in this study. The two subjects who suffered from poorly controlled diabetes and were diagnosed as mildly demented would have been detected with routine laboratory investigations, which would be undertaken in clinical practice. They should perhaps always be arranged in epidemiologic studies in all cases in which physical examination and/or other observations point to causes liable to cause clouding, memory impairment, and confusion in the elderly.

Depression was missed in a number of minimally demented subjects, probably because depressive psychomotor retardation was mistaken for inertia, the apathy of dementia. The depressions of the aged are frequently "silent," just as many of their physical diseases which are acute and florid in presentation in early life are liable to be muted in the elderly. Psychomotor retardation has recently emerged as a highly specific feature of endogenous depressions in particular. It is also found in a proportion of nonendogenous cases. Specific scales have been developed in France to measure this dimension (14,15).

The discriminating and prognostic value of this dimension has recently been confirmed by the studies of Parker and his colleagues in Australia (16). Items from these scales should perhaps be incorporated into future editions of CAMDEX, to assist in the differentiation of depressive psychomotor retardation from the apathetic and torpid state of many demented patients.

A depressive illness may pose further difficulties for diagnosis as a result of agitation, lack of concentration and, in acute and severe cases, a period of clouded consciousness. However, when history-taking and objective observation confirm the presence of progressive and unremitting failure of performance in the activities of daily life over a period of months, as well as consistent failure in cognitive tests, the presence of severe depression should not preclude a diagnosis of dementia. True depressive pseudodementia is a rare condition. Depressive symptoms form part of the clinical picture of early primary dementias and also of multiinfarct dementia.

The most important finding in the context of this conference has been the impressive validation of the diagnosis of mild dementia as performed with the aid of the CAMDEX schedule. Reexamination after a year confirmed this diagnosis in 64 of 67 cases (94.5%). There was a significant decline in mean score on the MMSE after 1 year, both in those patients initially judged as suffering from "mild" dementia and in those suffering from "moderate" dementia. Two unconfirmed patients were "minimal" cases and they remain at a certain risk of undergoing further deterioration. Differentiation of mild dementia from normal aging has been regarded in the past as an unreliable exercise (17,18). If the results of this study can be confirmed in subsequent inquiries, the CAMDEX will have been shown to represent a significant advance in the identification of dementia at an early stage of development.

REFERENCES

1. American Psychiatric Association. *Diagnostic and statistical manual of mental disorders. DSM-III-R,* 3rd ed, revised. Washington, DC: Division of Public Affairs, APA; 1987.
2. World Health Organization. *ICD-10 1987. 1987 Draft of Chapter V Categories F00–F99 Mental, Behavioural and Developmental Disorders. Clinical Descriptions and Diagnostic Guidelines.* Geneva: WHO Division of Mental Health; 1987.
3. Roth M, Tym E, Mountjoy CQ, et al. CAMDEX: a standardised instrument for the diagnosis of mental disorder in the elderly with special reference to the early detection of dementia. *Br J Psychiatry* 1986;149:698–709.
4. Kendrick DC, Moyes ICA. Activity, depression, medication and performance on the revised Kendrick Battery. *Br J Soc Clin Psychol* 1979;18:341–50.
5. Roth M, Hopkins B. Psychological test performance in patients over 60. I. Senile psychosis and the affective disorders of old age. *J Ment Sci* 1953;99:439–50.
6. Blessed G, Tomlinson BE, Roth M. The association between quantitative measures of dementia and of senile change in the cerebral grey matter of elderly subjects. *Br J Psychiatry* 1968;114:797–811.
7. Copeland JRM, Kelleher MJ, Kellett JM, et al. A semi-structured clinical interview for the assessment of diagnosis and mental state in the elderly: The geriatric Mental State Schedule I. Development and reliability. *Psychol Med* 1976;6:439–49.
8. Wing JK, Cooper JE, Sartorius N. *The measurement and classification of psychiatric symptoms.* London: Cambridge University Press; 1974.
9. Folstein MF, Folstein SE, McHugh PR. "Mini-mental State": a practical method for grading the cognitive state of patients for the clinician. *J Psychiatr Res* 1975;12:189–98.
10. Hachinski VV, Iliff LD, Zihlka E, et al. Cerebral blood flow in dementia. *Arch Neurol* 1975;32:632–7.
11. O'Connor DW, Pollitt PA, Roth M. A follow-up study of dementia diagnosed in the community using the Cambridge Mental Disorders of the Elderly examination. *Acta Psychiatr Scand* 1990;81:78–82.
12. Bergmann K, Kay DWK, Foster EM, McKechnie AA, Roth M. A follow-up study of randomly selected community residents to assess the effects of chronic brain syndrome and cerebrovascular disease. In: *Proceedings of the 5th World Congress of Psychiatry.* Amsterdam: Excerpta Medica; 1971:856–65.
13. O'Connor DW, Pollitt PA, Treasure FP, Brook CPB, Reiss BB. The influence of education, social class and sex on Mini-Mental State scores. *Psychol Med* 1989;19:771–6.
14. Widlöcher D, Allilaire JF, Frechette D. Systeme d'actions et histoire du concept. In: Widlöcher D, ed. *Le ralentissement dépressif.* Paris: PUF 1983:7–25.
15. Lecrubier Y. Une "limite biologique" des états dépressifs? In: Widlöcher D, ed. *La ralentissement dépressif.* Paris: PUF; 1983:71–86.
16. Parker G, Hadzi–Pavlovic D, Boyce P, et al. Classifying depression by mental state signs. *Br J Psychiatry* 1990;157:55–65.
17. Henderson AS, Huppert FA. The problem of mild dementia. *Psychol Med* 1984;14:5–11.
18. Brayne C, Calloway P. Normal ageing, impaired cognitive function, and senile dementia of the Alzheimer's type: a continuum? *Lancet* 1988;2:1265–6.

Guidelines for Drug Trials in Memory
Disorders, edited by N. Canal, et al.
Raven Press, Ltd., New York © 1993.

24

Selection Methodologies

Steven H. Ferris

*Aging And Dementia Research Center, New York University Medical Center,
New York, New York 10016*

The selection of subjects to participate in clinical trials for memory disorders [most commonly patients with Alzheimer disease (AD) or normal elderly persons with age-associated memory impairment (AAMI)] must be based on a comprehensive state-of-the art diagnosis. The clinical diagnosis of AD requires that patients exhibit cognitive impairment (dementia) of sufficient magnitude to affect functioning in daily life. The specific aspects of cognition that typically decline in the early stages of AD include memory (the "cardinal" symptom), language, praxis, visuospatial function, abstraction, attention, and psychomotor function. When the cognitive symptoms are severe, experienced clinicians can easily confirm these impairments. However, in the early to moderate stages of AD, a comprehensive cognitive assessment is required to document objectively the nature and magnitude of impairment. Objective psychometric evaluation is crucial for identifying mild or borderline dementia because the patterns of cognitive decline associated with AD and aging are qualitatively similar. Objective cognitive tests are also essential for identifying subjects who meet research diagnostic criteria for AAMI (1). The general types of measurements available for assessment of cognitive status include global scales [e.g., Global Deterioration Scale (GDS), Clinical Dementia Rating Scale (CDR)], composite cognitive evaluations [e.g., Mini-Mental State Examination (MMSE), Alzheimer Disease Assessment Scale (ADAS)], psychometric/neuropsychological test batteries, and assessments of activities of daily living (ADL). Each category of assessment can play a useful role in the diagnostic process. The specific rationale and current state of the art for performance-based cognitive assessment domains are reviewed in this chapter. The utility of face-valid, computerized psychometric tests is also discussed, including their potential value for very early diagnosis.

DIAGNOSTIC EVALUATION OF ALZHEIMER'S DISEASE

There are three major goals in performing a diagnostic evaluation for possible AD. The first goal is to confirm the clinical symptoms, onset, and course

TABLE 1. *Documenting AD symptoms*

Impairment of recent memory
Impairment in *one or more* of the following
Language (aphasia)
Psychomotor (apraxia)
Perception (agnosia)
Abstraction
Judgment
Spatial orientation
Impairment of ADL sufficient to affect work or social function
Noncognitive behavioral symptoms
Personality change
Depression
Delusions/hallucinations
Agitation
Sleep disturbance
Wandering

of AD according to well-established inclusion criteria, such as the NINCDS-ADRDA work group criteria (2) and the DSM-III-R (3). A complete documentation of AD symptoms includes evaluating and confirming the presence of the symptoms outlined in Table 1. Current criteria for AD require the presence of impairment in memory and at least one other area of cognition, and require a severity of impairment sufficient to affect activities of daily living (e.g., work or social function). Current criteria for AAMI require memory performance that is at least one standard deviation below the mean performance of young subjects. The second diagnostic goal is to rule out other possible causes of dementia or age-associated memory decline through a detailed history and a complete medical evaluation. Finally, when patients are being selected for research protocols (including clinical trials), an additional goal is to apply more specific study inclusion and exclusion criteria. Such criteria for AD trials usually call for inclusion of patients with particular characteristics (e.g., specific stages or severity of dementia) and exclude patients with certain contraindicated medical conditions (e.g., significant heart disease or concomitant medications).

The recommended components of a complete diagnostic evaluation that enable a clinician to achieve these goals include the following: a complete history (medical, psychiatric, cognitive, and social); a cognitive/neuropsychological assessment (see below); laboratory tests (SMA 6/12, CBC with differential, urinalysis, vitamin B_{12} and folate, T_3, T_4 and TSH, VDRL); electrocardiogram and chest x-ray; physical, neurologic and psychiatric exams; and neuroradiology [computed tomography (CT) or magnetic resonance imaging (MRI) scan]. Other ancillary tests may be called for or can be included for research purposes, such as lumbar puncture (LP) for cerebrospinal fluid (CSF) studies, clinical or computer electroencephalography (EEG), and single photon emission tomography (SPECT) or position emission tomography (PET).

DEMENTIA ASSESSMENT DOMAINS

In evaluating the clinical symptoms of AD, the various evaluation methods available can be conveniently categorized into the five assessment domains listed in Table 2 (4). As the initial diagnostic goal is to confirm cognitive impairment, the remainder of this chapter will focus on composite cognitive scales and objective psychometric batteries. However, ADL assessment, global staging, and noncognitive behavioral assessment are essential components of a complete dementia evaluation. ADL assessment provides valuable information about the range of daily activities required for personal self-maintenance and independent, productive community residence. Such information indicates whether the degree of impairment is sufficient to warrant a clinical diagnosis of dementia and assesses the clinical impact of cognitive decline or the clinical significance of treatment effects. Global staging enables the clinician to specify the overall symptom severity of a patient or patient group. Staging provides a basic measure of global severity and provides a useful index for selecting or comparing patients. Noncognitive behavioral symptom assessment is important because symptoms such as depression, delusions, hallucinations, agitation, and aggressiveness can compound the cognitive symptoms, can have a great impact on a caregiver's ability to maintain a patient at home, and are the symptoms of AD that are most amenable to treatment.

COMPOSITE COGNITIVE ASSESSMENTS

These measurements use multiple rating items or performance subtests to assess a variety of relevant cognitive symptoms and provide a total score

TABLE 2. *Assessing of AD symptoms*

Composite cognitive assessments
  MMSE
  Blessed DS
  Mattis DRS
  ADAS
  BCRS
Objective psychometric batteries
  NYU Test Battery
  MAC Test Battery
  SKT Battery
ADL assessment
  ADL and IADL scales
Global staging
  GDS
  CDR
Behavioral assessment
  Cornell Depression Scale
  BEHAVE-AD
  ADAS (noncognitive)

that represents a composite index of the magnitude of cognitive impairment. With these scales, cutoff scores are usually established that differentiate dementia from normal cognitive function. These instruments can be used to confirm the presence of dementia, to select cases for research protocols, and to monitor change in clinical trials or longitudinal studies.

The MMSE (5,6) is a widely used dementia screening instrument which assesses orientation, recall, praxis, calculation, and language. It has a score range of 0–30 and takes 8 to 15 min to administer. Although the usual dementia cutoff score is 23 or less, scores are known to be influenced by level of education (6). The Mattis Dementia Rating Scale (MDRS) (7,8) was designed to screen for brain pathology in geriatric patients. Cognitive functions assessed hierarchically include attention, praxis, memory, perseveration (verbal and motor), and abstraction (verbal and nonverbal). The score range is 0–144 and it takes 15 to 45 min to administer.

The Blessed dementia instruments (9,10) consist of two major subscales, the Blessed Dementia Scale (DS), which evaluates functional and emotional impairment, and the Blessed Information–Memory–Concentration (IMC) Test. The Blessed DS (score range 0–28) is not an ideal instrument for assessing cognitive status because it includes noncognitive behavioral items. However, the Blessed IMC (score range 0–37) provides a good overall estimate of intellectual functioning. The ADAS (11,12) has become widely used both as a cognitive screening instrument and as an outcome measurement in clinical trials. This instrument, which takes 30 to 60 min to administer, was designed to provide a composite assessment of all major symptoms of AD. It consists of a cognitive subscale (11 subtests of memory, language, and praxis; score range 0–70) and a noncognitive subscale (10 items rating mood, vegetative functions, agitation, delusion, hallucinations, concentration, and distractibility; score range 0–50). Although the cognitive subscale alone is typically used as a primary outcome measurement in research protocols, a potential limitation is the lack of concentration assessment (concentration is inappropriately part of the noncognitive subscale).

The Brief Cognitive Rating Scale (BCRS) (13,14) assesses cognition on five axes: concentration, recent memory, past memory, orientation, and functioning and self-care. Each axes is rated by a clinician on a 1 to 7 scale. There are guidelines for rating each area based on the clinical symptoms identified in a semistructured interview. The BCRS has been widely used in longitudinal studies and clinical trials with AD patients.

NEUROPSYCHOLOGICAL/PSYCHOMETRIC TESTS

Objective performance tests are a routine component of the diagnostic process for AD and AAMI because of the need to document relevant disturbances in higher cortical function. The general requirements for cognitive

TABLE 3. *Requirements for cognitive assessment batteries*

Sample full range of relevant cognitive functions
Sensitivity to deficits of aging and dementia
Sensitivity to longitudinal change
Difficulty range appropriate to severity of patient sample
Equivalent forms for repeated administration
Reasonable duration (e.g., less than 1 h)
Sensitivity treatment effects
Good reliability
Good validity (relation to brain pathology or ADL symptoms)
Additional useful features
  Face-validity
  Test computerization
  Animal model relevance

test batteries are listed in Table 3. Such tests, especially those with well-developed, age-specific norms, can be useful in documenting significant decline in cognition, determining patterns of cognitive dysfunction, evaluating the rate and manner of cognitive decline, and assessing the effects of treatment. Because the patterns of cognitive decline in normal aging and early dementia primarily differ quantitatively rather than qualitatively (15), objective tests are particularly useful for evaluating very early, mildly impaired patients. The greater breadth and sensitivity of these tests, in comparison with more global composite scales, also makes objective cognitive batteries useful in early clinical trials when the nature and effect size of a new drug are not clearly known.

The New York University (NYU) Test Battery is a computerized evaluation that was designed to optimize the assessment of cognitive changes in normal elderly subjects, subjects with age-associated memory impairment, and elderly patients with dementia (16). This battery contains 12 subtests that evaluate immediate memory, recent memory, language, concept formation, and psychomotor speed and attention. It was specifically constructed to provide an appropriate range of difficulty, to increase reliability through computerization, and to have reasonable face validity (i.e., similarity to real-life cognitive difficulties). Two of the subtests also were designed to parallel tests used in animals during the preclinical evaluation of putative cognition-enhancing compounds (17,18). Several manual subtests have been employed with the NYU test battery to expand the range of cognitive functions assessed (16). It has been used to track longitudinal change (19,20) and psychopharmacologic response (21,22) in aging and in patients with dementia. The provision of multiple equivalent forms permits repetitive testing. Measurements in the battery have shown sensitivity to cholinergic disruption (21,22) and may be useful for early prediction of dementia in mildly impaired subjects (19). The potential ability to select cases with mild impairment who are at high risk for developing dementia will prove particularly useful for evaluating future pharmacologic agents that may delay the onset of dementia.

The Memory Assessment Clinics Test Battery utilizes 13 face-valid computerized subtests to evaluate thoroughly various aspects of memory function (including everyday verbal and visual memory) as well as attention and psychomotor speed in normal elderly subjects and in patients with AD (23). It was designed for evaluation of potential cognition-enhancing compounds, has norms based on very large samples across wide ranges of age, is available in five alternate forms, and has equivalent versions in five foreign languages, with more versions presently under development. This test battery has been widely used for assessing pharmacologic effects on cognition in multicenter trials in the United States and Europe.

The SKT Test Battery contains nine manually administered subtests that are designed for the measurement of recent memory and attention in patients with mild to moderately severe cognition impairment (24). The SKT is available in five alternate forms and can be administered quickly (10 to 15 min). It has been used in multicenter clinical drug trials, including those involving patients with AD.

Many other neuropsychological tests have been used for evaluating patients with Alzheimer disease and for studying the cognitive impairment that occurs in this condition. For example, the Guild Memory Test (25) includes tests of immediate and delayed recall of paragraphs and paired associates and immediate recall of designs. The test has age-specific norms and has been used to study cross-sectional and longitudinal changes in normal aging and in AD. The Wechsler Memory Scale-Revised (WMS-R) (26), which contains nine subtests of a very broad range of memory function and has excellent age norms, has been used to differentiate amnestic patients and patients with AD.

CONCLUSIONS

As reviewed above, there are many composite scales and psychometric tests available for confirming and studying the cognitive impairments associated with AD. The specific measures selected depend on the nature of the subjects to be evaluated and on the particular goals of the clinician or researcher. These measurements are particularly useful for selecting subjects for clinical trials and for evaluating the efficacy of pharmacologic agents.

REFERENCES

1. Crook T, Bartus RT, Ferris SH, Whitehouse P, Cohen GD, Gershon S. Age-associated memory impairment: proposed diagnostic criteria and measures of clinical change—report of a NIMH Work Group. *Dev Neuropsychol* 1986;2:261–76.
2. McKhann G, Drachman D, Folstein M, Katzman R, Price D, Stadlan EM. Clinical diagnosis of Alzheimer's disease: report of the NINCDS-ADRDA work group under the auspices of Department of Health & Human Services Task Force on Alzheimer's disease. *Neurology* 1984;34:939–44.

3. American Psychiatric Association. *Diagnostic and Statistical Manual of Mental Disorders-Revised,* 3rd ed. Washington, DC: American Psychiatric Association; 1987.
4. Kluger A, Ferris SH. Scales for the assessment of Alzheimer's disease. *Psychiatr Clin North Am* 1991;14:309–26.
5. Folstein MF, Folstein SE, McHugh PR. Mini-mental state: a practical method for grading the cognitive state of patients for the clinician. *J Psychiatr Res* 1975;12:189–98.
6. Cockrell JR, Folstein MF. Mini-mental state examination (MMSE). *Psychopharmacol Bull* 1988;24:689–92.
7. Mattis S. Mental status examination for organic mental syndrome in the elderly patient. In: Bellack R, Karasu B, eds. *Geriatric psychiatry.* New York: Grune & Stratton; 1976: 77–121.
8. Mattis S. *Dementia rating scale professional manual.* Odessa FL: Psychological Assessment Resources; 1988.
9. Blessed G, Tomlinson BE, Roth M. The association between quantitative measures of dementia and senile change in the cerebral gray matter of elderly subjects. *Br J Psychiatry* 1968;114:797–811.
10. Blessed G, Tomlinson BE, Roth M. Blessed-Roth dementia scale (DS). *Psychopharmacol Bull* 1988;24:705–8.
11. Rosen WG, Mohs RC, Davis KL. A new rating scale for Alzheimer's disease. *Am J Psychiatry* 1984;141:1356–64.
12. Mohs RC, Cohen L. Alzheimer's disease assessment scale (ADAS). *Psychopharmacol Bull* 1988;24:627–8.
13. Reisberg B, Schneck MK, Ferris SH, Schwartz GE, de Leon MJ. The brief cognitive rating scale (BCRS): findings in primary degenerative dementia (PDD). *Psychopharmacology Bulletin* 1983;19:47–50.
14. Reisberg B, Ferris SH. The Brief Cognitive Rating Scale (BCRS). *Psychopharmacol Bull* 1988;24:629–36.
15. Ferris SH, Flicker C, Reisberg B, Crook T. Age-associated memory impairment, benign forgetfulness and dementia. In: Bergener M, Reisberg B, eds. *Diagnosis and treatment of senile dementia.* Berlin: Springer-Verlag; 1989:72–82.
16. Ferris SH, Flicker C, Reisberg B. NYU computerized test battery for assessing cognition in aging and dementia. *Psychopharmacol Bull* 1988;24:699–702.
17. Flicker C, Bartus RT, Crook T, Ferris SH. Effects of aging and dementia upon recent visuospatial memory. *Neurobiol Aging* 1984;5:275–83.
18. Flicker C, Ferris SH, Crook T, Bartus RT. A visual recognition memory test for the assessment of cognitive function in aging and dementia. *Exp Aging Res* 1987;13:127–32.
19. Flicker C, Ferris SH, Reisberg B. Mild cognitive impairment in the elderly: predictors of dementia. *Neurology* 1991;41:1006–9.
20. Flicker C, Ferris SH, Reisberg B. A two-year longitudinal study of cognitive function in normal aging and dementia. *J Geriatr Psychiatr Neurol* (in press).
21. Flicker C, Serby M, Ferris SH. Scopolamine effects on memory, language, visuospatial praxis, and psychomotor speed. *Psychopharmacology,* 1990;100:243–50.
22. Flicker C, Ferris SH, Serby M. Hypersensitivity to scopolamine in the elderly. *Psychopharmacology* 1992;107:437–41.
23. Larrabee GJ, Crook T. A computerized everyday memory battery for assessing treatment effects. *Psychopharmacol Bull* 1988;24:695–7.
24. Erzigkeit H. The SKT—a short cognitive performance test as an instrument for the assessment of clinical efficacy of cognition enhancers. In: Bergener M, Reisberg B, eds. *Diagnosis and treatment of senile dementia,* Berlin: Springer-Verlag; 1989:164–74.
25. Gilbert JG, Levee RF. Patterns of declining memory. *J Gerontol* 1971;26:70–5.
26. Wechsler D. *Wechsler Memory Scale—Revised.* San Antonio: Psychological Corporation/Harcourt Brace Javanovich, 1987.

Guidelines for Drug Trials in Memory
Disorders, edited by N. Canal, et al.
Raven Press, Ltd., New York © 1993.

25

Discussion

Dr. Drachman: We are all handicapped by the way in which we use diagnostic criteria that are not perfect. If a diagnostic instrument is not rated 100% sensitivity and specificity to zero, it is difficult to use because we tend to think in terms of a disease state either being present or not. I would like to recommend the use of criteria that are *not* perfect, that are not always present, but rather that are sometimes present within the framework of the Bayesian statistical methods, to improve diagnoses. These are not absolute criteria, but they are contributory and useful.

Dr. Erkinjuntti: Those criteria are very good if you compare them with other criteria, such as the criteria for multi-infarct dementia. The most important point is for the patient to exhibit dementia by definition. Many studies quote the DSM-III criteria, perhaps not noting that there is stated short-term and long-term memory, which is a crucial point. Those criteria exclude most of the early cases, and this is not Alzheimer disease.

Dr. McKhann: Dr. Levy, after choosing the best criteria possible, did any of your patients turn out not to have Alzheimer disease? It seems to be to be inevitable that you would include some wrong patients, but might be able to distinguish them after the fact.

Dr. Levy: That is not very easy to answer because we have only one postmortem to date. We saw no reasons to change the diagnosis in any patients during the follow-up period. The one patient who has come to postmortem was a "responder" who exhibited a 5-point increase in Mini-Mental State Examination (MMSE) score. This patient had classic Alzheimer pathologic changes, with plaques and tangles in the temporal lobe, hippocampus, and near cortex, but he also had some Lewy bodies.

Dr. McKhann: In other diseases with which I am familiar, for example, some of the studies of multiple sclerosis, the most productive strategy has been to determine time to reach a particular outcome, rather than just choosing an arbitrary time to compare two populations. Would different findings have developed in your study if you could have picked particular outcomes and determined how long it took each group to reach these outcomes? This is really an extension of survival data, except with a different type of end point.

Dr. Levy: Survival itself would not be a useful end point, and there is no evidence that any of the drugs in use extend survival time, but your approach is interesting.

Dr. Wilcock: Dr. Roth, how does the CAMDEX handle dementia scores for conditions other than Alzheimer disease and multi-infarct dementia? The prevalence of the other dementias in your presentation was very much lower than many of us would have expected.

Dr. Roth: There is a specific scale for multi-infarct dementia. The epidemiologic study included both multi-infarct dementia and Alzheimer disease in the total number of dementia figures. Other dementias were referred to as the secondary dementias in a population of 75 years and more, and we did not find this to be more than a very rare condition.

Dr. Thal: You suggested that the CAMDEX would be very useful as an epidemiologic screening instrument. What would happen if you applied this type of scale to Third World countries where the education level is very low?

Dr. Roth: The CAMDEX is not a screening instrument; it is an instrument for arriving at a diagnosis. The screening instrument would be the abridged form. There is a minimal, insignificant effect of education and social class in the CAMDEX. In fact, many of the patients who had dementia in this study were individuals who had academic careers. Poorly educated people of low social class were more likely to score below the accepted cutoff point on the MMSE in our Cambridge study, but no more likely to be diagnosed as demented in light of detached clinical investigation.

Dr. Korczyn: Dr. Ferris, you have emphasized the importance of early recognition of demented patients or Alzheimer disease, and while fully agreeing with you academically and theoretically, I wonder about the practicality of this. If you are referring to patients in GDS stage 3, it would be very difficult to show that a drug is helpful symptomatically. To show that a prospective drug is helpful in preventing deterioration would require a very long time because it takes 4 years for 50% of patients to deteriorate significantly.

Dr. Ferris: Eventually I would like to prevent people from developing the disease. Early markers are possible, and if the next generation of drugs, for example, slows amyloid deposition, we will want to identify people very early because the target will be to slow the disease course or to prevent or delay disease onset.

Guidelines for Drug Trials in Memory Disorders, edited by N. Canal, et al.
Raven Press, Ltd., New York © 1993.

26

Assessment of Drug Effects in Age-Associated Memory Impairment

Thomas H. Crook

Memory Assessment Clinic, Bethesda, Maryland 20814

Nearly 20 years ago, Steve Ferris and I began thinking about the question of assessing efficacy in trials of drugs designed to treat memory disorders of later life. Our first study was a clinical trial of hyperbaric oxygen (1) in patients who would be diagnosed today as suffering from Alzheimer disease (AD). In looking for neuropsychological tests to assess the efficacy of this treatment we found what one would find today, i.e., tests that have obvious technical problems and one obvious conceptual problem. The conceptual problem is that the task of the subject in testing usually has almost nothing to do with the clinical problems that bring the patient for treatment.

In view of these problems, we undertook an effort to develop new tests, and this effort began with consideration of the problems that occur in everyday life as an individual ages. Of course, these problems are greatly exaggerated in neurologic disorders such as AD. An obvious case is the problem of remembering the name of an individual to whom one is introduced. This is the most common memory problem throughout Western cultures (2), and of course clinicians immediately recognize the problem in AD where a patient often cannot remember even a single new name despite repeated introductions. Another obvious example is the problem of remembering what one has read. Again, this is an increasingly prevalent problem with advancing age and a problem that is often disabling in the case of neurologic disease and trauma.

We reasoned that if we were to take these kinds of tasks on which problems are seen clinically and attempt to simulate them in the laboratory, based on useful paradigms from experimental psychology, we might be able to develop a series of tests that would be useful in assessing efficacy in clinical trials (3). Within the past 7 years we have adapted personal computers, computer graphics, touch-screen, and laser-disc technology to the task. Many of the tasks that we adapted to this technology are similar to those used in clinical practice. For example, a standard digit-span task is presented on a computer screen but the task is made more realistic because the subject is required to dial the digits on a touchtone phone interfaced with the computer (4). Similarly, we have a task in which the subject is presented with objects on the computer screen and asked to place the objects in various rooms in a computer representation of a house (5). After 40 min the subject is asked to recall the location of each object by touching the room in which the object was placed.

Another example of the test is topographic memory (6). This test was developed in collaboration with Dr. Raymond Bartus and several other colleagues involved in studying the effects of drugs on models of learning and memory in animals. For example, we were interested in spatial tasks comparable to maze learning tasks used in preclinical studies. In this effort we first filmed every possible route through downtown San Diego. The subject was shown the route on the computer monitor and then taken along the route again. On this second "trip," the subjects were asked at each intersection which way they turned previously when driven through the city. We have some psychometric problems with this test (7) and have since gone to a somewhat less ecologically appealing test, but one that we believe will be more useful in drug trials, again retracing a route on a map but this time using a task much like a standard maze learning task (8).

We also use measurements that are standard psychometric measurements in which we simply use the computer for administration. For example, one measurement requires subjects to learn a series of first and last names and then to recall each first name when presented with the corresponding last name (9). We employ a number of different paradigms modeled on other everyday memory tasks such as facial recognition (10), name–face association (11), recall of verbal information under variable conditions of distraction (12), and recall of verbal and visual information from daily life (13).

One specific example is a test in which the subject is "introduced" to persons on live video (11). Under one condition, 14 persons appear and introduce themselves. They then reappear on the screen in a different order from that in which they appeared originally. The task of the subject is to provide the name of each individual. Performance is scored for this first acquisition trial, and then a second and a third acquisition trial are conducted. Approximately 40 min after this third and final acquisition trial, a delayed recall trial is conducted in which the names are not presented but the subject is asked to recall each name when presented with each individual on the computer screen. We have administered these tests to more than 3,000 carefully screened normal subjects in the United States and have found clear and highly significant differences in performance among persons of different ages. A striking age-related decline was seen on many measurements, even though the older subjects were particularly well educated and scored above

TABLE 1. *Name–face association test demographic data, Progetto Memoria, San Marino data (n = 309)*

	Age group (years)					
	20–29	30–39	40–49	50–59	60–69	70 +
Age						
Mean	24.06	34.29	44.29	54.41	64.62	74.64
SD	2.76	2.92	2.81	2.19	2.91	3.02
Education						
Mean	11.06	10.84	7.15	5.13	3.89	2.64
SD	3.31	4.28	3.79	2.86	2.27	1.65
MMSE						
Mean	28.79	28.89	28.02	26.67	25.15	23.55
SD	1.17	1.38	1.59	2.73	2.99	4.01
n	72	62	52	54	47	22
% Female	48.6	51.6	55.8	48.1	57.4	45.5

average, and well above younger subjects, on a standard test of verbal intelligence (e.g., refs. 9,11).

An even more striking effect of age is seen in the general population. A random sample was drawn from the normal population of the Republic of San Marino (14). Demographic characteristics of study subjects are shown in Table 1, performance scores are shown in Table 2, and changes in performance as a function of age are illustrated in Fig. 1.

In our treatment studies in age-associated memory impairment (15), this is this sort of deficit that is the target of treatment. The question is, can we take healthy people in their fifties, sixties, and seventies who are performing in this range and improve their performance so that it comes closer to the

TABLE 2. *Name–face association test performance differences among age groups, Progetto Memoria, San Marino data (n = 309)*

Presentation of 14	Age group (years)						F value (sig. of F)	TukeyB
	20–29	30–39	40–49	50–59	60–69	70 +		
First								1–2,3,4,5,6
Mean	3.81	2.72	2.42	1.35	1.00	0.77	24.34	2–4,5,6
SD	2.13	2.00	1.63	1.32	1.23	0.97	0.00	3–4,5,6
Second								1–2,3,4,5,6
Mean	8.96	7.30	6.33	3.91	2.98	2.05	43.50	2–4,5,6
SD	2.93	3.51	2.87	2.52	2.29	1.89	0.00	3–4,5,6
Third								1–2,3,4,5,6
Mean	11.92	10.08	9.29	6.37	4.68	3.68	59.47	2–4,5,6
SD	2.24	3.33	3.07	3.10	2.65	2.83	0.00	3–4,5,6
								4–5,6
Delayed								1–2,3,4,5,6
Mean	11.35	9.38	8.27	5.56	4.15	2.45	51.86	2–4,5,6
SD	2.61	3.74	3.50	3.35	2.65	2.70	0.00	3–4,5,6
								4–6

Sig., significance.

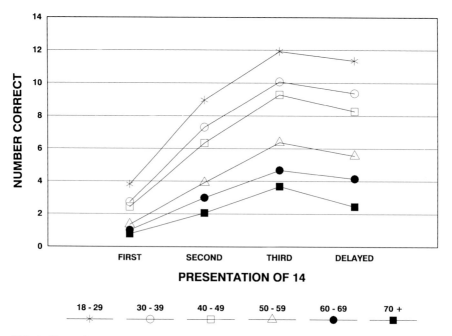

FIG. 1. Name–face association test performance differences among age groups, Progetto Memoria, San Marino data (*n* = 309).

performance associated with younger people? We ask the same question in the case of our cardiac bypass work and other work, i.e., can we reverse or diminish this deficit? The answer, in the first dozen or so clinical trials we conducted, was no (e.g., 16). We failed repeatedly in age-associated memory impairment and other indications to pharmacologically reverse the deficits that are so clear on these tasks of daily life.

Our first positive findings were reported in 1991 (17), concerning the effects of 300 mg of the phosphatidylserine formulation derived from bovine cortex. This was a 12-week, placebo-controlled, randomized trial in which we found in 150 AAMI subjects a relatively modest effect favoring drug. What we found particularly interesting is that when one examines those patients who are relatively impaired, whom we believe to be at increased risk for dementia (about 40% of our sample), the magnitude and the consistency of the drug effect become more apparent. We saw an effect on the clinical global measures that was consistent with the changes on performance tests. Thus, clinicians detected the same changes that were seen in testing. The effects seen on both testing and clinical ratings were not overwhelming, but they appear reliable and may be of interest in that age-related changes accepted as inevitable were shown, in this case, to be modifiable through pharmacologic treatment.

We do not believe for a moment that this is the only means of pharmacologically treating AAMI. Indeed we, following the much earlier lead of pioneers such as Professors Gottfries and Carlson, have argued that multiple neurochemical abnormalities underlie AAMI and that multiple strategies for treatment may be identified (18,19).

REFERENCES

1. Raskin A, Gershon S, Crook T, Sathananthan G, Ferris S. The effects of hyper- and normobaric oxygen on cognitive impairment in the elderly. *Arch Gen Psychiatr* 1978;35:50–6.
2. Crook TH, Youngjohn JR, Larrabee GJ, Salama M. Aging and everyday memory: a cross-cultural study. *Neuropsychology* 1992;6:123–36.
3. Crook T. Cognitive assessment in the year 2000. In: Gaitz C, Niederehe G, Wilson N, eds. *Aging 2000 our health care destiny: psychosocial issues.* New York: Springer-Verlag; 1985: 119–25.
4. West RL, Crook TH. Age differences in everyday memory: laboratory analogues of telephone number recall. *Psychol Aging* 1990;5:520–9.
5. Crook TH, Youngjohn JR, Larrabee GJ. Misplaced Objects Test: a measure of everyday visual memory. *J Clin Exp Neuropsychol* 1990;12:808–22.
6. Flicker C, Ferris SH, Crook T, Bartus RT. Equivalent spatial-rotation deficits in normal aging and Alzheimer's disease. *J Clin Exp Neuropsychol* 1988;10:387–99.
7. Zappala G, Martini E, Crook T, Amaducci L. Ecological memory assessment in normal aging. *New Dev Neuropsychol Eval* 1989;5:583–94.
8. Crook TH, Youngjohn JR, Larrabee GJ. The influence of age, gender, and cues on computer simulated topographic memory. *Dev Neuropsychol* 1993;9:41–53.
9. Youngjohn JR, Larrabee GJ, Crook TH. First–Last Names and the Grocery List Selective Reminding Test: two computerized measures of everyday verbal learning. *Arch Clin Neuropsychol* 1991;6:287–300.
10. Crook TH, Larrabee GJ. Changes in facial recognition memory across the adult life span. *J Gerontol Psychol Sci* 1992;47:138–41.
11. Crook TH, West RL. Name recall performance across the adult life span. *Br J Psychol* 1990;81:335–49.
12. Crook TH, West RL. The driving-reaction time test: assessing age declines in dual-task performance. *Dev Neuropsychol* 1993;9:31–9.
13. Crook TH, Youngjohn JR, Larrabee GJ. The TV News Test: a new measure of everyday memory for prose. *Neuropsychology* 1990;4:135–45.
14. Crook TH, Zappala G, Cavarzeran F, Measso G, Pirozzolo F, Massari D. Recalling names after introduction: changes across the adult life-span in two cultures. *Dev Psychol* 1993.
15. Crook TH. Diagnosis and treatment of normal and pathologic memory impairment in later life. *Semin Neurol* 1989;9:20–30.
16. McEntee WJ, Crook TH, Jenkyn LR, Petrie W, Larrabee GJ, Coffey DJ. Treatment of age-associated memory impairment with guanfacine. *Psychopharmacol Bull* 1991;27:41–6.
17. Crook TH, Tinklenberg J, Yesavage J, Petrie W, Nunzi MG, Massari D. Effects of phosphatidylserine in age-associated memory impairment. *Neurology* 1991;41:644–9.
18. McEntee WJ, Crook TH. Serotonin, memory, and the aging brain. *Psychopharmacology* 1991;103:143–9.
19. McEntee WJ, Crook TH. Age-associated memory impairment: a role for catecholamines. *Neurology* 1990;40:526–30.

Guidelines for Drug Trials in Memory Disorders, edited by N. Canal, et al.
Raven Press, Ltd., New York © 1993.

27

Clinical Assessment of Efficacy for Drug Trials in Memory Disorders

*Mary Sano and †Richard Mayeux

*Departments of *†Neurology and †Psychiatry, Columbia University, College of Physicians and Surgeons, New York, New York 10032; *†The New York State Psychiatric Institute Memory Disorders Clinic, and the *†Center for Alzheimer's Disease Research, New York, New York*

The development of drugs for the treatment of memory disorders is complicated by many issues, including assessment of the clinical impact of the problem. Clinical assessment requires standardized evaluation and should not be confused with clinical judgment. Although the difference may seem obvious, the dilemma arises in drug trials that attempt to use a "clinical global impression of change." Typically, these outcome measurements ask the clinician to evaluate a drug response in terms such as improved, no change, or worse. This is usually done in the absence of a priori criteria for making the judgment. This technique is not new and is not restricted to drug trials. The controversy over clinical versus actuarial judgment can be traced back to the 1950s. In 1989, a review of comparative studies, in which "judgments" could be independently verified, was published in *Science*. The review examined studies of the prediction of survival time, of disease etiology, and of treatment outcomes. The clinical judgment was never superior to actuarial methods. In fact, clinical judgment was not improved by practice, experience of the clinician, or additional sources of information.

The authors warn

> "A unique capacity [of the clinician] to observe is not the same as a unique capacity to predict on the basis of integration of observation. . . . virtually any observation can be coded quantitatively and thus subjected to actuarial analysis." (1)

However, the clinician, through standardized clinical assessments, has the unique capacity to observe. The task lies in choosing useful aspects of clinical status to evaluate. The following will focus on issues of clinical assessment for drug trials for memory disorders in aging. Specifically we will describe Alzheimer disease (AD), for which criteria have been set to establish the diagnosis. There will be an occasional reference to age-associated memory impairment (AAMI) for which criteria have also begun to appear (2).

The criteria of the DSM-III-R (3) describe impairment severe enough to interfere with social and occupational functioning. The same domains are used to rate the severity of the disease as well as to make the diagnosis. For example, NINCDS-ADRDA criteria (4) specifically mention impairments in language, motor skill, perception, and activities of daily living as supportive of the diagnosis. The Clinical Dementia Rating Scale (CDR) (5), which marks the severity of the disease, assesses similar domains, including memory, judgment, community affairs, personal care, and home and hobbies. Although these domains overlap, very different instruments can be used for diagnoses and to measure change. Finally as the disease progresses, indices of morbidity or mortality can be considered as outcome measures. For example, loss of independent function, loss of ambulation, institutionalization, and death may be outcomes.

The criteria for AAMI do not include occupational or functional impairment, but they are recognized as a likely concomitants (2).

ASSESSMENT OF FUNCTIONAL CAPACITY

Activities of Daily Living

Functional independence can be described by two categories of activities: activities of daily living (ADL) and instrumental activities of daily living (IADL). IADL describes activities needed to negotiate the environment, such as shopping, transportation, and housekeeping. ADL represent self-care. Although loss of independence can be demonstrated in both categories, patients with AD usually demonstrate very minimal IADL function even at the earliest stages of disease suggesting that ADL rather than IADL may be an appropriate category to assess in this group. IADL, on the other hand may be appropriate for assessing the functional impact of memory loss in nondemented elderly persons, as this domain does deteriorate with age (6) and with cognitive loss (7).

Quality of Life

Another method for evaluating function is through "quality of life" assessment (QLA). These outcome measurements assess the impact of disability on the degree of satisfaction that the person experiences. In choosing a QLA, there are four essential attributes to be considered. The first three are required of any instrument: they must be reproducible, valid, and responsive. In addition, for this population they must be easy enough to use in the presence of cognitive compromise.

In a review of QLA, Guyatt et al. (8) describes two types of instruments. Generic instruments that are applicable to many different populations may cover a range of function, disability, and distress. The advantage of such instruments is their ability to allow comparisons between interventions or conditions. In addition, they provide a single number representing net impact by summarizing effects on different aspects of health status. The major disadvantage of these instruments is their inadequate assessment of a specific area of interest. Their generic nature may make them unresponsive to a specific condition or problem. The Sickness Impact Profile (SIP) is a health profile used in many different medical settings (9). The scale contains five independent categories and two dimensions which can be summarized in a single overall score. It has been used in studies of diseases that have examined elderly patients, including studies of cardiac rehabilitation, total hip joint arthroplasty, and treatment of back pain. These studies suggest that the SIP may be responsive to a wide range of medical conditions.

In our experience, however, many of the domains do not reflect the impact of dementia although a few may be valuable. Table 1 demonstrates that among patients with AD there is little correlation between the dimensions of the SIP and change in memory scores in a 6-week clinical trial with a cholinesterase inhibitor. A second type of QLA focuses on a specific domain of function. The domain is chosen on the basis of clinical observation. For this reason, these instruments may be more responsive than generic instruments. However, their specific nature makes it more difficult to compare with other conditions. The Squires Memory Test was designed to measure memory complaints after electroconvulsive therapy (ECT) (10). We have used this instrument in clinical trials of patients with AD and have seen correlations between change in memory test scores and change in items that assess "attention," "alertness," and "moment to moment" recall (11).

TABLE 1. *Correlation between change on domains of the Sickness Impact Profile and change on a word list test after a 6-week double-blind trial of a cholinesterase inhibitor*

Domain	n	Correlation coefficient
Sleep and rest	27	0.28
Emotional behavior	27	0.22
Mobility	27	0.12
Body care and motion	27	0.07
Social interaction	27	0.12
Alertness behavior	27	0.17
Communication	27	0.03
Ambulation	27	0.12
Eating	27	0.20
Home management	27	0.25
Recreation and pastimes	27	0.01
Work	27	0.12
Total score	27	0.18

Functional Independence

Another method for assessment of function is to assess the degree to which the individual is independent across all activities, rather than to evaluate the specific activities. The Schwab and England (S&E) ADL scale was designed to measure independence in patients with Parkinson disease (PD) (12). Although the assumption in PD is that the loss of independence is due to physical disability, the evaluation is independent of motor function. In fact, the loss of independence does not always correlate with motor signs and symptoms, particularly in longitudinal studies. This may be due to the impact of other factors such as motivation, initiation, and cognitive disturbances.

To determine the utility of the S&E ADL scale in patients without PD, the baseline data for community-dwelling elderly patients were evaluated (13). These individuals were free of neurological problems, other than dementia. Both patient or informant and a clinician rated the S&E ADL scale. The correlation between subject/informant and physician was equal among both the demented and nondemented cases (for demented: $n = 350$, $r = 951$; nondemented: $n = 569$, $r = 0.965$). The S&E ADL scale was highly correlated with CDR ($r = 0.805$, $p < 0.001$), suggesting that it is sensitive to disease progression. Table 2 lists the mean and standard deviation of the S&E ADL scale for each CDR.

We also examined the utility of the S&E ADL scale in a nondemented population with various degrees of cognitive impairment. Three groups are described; the first consists of those who are not demented but have significant cognitive deficit and have functional complaints. The second group, also not demented, is less impaired than the first but has measurable cognitive impairment and may or may not have functional complaints. The third group has no significant impairment. These individuals may have a low score on an isolated cognitive test, but it is deemed "of no clinical significance" on the basis of functional and other information. Table 3 provides the mean and standard deviations of the S&E ADL scale for these nondemented patients. Overall, it appears that the S&E ADL scale is very sensitive for assessment of both demented and nondemented populations.

TABLE 2. *Mean and standard deviation of S&E by CDR rating in community dwelling elderly without other neurological disorders*

CDR	n	S&E ADL (%)
0.0	211	91.79 (15.45)
0.5	25	78.57 (21.15)
1.0	114	68.28 (24.19)
2.0	105	42.06 (18.16)
3.0	59	25.93 (19.13)

TABLE 3. *Mean and standard deviation of S&E by cognitive impairment in community dwelling elderly without other neurological disorders*

Group	n	S&E ADL (%)
Demented		49.4 (21.3)
Not Demented		
Scores near dementia	104	70.0 (22.9)
Possible significant deficit	146	81.8 (19.1)
No significant deficit	603	91.5 (13.9)

CHOOSING DOMAINS SENSITIVE TO A GIVEN DISEASE STAGE

Factors of the Blessed Dementia Rating Scale

In degenerative diseases, such as AD there may be a shift in the importance of one functional domain versus another domain as the disease progresses. The ability to evaluate clinical efficacy may depend on the use of certain domains at certain points in the natural history of the disease. This is supported by the differential sensitivity of IADL and ADL in patients with AD. We examined this question with a standardized version of the Blessed Dementia Rating Scale (BDRS) (14). This instrument is often used in AD because it demonstrates a correlation between postmortem biochemistry, neuropathology, and functional impairment. It includes items that assess the cognitive aspects of IADL, such as doing chores, making change, and getting around in the neighborhood. It also assesses ADL such as eating, dressing, and toileting, and personality factors that assess initiation and motivation. In other words, it captures cognitive and motivational aspects of IADL and ADL functions. A factor analysis of the 22 items in the BDRS, in 187 patients with AD, identified four independent factors: cognitive, personality change, apathy/withdrawal and basic self-care (15). Figure 1 lists the four factors and the items which were used to create them. These factors appear to describe clinically relevant constructs. Perhaps more importantly, they describe domains that represent change occurring at different points in the disease. Figure 2 describes the percent total score (i.e., maximum deficit) as a function of duration of illness for each factor. Factor 1 was sensitive to behavioral change early in the disease and the degree of impairment continued to rise as the disease progressed. In fact, 34% of the patients had near maximal scores on this factor at the first visit. Factor 4 was typically not affected in early stages of the disease (i.e., less than 10% had maximal scores at the first visit) but is sensitive to later stages. In this study, factor 4 began to be sensitive between 4 and 5 years after disease onset. Factors 2 and 3, which represent personality change, appear to increase over time but are not sensitive to duration of illness.

These factors were also examined using a survival analysis in a longitudi-

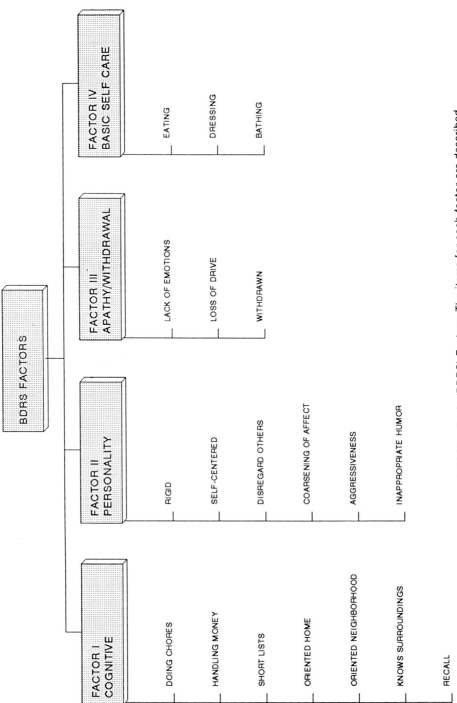

FIG. 1. Blessed Dementia Rating Scale (BDRS) Factors. The items for each factor are described.

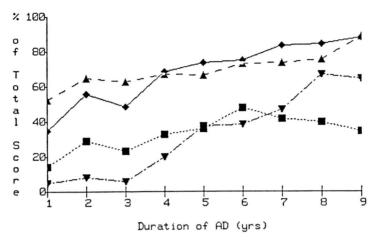

FIG. 2. Progression of the BDRS factors over time. Scores are expressed as percent of total possible score for each factor. Factor I, —◆—; factor II, - - -■- - -; factor III, – – –▲– – –; factor IV, – - -▼– - –.

nally followed cohort. A clinically meaningful end point was determined for each factor (15). Survival was examined in a cohort followed for up to 7 years (mean follow-up 3.1 ± 1.6 years). Survival curves for each factor were used to determine the time at which 50% of the patients reached maximum deficit. This is summarized in Table 4. Fifty percent of the patients reached an end point on factor 1 at 2.1 years after the initial visit; on factor 2 at 3.1 years; on factor 3 at 1.7 years, and on factor 4 at 3.3 years.

Clearly, the utility of assessing a given domain in a clinical trial depends on where the individual is in the progression of the disease.

Morbidity/Mortality as Outcome Measurements

Measurements of morbidity and mortality may be important in dementia although they may occur at in infrequent rate and very late in the disease.

TABLE 4. *Factor of the Blessed Dementia Rating Scale. Performance at first visit and survival time*

Factor	% With maximal deficit at first visit	Time to 50% survival (no. years)
1. Cognitive	34.3	2.2
2. Personality change	13.4	3.1
3. Apathy/withdrawal	77.1	1.7
4. Basic self-care	10.4	3.3

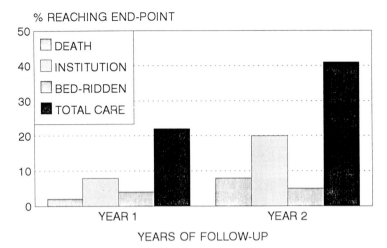

FIG. 3. Hypothetical rate of incidence of "clinically meaningful" outcome measures. Estimates are based on reports of multicenter studies describing similar but not identical types of outcomes.

Figure 3 presents hypothetical data that estimate the incidence of indicators of mortality and morbidity in patients with AD. Although each variable (death, institutionalization, becoming bedridden, and loss of self-care) is important and all increase over time, the overall incidence remains low and therefore requires a large sample to study.

ASSESSMENT OF PREDICTORS OF CLINICAL OUTCOMES

Neurobehavioral Signs Predict Cognitive Decline

We have noted that certain clinical signs appear to be associated with more rapid deterioration in cognitive and functional domains. The original observation suggested that the presence of extrapyramidal signs (EPS), myoclonus, and psychosis in AD suggested a more aggressive progression of disease (16).

The presence of each sign at first visit was associated with poorer performance on a mental status examination. EPS was associated with poorer performance in functional activities. Because this only demonstrates more severe disease, we compared patients with and without these predictive signs at first visit using a survival analysis with end points that represent significant cognitive and functional impairment (17). Table 5 displays the characteristics of patients with and without these signs. The cognitive end point used was a Modified Mini-Mental State Examination (mMMSE) score of less than 20 (18). This is approximately equivalent to an (original) MMSE score (19) of

TABLE 5. *The impact of the presence of extrapyramidal signs (EPS) and psychosis at first visit on cognitive and functional deterioration*

Group	Cognitive		Functional	
	% Reaching end point	Time to end point	% Reaching end point	Time to end point
EPS present	90	4.0 Yrs	80	5.5 Yrs
EPS absent	54	7.0 Yrs	54	5.8 Yrs
Psychosis present	70	5.5 Yrs	76	5.6 Yrs
Psychosis absent	59	7.0 Yrs	61	5.9 Yrs

10. There was a significant difference in the number of patients reaching the cognitive end point between those with and without EPS at the first visit. The approximate time for 50% of the EPS group to reach this cognitive end point was 4 years from disease onset whereas the time for the group without EPS was approximately 7 years. The functional end point was defined as a BDRS score of greater than 15. Although more patients with EPS reached this end point, compared with those without EPS, the survival time was no different. Patients with psychosis reached the cognitive end point faster than those without this sign. Functional impairment, as measured by the BDRS end point, was not predicted by the presence of psychosis.

Neurobehavioral Signs Predict Decline of Functional Factors

We were surprised by the lack of predictive value for either sign regarding functional decline, and we therefore chose to examine the predictive value of these signs for each of the functional factors described above. Survival analysis demonstrated that both EPS and psychosis predicted a faster decline in two of the four factors. We set end points that represented near maximal deficit for each factor, as described above and performed the survival analysis using time from the first visit rather than duration of illness, although we found the same result with both measures. Patients with psychosis at first visit reached an end point on factor 1 (i.e., cognitive aspects of function) faster than those without EPS at first visit. Fifty percent of the patients with psychosis reached the end point on factor 1 0.8 years after first visit, whereas those without this sign reached this end point 2.3 years after first visit. The presence of EPS at first visit was also predictive of faster decline on this factor. Patients with EPS also reached end point for factor 4, the self-care factor significantly faster than those without (with EPS, 1.8 years; without EPS, 4.2 years). The presence of psychosis did not predict a differential decline on this factor.

Myoclonus was not examined in these analyses because the patients represented too small a group with adequate follow-up before reaching end point.

TABLE 6. *Mean (± s.d.) of age and duration of illness in patients with and without clinical signs at first visit*

	Age at first visit	Duration of illness
Extrapyramidal signs		
Present	73.1 (± 10.9)	3.7 (± 2.1)
Absent	72.1 (± 8.4)	2.9 (± 1.6)
Psychosis		
Present	76.3 (± 9.0)	3.2 (± 1.2)
Absent	71.5 (± 9.4)	2.9 (± 1.8)
Myoclonus		
Present	63.0 (± 9.0)	4.5 (± 2.9)
Absent	73.5 (± 9.1)	3.0 (± 1.7)

Neurobehavioral Signs Predict Death

The next analysis examined the ability of these signs to predict death (20). Seventy-two patients were followed for an average of 5.05 (± 2.3) years. Survival analyses were conducted for patients with and without EPS, myoclonus, and psychosis. Patients with EPS or myoclonus at the initial visit died sooner (time from first visit) than those without. Table 6 lists the age at first visit and duration of illness for patients with these signs. Patients with and without EPS and psychosis were comparable. Those with myoclonus were younger than those without. Among those with EPS, the time by which 25% of the patients died was 2.7 years. In the group without EPS, 25% died within 5.2 years of first visit. The risk of death in patients who developed EPS was twice that of those who did not have the sign.

Among those with myoclonus at first visit, 50% died within 2.7 years of first visit. Among those without myoclonus 50% died 8.1 years from first visit. The risk of death in those with myoclonus was 3.5 times greater that in those without the sign. Clearly these signs are potent predictors of mortality in AD.

Finally, these measures are useful only when they occur with adequate frequency and before the other outcome measurements with which they are associated. We estimated the cumulative risk of developing EPS, psychosis and myoclonus in patients with AD (21). The same cohort described above was used in this analysis. Patients were followed for 5.05 years and evaluated at least twice with a minimum of 6 months between evaluations. EPS and psychosis emerged earlier than myoclonus. These results suggest that these predictive signs are evidence of progression rather than evidence of subtypes of disease. The incidence rate during the follow-up period was 32.9% for EPS, 29.63% for psychosis, and 34% for myoclonus. This suggests that the relative frequency of occurrence is high enough to observe in a clinical trial of 12 months or longer.

To summarize, the presence of EPS, psychosis, and myoclonus predicts a more rapid deterioration in specific domains. Psychosis is a transient sign, which makes it more difficult to assess. However, it predicts more rapid deterioration of cognitive and functional capacity. Specifically, it predicts the cognitive aspects of functional deterioration, which parallel IADL functions. However, the presence of psychosis is not associated with mortality in AD. EPS is a persistent sign which predicts a more rapid cognitive decline and a more rapid decline of basic self-care functions. In addition, the presence of EPS predicts earlier mortality. Finally, myoclonus is associated with more severe impairment in both cognitive and functional status, but its predictive utility is difficult to assess in these domains because it occurs relatively late in the disease and we have not had adequate follow-up in the past. However, it is a potent predictor of mortality.

Utility of Neurobehavioral Signs in Clinical Trials

To illustrate the utility of these predictive signs as outcome measures in clinical trials, I would like to suggest the following calculations. Among patients without EPS at the initial visit, the 2-year projected rate of inception of EPS was 0.21. To observe a similar effect size in factor 4 of the BDRS (self-care factor), one would need to observe for 3.5 years. To observe a similar effect size in reaching a cognitive end point (i.e., mMMSE scores) one would need to observe for 3.1 years. An alternate way to compare the utility (as outcome measurements in clinical trials) of these predictor signs with direct clinical assessment of function and cognition is to determine the power one would have to observe an effect of equal size and an equivalent observation period for each measurement. With the present results, using an n of 60 and 2 years of observation, it is projected that the power to observe a median effect in incidence of EPS is 65%; in the mMMSE the end point is 22% and in self-care the end point is 10%. Table 7 describes the number of subjects required to reach 80% power for these outcome measures. It is estimated that the number of subjects needed would be 100, 250, and >400 for EPS, mMMSE, and self-care factors, respectively (22).

TABLE 7. *Predicted power and required sample size to observe a median effect with a 2-year period of observation using three different outcome measures*

Measure	Power[a]	n[b]
EPS inception	65	100
Cognitive end point	22	250
Self-care end point	10	>400

[a] Power estimate for a study with an n = 60/group.
[b] Number required to achieve 80% power.

CONCLUSION

The clinical evaluation of patients with AD, and perhaps of those with other forms of memory loss, begins with standardized assessment, with the hope of avoiding non-criteria–based clinical judgments. The outcome measurements must capture domains of relevance to a given disease. In a progressive disease they must also be sensitive to the stage of the disease. Outcome measures may define abilities that underlie the performance of certain activities. For example, the analysis of the BDRS items identified factors that assessed the cognitive component and the motivational components of ADL and IADL performance. These factors are sensitive to change at different periods during disease progression. Finally, the evaluation of the presence of neurobehavioral signs such as EPS, psychosis, and myoclonus may also serve an important purpose in the assessment of dementia, as they appear to mark the initiation of a significant deterioration in the disease. The early appearance of these signs may permit a shorter observation period for clinical trials.

ACKNOWLEDGMENT

This work was supported by federal grants AG-08702 and RR00645 to the Clinical Research Center in the Presbyterian Hospital in the City of New York and The Charles S. Robertson Memorial gift for Research in Alzheimer's Disease. Dr. Sano is a Herbert Irving Assistant Professor in the Department of Neurology.

REFERENCES

1. Dawes RM, Faust D, Meehl PE. Clinical versus actuarial judgment. *Science* 1989;243: 1668–73.
2. Crook T., Bartus RT, Ferris SH, Whitehouse P, Cohen GD, Gershon S. Age-associated memory impairment. Proposed diagnostic criteria and measures of clinical change: report of a National Institute of Mental Health work group. *Dev Neuropsychol* 1986;2:261–76.
3. American Psychiatric Association, Diagnostic and Statistical Manual of Mental Disorders, 3rd edition, revised. APA: Washington, DC, 1987.
4. McKhann G, Drachman D, Katzman R, Price D, Stadlan EM, Clinical Diagnosis of Alzheimer's Disease NINCDS-ADRDA work group. *Neurology* 1984;34:939–44.
5. Burke WJ, Miller JP, Rubin EH, et al. The reliability of the Washington University Clinical Dementia Rating. *Arch Neurol* 1988;45:31–2.
6. Spector WD, Katz S, Murphy JB, Fulton JP. The hierarchical relationship between activities of daily living and instrumental activities of daily living. *J Chron Dis* 1987;40:481–9.
7. Aske D. The correlation between mini-mental state examination and Katz ADL status among dementia patients. *Rehabilit Nurs* 1990;15:140–3.
8. Guyatt GH, Sander JO, Veldhuyzen VZ, Feeny DH, Patrick DL. Measuring quality of life in clinical trials: a taxonomy and review. *CMAJ* 1989;140:1441–8.
9. Bergner M, Bobbitt R, Carter W, Gilson B. The sickness impact profile: development and final revision of a health status measure. *Medical Care* 1981;19:787–805.

10. Squire LR, Wetzel CD, Slater PC. Memory complaint after ECT, assessment with a new self-rating instrument. *Bio Psychiatry* 1979;14:791–801.
11. Bell K, Sano M, Stricks L, Marder K, Stern Y, Mayeux R. Physostigmine in Alzheimer's disease: risk/benefit considerations. *Neurology* 1990;40:229.
12. Schwab R, England A. Projection technique for evaluating surgery in Parkinson's Disease. In: Gillingham F, Donaldson I, eds. Third Symposium on Parkinson's Disease. Edinburgh: E&S Livingstone, 1969.
13. Sano M, Stern Y, Gurland B, Tatemichi T, Mayeux R. Schwab and England scale in community elderly: reliability and validity. *Neurology* 1992;42(suppl 3):226.
14. Blessed G, Tomlinson BE, Roth M. The association between quantitative measures of dementia and senile changes in the grey matter of elderly subjects. *Br J Psychol* 1968;225: 797–811.
15. Stern Y, Mayeux R, Hesdorfer D, Sano M. Measurement and prediction of functional change in Alzheimer's disease. *Neurology* 1990;40:8–14.
16. Mayeux R, Stern Y, Sano M: Heterogeneity and prognosis in dementia of the Alzheimer type. *Bull Clin Neurosci* 1985;50:7–10.
17. Stern Y, Mayeux R, Sano M, Hauser WA, Bush T: Predictors of disease course in patients with probable Alzheimer's disease. *Neurology* 1987;37:1649–53.
18. Stern Y, Sano M, Paulson J, Mayeux R: Modified Mini-Mental State Examination: validity and reliability. *Neurology* 1987;37(supp 1):179.
19. McHugh PR. "Mini-Mental State." A practical method for grading the cognitive state of patients for the clinician. *J Psychiatr Res* 1975;12:189–98.
20. Stern Y, Mayeux R, Sano M, Chenn J. Predictors of Mortality in Alzheimer's Disease. *Ann Neurol* 1989;26:132.
21. Chen J, Stern Y, Sano M, Mayeux R. Cumulative risks of developing extrapyramidal signs, psychosis or myoclonus in the course of Alzheimer's disease. *Arch Neurol* 1991;48:1141–3.
22. Fleiss JL. *Statistical methods for rates and proportions*, 2nd ed. New York: John Wiley and Sons; 1981.

Guidelines for Drug Trials in Memory Disorders, edited by N. Canal, et al.
Raven Press, Ltd., New York © 1993.

28

Neuropsychological Assessment in Patients with Memory Impairment and with Alzheimer Disease

François Boller, Michel Panisset, and *Judith Saxton

*INSERM U 324, Centre Paul Broca, 75014 Paris, France; and
*Alzheimer Disease Research Center, University of Pittsburgh,
Pittsburgh, Pennsylvania 15213*

The recent introduction of large scale longitudinal studies and therapeutic trials for patients with memory disorders, dementia, and Alzheimer disease (AD) has stressed the need for new approaches to the assessment of these patients. The role of neuropsychological assessment, once thought by some to be limited to helping establish a diagnosis, now serves additional purposes representing different approaches. This chapter reviews these different approaches and discusses the various techniques to be used, according to one's goal. A brief review of the neuropsychological changes associated with normal aging is included, together with some of the tests used for the informal assessment of cognitive functions in aging and dementia. This chapter also presents the neuropsychological findings typical of mild to moderate AD and addresses some aspects of testing in early and late phases of the disease. Finally, it discusses some of the problems of neuropsychological assessment in relation to therapeutic trials.

GOALS AND STRATEGIES

Many new techniques have modified the typical approach to the patient with dementia. Some of them, such as computed tomography (CT) and magnetic resonance imaging (MRI), have now become practically routine. Others, such as quantified electroencephalography (EEG) and spectral analysis, positron emission tomography (PET), and single photon emitting computed tomography (SPECT), are in less common use. Finally, some are still experimental (e.g., nuclear magnetic resonance spectroscopy and cerebrospinal fluid experimental analysis). These techniques have not made neuropsychology obsolete. On the contrary, some (particularly the PET and the SPECT) are consistently used in conjunction with cognitive tests. Other techniques may help in the clinical diagnosis, but none has replaced cognitive assessment. On the other hand, there is no question that because of their introduction the role of neuropsychological test performance in the assessment and management of demented patients has changed.

One can outline at least three different strategies in the neuropsychological evaluation of patients with dementia and probable AD. First of all, in the early phases of the disease, neuropsychological assessment plays a crucial role, clearly addressed by the NINCDS-ADRDA criteria (1), in confirming (or rejecting) the diagnosis of dementia and, to a lesser extent, in differentiating AD from other conditions that produce dementia. The validity of these criteria has been confirmed in the United States (2) and in France (3). Second, in more advanced stages of the disease, assessment may help the clinician to set up a realistic therapeutic plan and, if possible, to establish a prognosis concerning certain landmarks such as loss of competency or institutionalization. Finally, during therapeutic trials, performance on neuropsychological tests is an indispensable aid to assessment of the efficacy of treatment. The inadequacy of neuropsychological assessment instruments has represented a very sizable part of the criticisms raised by some recent reports of therapeutic trials in AD (4–7).

The first strategy (early phases) emphasizes what has been lost, whereas the second (more advanced stage) should aim particularly at showing what cognitive abilities are preserved. The main goal of the third strategy (therapeutic trials) is to define the current level of functioning of each subject so that a baseline can be set up against which any potential improvement can be compared. In addition, one has to ensure that any possible therapeutic effect is not restricted solely to improvement in neuropsychological test results obtained in the laboratory. It is important to stress at this point that whatever the strategy and the clinical context, neuropsychological test results should never be used alone for the diagnosis of dementia; in all cases, the judgment of the clinician remains indispensable.

NORMAL AGING

One important preliminary question is the differentiation of early dementia from normal aging. Our understanding of the neuropsychological changes that take place in normal aging has evolved considerably in the recent past [see (8) for a detailed discussion]. Most studies have found that, in general, verbal functions are relatively preserved in aging subjects, whereas nonverbal functions tend to show a decline. This is reflected in the results of classical intelligence tests such as the Wechsler Adult Intelligence Scale (WAIS): up to age 75, there tend to be few or no changes on verbal subtests, such as vocabulary or arithmetic. In contrast, digit–symbol substitution, object assembly, and other performance subtests often show changes starting at age 60 (9). Performances on more detailed neuropsychological tests show that, in general, the most important changes involve attention (particularly divided attention), some visuospatial functions, and some processes involved in learning and remembering. A particular entity called ''benign senescent forgetfulness'' (10) or age-associated memory impairment (AAMI) (11) has been identified, although its nosologic significance is still not completely clarified.

Some authors (reviewed in ref. 12) have found, however, that when assessment is restricted to elderly subjects who are completely free of any disease, the effect of aging on cognitive functions appears to be minimal. Furthermore, it has been demonstrated that many of these subjects do not show a decrease in cerebral metabolism as shown by PET scan (13). In conclusion, it is important to stress that a major loss of memory and a sizable intellectual decline are not part of normal aging and represent clear indications for further work-up.

NEUROPSYCHOLOGICAL FINDINGS IN AD

Neuropsychological Assessment in Aging and Dementia

The examination techniques for elderly subjects do not differ from those used for the assessment of younger adults, except for some problems related to the very frequent impairment of sensory organs, particularly vision and hearing.

As for any disease, it is essential to obtain a thorough and detailed history. However, unlike patients with other diseases, the AD patient is often unable to provide such a history and it is therefore essential to obtain the information from an independent source, such as the spouse or another person well acquainted with the patient's past and present daily life. Following the important concepts included in DSM-III-R (14), one must note and rate the severity and the significance of the changes that have occurred. In addition, one must establish the nature of the first and subsequent symptoms and the time at which they occurred. Memory deficits are the most frequent early symptom, but there may also be other more ''focal'' presenting symptoms (see below).

Examination

A series of domains must be examined in each case, particularly when dementia is suspected. Provided below are some brief examples of questions to be asked, based mainly on the DSM-III-R (14).

Attention and orientation can be assessed by asking about time and place. The examiner will note the degree of concentration during the interview.

Attention can be estimated more formally with the letter cancellation test (15), in which subjects are shown a series of letters presented in one or more rows, with a designated target letter randomly interspersed among them. The task consists of crossing out all target letters (e.g., all Bs). The number of errors and the time used can both be taken into account.

Language and language-related functions are assessed mainly by carefully noting how the subject answers questions. Are the subject's words and sentences correct in terms of grammar and syntax? Does the subject's language present the richness and variety to be expected from his/her socioeconomic background? Can the subject recognize and name objects and parts of objects? Perform simple and complex commands? Sign his/her name, but also write a full sentence describing the weather or his/her occupation? Can the subject read, both aloud and showing that he/she has grasped the meaning of what he reads? Perform simple calculations (16)? Can the subject imitate gestures and demonstrate the use of objects (e.g., "show me how you use a comb")? One must also ascertain that the subject is able to recognize colors, faces, and to interpret complex pictures.

Visuospatial behavior can be tested by noting the subject's right–left orientation, by asking the subject to draw a simple picture [e.g., a clock face with numbers and hands showing 11:10 (17)] or to copy drawings such as a cube. One should also observe the subject's ability to orient him/herself on a map or to dress.

Memory, both short-term and long-term, can be tested, respectively, by asking the subject to repeat some information that was provided a few moments before (e.g., three common objects), or to provide data on well-known events (e.g., dates or sport and political events).

Reasoning and abstract abilities, judgment, and overall intellectual level are usually tested by asking subjects to interpret proverbs or to provide similarities and differences (e.g., "what is the difference between a bus and a truck?"). The best way to assess these abilities, however, is to see how subjects react to the crises, small and large, of everyday life (i.e., their capacity to judge and to adapt). To get reliable information on this specific point, it is usually indispensable to talk to a relative well acquainted with the patient.

"Frontal lobe" functions is the general term used for aspects of behavior that are responsible for the organization of other cognitive functions. These are assessed mainly through questions and observations about the appropriateness of mood and social habits, the level of motivation, the ability to plan ahead, and about sexual and eating behaviors. Observation of the types of answers given on tests that measure different cognitive functions gives a qualitative assessment of perseveration, vulnerability to interference, and difficulty in inhibiting inappropriate responses. Luria's three consecutive hand movements and copying of alternating m's and n's (or squares and triangles), and the go–no-go paradigm are tests of perseveration and of the ability to inhibit inappropriate response tendencies.

The Mini-Mental State Examination (MMSE) introduced by Folstein et al. (18) provides an easy, short, and reliable way of assessing cognitive functions. Scores range from 0 to 30. Actual scores must be weighed against the socioeconomic status and the age of the subject (19). It is important to be aware that the instructions provided with the original publications by Folstein and his group (18,20) are not complete and are sometimes equivocal. The most striking example is the choice left to the examiner between spelling "world" backwards and the "serial sevens" task. The different methods of administration that have come into use are therefore not always of comparable difficulty, and different scores and thresholds can be obtained (20–23).

Another useful and widely used tool for quantification of dementia is the Clinical Dementia Rating scale (CDR) (24), which is based on clinicians' global ratings of subjects according to their abilities. This scale ranges from 0 (unimpaired) to 3 (severely demented).

An interesting result of the coordination among the Alzheimer Disease Research Centers (ADRC) acreated by the National Institute on Aging has been the formation of the Consortium to Establish a Registry for Alzheimer's Disease (CERAD). The CERAD protocol (25) includes clinical assessment (requiring the administration of both the MMSE and the CDR) as well as a short standardized neuropsychological battery. It has been translated into several languages, and the French version is now in use in French-speaking Canada and in France. Although it has not yet been evaluated in therapeutic trials, the CERAD protocol would fulfill many of the requirements expected for such a use (26).

Changes Observed in AD

Early Stage

As mentioned above, the earliest sign of AD is often memory loss. Occasionally, however, the first sign is aphasia (27) or a visuospatial disorder (28). These asymmetrical clinical pictures of the early stage of the disease have been shown to be associated with corresponding asymmetries of cerebral metabolism (29). Their subsequent evolution and neuropathologic significance may sometimes differ from typical AD (30). The first sign may also be a personality change (irritability, apathy) or a picture that simulates a psychiatric disorder (depression, paranoid syndrome). There may also be other changes (e.g., striking sleep disorders, changes in appetite, disorders of gait, incontinence). These behavioral or noncognitive changes are infrequent as a presenting sign but are almost the rule in later stages of the disease. Even though they often contribute very significantly to the burden imposed on caregivers, these changes have received relatively little attention in the literature (31).

Middle Stage

In patients with early to middle stage AD (roughly corresponding to a CDR of 1 or 1–2), attention tends to be relatively maintained; if these are impaired, one should normally think in terms of delirium rather than dementia, particularly if the changes have occurred rapidly. On the other hand, orientation is almost universally impaired.

Language, as assessed by classical tests or batteries, is often said to be unimpaired in early AD, but careful testing often shows that in fact there is difficulty coming up with names and, in general, a paucity of thought and a simplification of phrase structure. On occasion language is much more strikingly impaired, even in the early phases of the disease. Mutism occurs universally in the later stages but can sometimes occur even in the early phase. This typically occurs in the early stages of Pick's disease, a condition even less well known than AD and encountered infrequently, at least in North America (32). Another characteristic of AD is the frequency of responses that do not fit the questions that have been asked, such as simple repetition of a command rather than its execution, writing "clock" when asked to draw a clock or commenting on the phrase presented rather than repeating it (33).

The performance of gestures on command or by imitation, and the demonstration of the use of objects, are often impaired in AD (34). Other disorders of gestures include motor impersistence, an inability to sustain simple acts such as keeping one's tongue protruded (35,36), and Lhermitte's utilization behavior, a tendency to manipulate and use every object seen or touched by the patient (37), probably seen more often in Pick's disease than in AD.

Visuospatial behavior is almost always impaired, even in the early phases of AD. It may be one of the reasons for the tendency to wander and get lost, often seen (and dreaded) by the patient's family.

Memory impairment is, of course, the presenting symptom in the majority of cases of AD. It is characterized clinically by inability to learn new material of whatever kind and by difficulty recalling previously learned material. In fact, the diagnosis of "probable AD" (1) can hardly be justified in the absence of a memory disorder. Experimental studies indicate that even though memory for old events often appears to be less impaired, it is nevertheless also affected. Current research has shown that memory deficits in AD are actually the product of several different processes (38–40), some of which are more impaired than others. Nevertheless, it can be stated that in AD the deficit is particularly severe, affecting even recognition of recently learned material. Although this is not pathognomonic for AD, it differs from what is found in normal aging and in some other dementia-producing diseases, such as Huntington's disease.

Overall intellectual abilities, as measured by standard batteries such as the WAIS, show a marked decline in AD, characterizing the passage from an early (amnestic) to a later (demented) stage of the disease. One often finds a striking dissociation between verbal abilities, which are relatively preserved, and nonverbal abilities (as measured by the performance scale of the WAIS). In some cases, however, verbal abilities are more impaired.

Late Stages

The classical neuropsychological tests used in AD tend to lose their utility in the more advanced stages of the disease because performance often "bottoms out" (i.e., it can no longer be measured by tests that have been designed for moderately impaired patients). Researchers from the Pittsburgh ADRC (41) have recently described a "Severe Impairment Battery" (SIB) which allows quantifiable evaluation of the cognitive deficits typically seen in severely impaired patients. The battery, which is also used in other countries, particularly Italy and France (42,43), requires only 20 or 30 min to administer and is designed to resemble an interview rather than an actual test. Credit can be given for nonverbal and partially correct responses. The SIB enables the examiner to assess attention, orientation, language, memory, visuoperception, and constructional abilities. In addition, there is an assessment of social skills, praxis, and responding/orienting to name. Possible scores range from 0 to 133. Figure 1 shows that the results of the SIB for 15 patients with

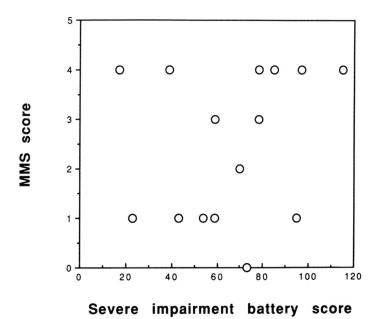

Severe impairment battery score

FIG. 1. Scores at the Mini-Mental State Examination (MMS) and at the Severe Impairment Battery for 15 subjects with probable Alzheimer disease and with MMS below 5. Data derived from (41).

MMSE scores of less than 5 have a wide range, which presumably allows documentation of worsening or improvement of cognition. Results thus far show that on a follow-up extending over a period of 1 year, the SIB demonstrated that even at the later stages of the disease AD patients show an important variability in their cognitive performances. The SIB was also able to show a deterioration in all cognitive domains. Orientation, praxis, and memory were the most affected, whereas social interactions were better preserved (43).

There are several advantages of such a battery. By highlighting preserved abilities, the SIB can provide information relevant to the subject's placement in a care facility. It can also provide cognitive data closer in time to neuropathologic examination, thus giving more meaning to clinicopathologic correlations. In addition, by allowing quantification of changes in ways not possible before, the SIB opens the way to therapeutic trials extended to more severely affected patients.

Prognosis: Markers of Fast Decline in AD

In a recent study by Boller et al. (44), we compared probable AD patients who had deteriorated rapidly to a group that had deteriorated much more slowly. At the time of the initial visit, there was no statistical difference between the two groups in the severity of dementia or, interestingly, in age. We compared the predictive value of verbal, nonverbal, and attention tasks and found that performance on verbal tests, particularly on naming tasks, was the best predictor of cognitive decline, even after the influence of the overall degree of dementia had been accounted for. If confirmed, this finding indicates that the physician has a way of meaningfully answering the questions always asked by the families (and sometimes by the patients themselves) concerning prognosis for the time of occurrence of major events, such as loss of competency or death. In addition, in therapeutic trials, particularly if they are protracted, knowledge that the natural course differs from patient to patient and can be estimated in each case would constitute a considerable advantage. In patients with rapid decline, a significant slowing of deterioration would represent a major therapeutic success (45).

Neuropsychological Tests and Therapeutic Trials

A number of specific problems are associated with the neuropsychological assessment of patients entered into therapeutic trials or into prospective studies. The main problems are related to their test–retest reliability, i.e., with the learning and the familiarization effects of the tests used. Such effects have been shown to be a particular feature of tests that have a large speed component, require an unfamiliar or infrequently practiced mode of response, and have a single solution (particularly if it is easily conceptualized once it is attained) (46,47). Interestingly, it has also been shown that in the elderly population cognitive impairment makes performance sensitive to repetition (48). Study designs such as "crossover" placebo–drug trials can alleviate this effect, and the use of different equivalent versions of the same test, or obtaining the maximal performance at baseline by repetitive administrations of the same tests (49,50), can also help to control of these effects.

Another problem is related to the fact that improvement during therapeutic trials is likely to be subtle, and therefore may require large multicenter, placebo-controlled, double-blind studies to arrive at objective results (7).

One additional problem is finding tests that establish a meaningful relationship between the test results and the clinical outcome as perceived by the patients and their families (and can therefore be considered "ecological"). In a few therapeutic trials of AD, behavioral scales have been used in conjunction with conventional neuropsychological tests (50,51). In many of these studies, an improvement was noted only on behavioral scales. There are several potential reasons for a possible discrepancy between neuropsychological test results obtained in the laboratory and clinical improvement as perceived by the families. First of all, each patient and each family have different expectations concerning the outcome of treatment. Second, families are often more disturbed by the noncognitive changes mentioned earlier and not taken into account by the tests. Finally, the neuropsychological tests used to determine the outcome may not be sufficiently related to the patients' activities of daily living (ADL). Results from research in progress at the Pittsburgh ADRC (Saxton J, personal communication) show data relevant to this issue. ADL are usefully divided into instrumental and physical ADL. Examples of instrumental ADL include use of the telephone, ability to shop, do housework, or take one's medications. On the other hand, physical ADL refer to routine overlearned activities such as eating, dressing, walking, or taking a bath. Not surprisingly, instrumental ADL decline faster than physical ADL. During investigation of which neuropsychological test was the best predictor of ADL competence, it was found that the best predictors were reaction times, ability to draw, visual form discrimination, and facial recognition. The common feature of all these tests is that they are nonverbal. This stands in contrast to some of the most commonly used tests: for example, in the MMSE the verbal component comprises a very sizeable portion of the test. The results of the Pittsburgh study emphasize the need to include a greater number of nonverbal tests than is usually the case among the tests used to assess the efficacy of therapeutic attempts.

ACKNOWLEDGMENT

This research was supported in part by funds from the Institut National de la Santé et de la Recherche Médicale (INSERM), by a grant from the

Medical Research Council of Canada/Canadian Alzheimer Society/Price Daxion (Dr. Panisset), and by grants AG05133 and AG03705 from the National Institutes of Health, National Institute on Aging, Bethesda, Maryland. Catherine Tzortzis and Gianfranco Dalla Barba provided useful suggestions for the manuscript.

REFERENCES

1. McKhann G, Drachman D, Folstein M, Katzman R, Price D, Stadlan EM. Clinical diagnosis of Alzheimer's disease: report of the NINCDS-ADRDA Work Group under the auspices of the Department of Health and Human Services Task Force on Alzheimer's Disease. *Neurology* 1984;34:939–44.
2. Huff FJ, Becker JT, Belle SH, Nebes R, Holland A, Boller F. Cognitive deficits and diagnosis of Alzheimer's Disease. *Neurology* 1987;37:1119–24.
3. Forette F, Henry JF, Orgogozo JM, et al. The reliability of clinical criteria for the diagnosis of dementia: a longitudinal multicentric study. *Arch Neurol* 1989;46:646–8.
4. Pirozzolo FJ, Baskin DS, Swihart AA, Appel SH. Oral tetrahydroaminoacridine in the treatment of senile dementia, Alzheimer's type. *N Engl J Med* 1987;316:1603.
5. Thal LJ. Pharmacological treatment of memory disorders. In: Boller F, Grafman J, eds. *Handbook of neuropsychology.* Amsterdam: Elsevier; 1989:247–67.
6. Boller F, Forette F. Alzheimer's disease and THA: a review of the cholinergic theory and of preliminary results. *Biomed Pharmacother* 1989;43:487–91.
7. Forette F, Panisset M, Boller F. Clinical trials in cognitive impairment of the elderly. *Aging* 1992;4:239–50.
8. Becker JT, Nebes R, Boller F. Neuropsychologie du vieillissement. In: Botez, MI, ed. *Neuropsychologie clinique et neurologie du comportement.* Paris: Masson & Presse Universitaire du Québec; 1987:371–9.
9. Hochanadel G, Kaplan E. Neuropsychology of normal aging. In: Albert ML, ed. *Clinical neurology of aging.* Lexington, MA: Lexington Books; 1984:121–32.
10. Kral VA. Senescent forgetfulness: benign and malignant. *J Can Med Assoc* 1962;86:257–60.
11. Crook T, Bartus RT, Ferris SH, Whitehouse P, Cohen GD, Gershon S. Age-associated memory impairment: proposed diagnostic criteria and measures of clinical change. Report of a National Institute of Mental Health work group. *Dev Neuropsychol* 1986;2:261–76.
12. Albert MS. Cognitive function. In: Albert MS, Moss MB, eds. *Geriatric neuropsychology.* New York: The Guilford Press; 1988:33–53.
13. Creasey H, Schwartz M, Frederickson H, Haxby J, Rapoport S. Quantitative computed tomography in dementia of the Alzheimer type. *Neurology* 1986;36:1563–8.
14. American Psychiatric Association. *Diagnostic and statistical manual of mental disorders.* 3rd ed. revised. Washington, DC: American Psychiatric Association; 1987.
15. Talland GA, Schwab RS. Performance with multiple sets in Parkinson's disease. *Neuropsychologia* 1964;2:45–53.
16. Parlato E, Lopez O, Panisset M, Iavarone A, Grafman J, Boller, F. Calculation disorders in Alzheimer's disease. *Int J Geriatr Psychiatry* 1992;7:599–602.
17. Ganansia–Ganem A, Parlato V, Tzortzis C. Visuo-spatial ability in aging [Abstract]. *Ital J Neurol Sci* 1991;12(suppl 5):49.
18. Folstein MF, Folstein SE, McHugh PR. "Mini Mental State" a practical method for grading the cognitive state of patients for the clinician. *J Psychiatr Res* 1975;12:189–98.
19. Bleeker ML, Bolla–Wilson K, Kawas C, Agnew J. Age-specific norms for the Mini-Mental State Exam. *Neurology* 1988;38:1565–8.
20. Anthony JC, LeResche L, Niaz U, Von Körff MR, Folstein MF. Limits of the MMS as a screening test for dementia and delirium among hospital patients. *Psychol Med* 1982;12:397–408.
21. Gagnon M, Letenneur L, Dartigues JF, et al. Validity of the Mini-Mental State Examination as a screening instrument for cognitive impairment and dementia in French elderly community residents. *Neuroepidemiology* 1990;9:143–50.

22. Ganguli M, Ratcliff G, Huff J, et al. Serial seven versus world backwards: a comparison of the two measures of attention from the MMSE. *J Geriatr Psychiatr Neurol* 1990;3:203–7.
23. Tzortzis C, Boller F. Le "Mini Mental State": interêt et limites d'un test d'évaluation rapide des fonctions cognitives. *Rev Neuropsychol* 1991;1:55–71.
24. Berg L. Clinical dementia rating (CDR). *Psychopharmacol Bull* 1988;24:637–9.
25. Morris JC, Heyman A, Mohs RC, et al. The Consortium to Establish a Registry for Alzheimer's Disease (CERAD). Part I. Clinical and neuropsychological assessment of Alzheimer's disease. *Neurology* 1989;39:1159–65.
26. Jarvik LF, Berg L, Bartus R. Clinical drug trials in Alzheimer disease. What are some of the issues. *Alzheimer Dis Assoc Disord* 1990;4:193–202.
27. Kirshner H, Webb W, Kelly M, Wells CE. Language disturbance: an initial symptom of cortical degeneration and dementia. *Arch Neurol* 1984;41:491–6.
28. Saxton JA, Keefe NC, Ratcliff GG, Boller F. Different presentations of early dementias. In: Wurtman RJ, Corkin SH, Growdon JH, eds. *Alzheimer's disease: advances in basic research and therapies. Proceedings of the Third Meeting of the International Study Group on the treatment of memory disorders associated with aging.* Zurich, Switzerland: 1984.
29. Foster NL, Chase TH, Fedio P, Patronas NJ, Brooks RA, Di Chiro G. Alzheimer's disease: focal cortical changes shown by positron emission tomography. *Neurology* 1983;33:961–5.
30. Mesulam M-M, Weintraub S. Relatively focal cortical degenerations. In: Boller F, Grafman J, eds. *Handbook of neuropsychology,* vol 8. Amsterdam: Elsevier; 1993:251–80.
31. Absher JR, Cummings J. Noncognitive behavioral alterations in dementia syndromes. In: Boller F, Grafman J, eds. *Handbook of neuropsychology,* vol 8. Amsterdam: Elsevier; 1993:313–36.
32. Morris JC, Cole M, Banker BQ, Wright D. Hereditary dysphasic dementia and the Pick–Alzheimer spectrum. *Ann Neurol* 1984;16:455–66.
33. Holland A, Boller F, Bourgeois M. Repetition in Alzheimer's disease: a longitudinal study. *J Neurolinguist* 1986;2:163–77.
34. Lucchelli F, Lopez O, Faglioni P, Boller F. Ideational apraxia in Alzheimer's disease. *Int J Geriatr Psychiatry* 1993 (in press).
35. Lopez OL, Becker JT, Boller F. Motor impersistence in Alzheimer's disease. *Cortex* 1991; 27:93–9.
36. Neuman E, Boller F. Etude neuropsychologique de l'impersistance motrice dans la maladie d'Alzheimer. *Rev Neuropsychol* 1992;2:207–25.
37. Lhermitte F, Pillon B, Serdaru M. Human autonomy and the frontal lobes. *Ann Neurol* 1986;19:326–34.
38. Boller F, Deweer B. Les troubles de mémoire dans les démences. In: Vander Linden M, Bruyer R, eds. *Neuropsychologie de la mémoire humaine.* Grenoble, St. Hyacinthe, Québec: Presses Universitaires de Grenoble & Edisem; 1991:89–107.
39. Shimamura AP. Disorders of memory; the cognitive science perspective. In Boller F, Grafman J, eds. *Handbook of neuropsychology.* Amsterdam: Elsevier; 1989:35–73.
40. Dalla Barba G, Boller F. Alzheimer's disease. *Curr Opin Neurol Neurosurg* 1991;4:80–5.
41. Saxton J, McGonigle–Gibson K, Swihart A, Miller M, Boller F. Assessment of the severely impaired patient: description and validation of a new neuropsychological test battery. *Psychol Assess J Consult Clin Psychol* 1990;2:298–303.
42. Parlato V, Galeone F, Iavarone A, Colombo A, Carlomagno S, Bonavita V. The Italian version of the Severe Impairment Battery for demented patients [Abstract]. *Ital J Neurol Sci* 1991;12(suppl 5):49.
43. Panisset M, Roudier M, Saxton J, Boller F. Validation d'une batterie d'évaluation neuropsychologique pour des patients avec démence grave. *La Presse Méd* 1992;27:1271–4.
44. Boller F, Holland A, Forbes M, Hood P, McGonigle–Gibson K, Becker JT. Predictors of decline in Alzheimer's disease. *Cortex* 1991;27:9–17.
45. Ferris SH. Therapeutic strategies in dementia disorders. *Acta Neurol Scand* 1990;82(suppl 129):23–6.
46. Quereshi MY. The comparability of WAIS and WISC subtest scores and IQ estimates. *J Psychol* 1968;68:73–82.
47. Dodrill CB, Troupin AS. Effects of repeated administration of a comprehensive neuropsychological battery among chronic epileptics. *J Nerv Ment Dis* 1975;161:185–90.
48. Lehman HE, Ban TA, Kral VA. Psychological tests: practice effect in geriatric patients. *Geriatrics* 1968;23:160–3.

49. Peters BH, Levin HS. Effects of physostigmine and lecithin on memory in Alzheimer's disease. *Ann Neurol* 1979;6:219–21.
50. Etienne P, Dastoor D, Gauthier S, Ludwick R, Collier B. Alzheimer's disease: lack of effect of lecithin treatment for 3 months. *Neurology* 1981;31:1552–4.
51. Gauthier S, Bouchard R, Lamontagne A, et al. Tetrahydroaminoacridine–lecithin combination treatment in patients with intermediate stage Alzheimer's disease. *N Engl J Med* 1990; 322:1272–6.

Guidelines for Drug Trials in Memory Disorders, edited by N. Canal, et al. Raven Press, Ltd., New York © 1993.

29

Issues of Design and Assessment May Affect the Determination of Efficacy in Cholinergic Treatment Studies in Alzheimer Disease

Brian A. Lawlor and *Bonnie M. Davis

*Section on Old Age Psychiatry, Department of Psychiatry, University of Dublin, Dublin, Ireland; and *Department of Psychiatry, Mount Sinai School of Medicine, New York, New York 10029-6574*

Despite the many theories about the etiology and pathogenesis of Alzheimer disease (AD), the cholinergic hypothesis remains at the forefront of the experimental therapeutics of this common and devastating illness. Post-mortem studies of Alzheimer brains demonstrate significant decreases in cortical cholinergic markers, together with loss of neurons in the nucleus basalis of Meynert (nbM), the principal cholinergic projection to the cortex from the basal forebrain (1,2). These findings, in addition to the wealth of pharmacologic and animal data supporting the importance of the cholinergic system in normal memory function (3,4), have led to continued support for the development of cholinomimetic agents that can definitively assess whether enhancement of cholinergic function can produce meaningful symptomatic improvement in AD.

In the past decade, many different cholinergic agents have been tried, including precursor agents, postsynaptic agonists, and cholinesterase inhibitors. To date, only the cholinesterase inhibitors have produced positive findings which have withstood the test of time and replication (5–7). However, the modest beneficial cognitive effects of these agents have been of doubtful clinical significance, and may occur only in a subgroup of patients.

The ideal agent to test the cholinergic hypothesis of AD may not be developed. Many of the drugs studied to date have unfavorable bioavailability characteristics, such as variable absorption and short half-life, poor brain penetration, and the occurrence of problematic side effects at doses that are too low to produce adequate central cholinesterase inhibition (3).

If we can assume that in the near future a more ideal cholinergic agent will be available to us, and that enhancement of central cholinergic transmission will improve cognition in at least a subpopulation of AD sufferers, certain issues that relate to the design and assessment of therapeutic trials in AD remain problematic and could affect whether or not a cholinergic agent can be shown to be efficacious. These issues are discussed in this chapter from the perspective of how they might be addressed in future clinical trials of cholinergic and other agents in AD.

POSSIBLE NEUROCHEMICAL HETEROGENEITY OF AD

In the older psychiatric nosology, presenile dementia and senile dementia were treated as two separate and distinct diseases, on the basis of clinical features and course. Presenile dementia (onset before 65 years) was characterized by prominent aphasia, apraxia, extrapyramidal features, and behavioral disturbance, with a more rapid course (8,9) in comparison with senile dementia, which was typified by a more pedestrian rate of progression and primarily by memory loss.

These different subtypes of AD may have different underlying neurotransmitter deficits. For instance, it has been suggested that the younger cases have a more widespread involvement of different neurotransmitter systems, including the noradrenergic and serotonergic, in addition to the cholinergic. Patients dying before age 80 have significantly greater brain norepinephrine losses (up to one-half the brain norepinephrine levels) (10) and greater locus coeruleus cell count losses (11,12) than those dying after 80. Furthermore, younger patients appear to have greater serotonergic GABAergic and noradrenergic deficits than do the older-onset patients, who reportedly suffer from a more pure "cholinergic" deficit (13). Interestingly, younger patients also have significantly greater losses of cells in the nbM and greater decreases in cholinergic markers than older patients; therefore, this neurochemical difference may not represent a difference in neurotransmitter deficits in younger versus older subjects but simply a more severe illness. A major question revolves around what constitutes early versus late-onset cases, because the only neuropathologic correlate addressing this question refers to onset at age 71 compared with onset at age 75.

Recent animal work that has attempted to model combined cholinergic/ noradrenergic, and cholinergic/serotonergic lesions suggests that although physostigmine can reverse the cognitive impairment produced by an nbM (cholinergic) lesion in the rat, physostigmine alone cannot improve the memory impairment when the animal has both a cholinergic/serotonergic and a cholinergic/noradrenergic lesion (14). Interestingly, noradrenergic or serotonergic lesions on their own do not produce learning impairment. The same conditions could operate in patients with AD: if there is a combined cholinergic/noradrenergic (or serotonergic) lesion, then a cholinergic strategy alone may fail because of the presence of a second neurotransmitter deficit.

Therefore, in a given sample of AD patients in a clinical trial, a cholinergic agent may not demonstrate efficacy in the group as a whole because of heterogeneous brain neurochemical changes in the group, but could be effective in a subgroup of patients who have a relatively pure cholinergic lesion. If this subgroup of responders exists, they might be differentiated on the basis of age of onset, illness duration, family history, clinical features, or by more biologic attributes such as cerebral blood flow pattern on single photon emission computed tomography (SPECT) or metabolic pattern on positron-emission tomography (PET) or, more simplistically, on the basis of whether they demonstrate a favorable response to a cholinomimetic. The currently available post-mortem data seem to indicate that older patients are more likely to respond to monotherapy with a cholinergic agent.

The recent multicenter tetrahydroaminacridine (THA) study may serve as a useful illustration of this point. In that study, 30–40% of patients showed a best dose, and approximately one third of patients demonstrated some beneficial effects during the replication phase. This multicenter patient population was composed of a heterogenous group of patients with onset >65 years and <65 years. One of the factors that could account for the finding that only a subgroup of patients show a beneficial response could be neurotransmitter heterogeneity, possibly defined by age of onset. Perhaps one of the most interesting secondary analyses of this large multicenter study could be the provision of further information on this interesting question.

CLINICAL HETEROGENEITY DEFINED BY RATE OF PROGRESSION

Another clinically heterogeneous subgroup of AD patients may exist that is defined by a variable rate of progression (15–17). In the group of patients identified by Berg with a slow progression rate, age of onset was variable and no clinical factors were clearly associated with slow rate of progression. Other studies have suggested that the presence of extrapyramidal symptoms or psychosis is associated with a more malignant course (17,18). As yet, no distinct neurobiology has been identified for those with slow or rapid progression. Furthermore, the majority of studies to date have not confirmed that onset before age 65 predicts a more rapid progression rate, and the finding that psychosis or behavioral symptoms influence rate of progression is not entirely consistent among studies.

If one accepts the fact that patients with AD can have very variable progression rates, problems could arise when a large sample of AD patients under study with an experimental agent is composed of different groups of patients, some of which progress at a very slow rate. The ''benign'' group may appear to respond to an experimental treatment when in reality they have not shown the expected progression over time. Much more needs to be known about the progression characteristics of study populations so that this aspect of variance can be identified and statistically adjusted for in treatment studies.

It will be interesting to examine the results of the recent multicenter trials with THA and HPO29 with these issues in mind, to determine whether these studies provide support for the thesis of heterogeneity of AD response and shed light on the clinical and other characteristics of responders versus nonresponders. If responders to THA or HPO29 have a particular profile (e.g., late age of onset), this would support the hypothesis of subtypes of responders and would generate interest in studies that may enrich the sample by including only patients who are likely to respond to that particular agent. It may also allow further study of the group of nonresponders to determine why they do not respond, and thus provide the impetus for studies on combination approaches in this subgroup. Along this line of thinking, a very preliminary report which studied the postural blood pressure decreases as a predictor of short-term drug response to the cholinesterase inhibitor HPO29 recently indicated that nonresponders to cholinomimetic therapy have greater pretreatment postural changes in blood pressure, suggesting that nonresponse may be linked to the presence of a noradrenergic deficit, in addition to the cholinergic dysfunction (19).

CONSOLIDATION OF MEMORY BY CHOLINESTERASE INHIBITORS AND THE CARRYOVER EFFECT

The issue of carryover effects in treatment trials of AD, particularly in relationship to cholinergic agents, may be an important factor in the determination of efficacy or the lack thereof in these studies. Anecdotally, investigators in this field have remarked that the beneficial effects of cholinesterase inhibitors are often best seen on first exposure in the "dose finding" phase and are not repeated on further treatment in the replication phase. Although carryover effects may be relevant to any pharmacologic agent in an AD trial, the effects of cholinesterase inhibitors on memory may have special implications for carryover effects. Why is this?

Cholinesterase inhibitors enhance consolidation in animals and humans within minutes, and this new learning remains accessible for an extended period of time without cholinergic influence. This can be demonstrated in animal and human experiments. For example, in nbM-lesioned animals tested on a passive avoidance task, improved learning is still apparent up to 3 days later, when the cholinesterase inhibitor is no longer present (14,20). In this passive avoidance paradigm, rats are shocked when they enter a dark compartment. Sixty seconds later they are given injections of physostigmine or saline. Testing occurs 72 h later. At this time, rats given physostigmine stay out of the dark compartment twice as long as rats given saline, despite the fact that there is no physostigmine in the animal at 72 h. Thus, the physostigmine "consolidated" the information, and once fixed in the memory engrams, it could be demonstrated 3 days later. Similarly, using a Morris Swim Maze task, when nbM-lesioned animals are treated with galanthamine, a long-acting cholinesterase inhibitor, 3.5 h before training, when tested 24 h later they can find the platform more quickly than after saline placebo (21).

Studies in humans also indicate that cholinesterase inhibitors such as physostigmine can enhance storage in long-term memory in cognitively intact young volunteers using a selective reminding task (22). These studies in animals and humans provide an explanation of how cholinergic treatment could affect test results at a point distant from treatment (i.e., during the placebo phase). It is therefore possible that testing performed during a placebo period after active drug treatment is contaminated by information learned during the treatment with cholinomimetic, thereby making it more difficult to demonstrate a drug/placebo difference.

Cholinergic dysfunction, as modeled by anticholinergic agents in normals, and as exists in AD patients (1,3,23,24), does not appear to affect the rate of forgetting in either normal volunteers or mildly affected AD patients (25,26). Although picture recognition differs between normal controls and AD patients at 10 min, retention at 24 h and at 7 days was proportional to that learned at 10 min, indicating problems in acquisition of information in AD subjects, but a normal rate of forgetting (25). Similar findings operate in complex figure and story passage recall (27). In a study where AD patients were allowed extended exposure time to test material to bring them up to a par with normal controls, AD patients had normal rates of forgetting (26). Thus, although mildly affected Alzheimer patients (these are the patients most often included in studies) have difficulty in acquiring information, with prolonged exposure time learning occurs, and the rate of forgetting of this information is no different than that of controls (28). Furthermore, one might expect that if cholinesterase inhibitors are effective in the acquisition and consolidation process, treatment with these agents, if effective in AD, would tend to normalize these defective processes.

The mechanism of memory consolidation of cholinesterase inhibitors, and the defect in acquisition but relatively normal retrieval in mild to moderately affected AD subjects, have a number of implications for current treatment trials and the use of psychological assessment instruments in these studies. An examination of recently completed cholinesterase treatment studies with THA provide some useful illustrations of how these issues may affect the determination of efficacy.

Dose-finding Studies

Many of the studies presently being carried out with cholinesterase inhibitors in AD use an "enrichment" paradigm, where patients first enter a dose-finding phase, and then a replication phase in which those that demonstrated a best dose receive that dose compared to placebo, or other comparison treatment condition, in a crossover design. A refinement of this design is to randomize best dose responders to either their best dose or placebo in a parallel design replication phase. Enrichment strategies have been championed because of the animal and human literature that has clearly demonstrated that there is a U-shaped curve in terms of response to cholinesterase inhibitors such as physostigmine; at low dose and at high dose, patients do not respond or actually worsen (29). Therefore, the idea behind the dose finding is that it will identify the dose at which that patient is most likely to respond. In the dose-finding phase, patients are typically exposed to at least two different doses of active drug and placebo for anything from 2 to 3 days up to 1 to 2 weeks. Best dose is defined as the dose on which a particular criterion defined a priori is attained or the dose associated with the best performance on cognitive testing compared with placebo. The problem with dose-finding paradigms has been that many patients do not demonstrate a best dose, and in studies where best dose has been defined in a dose-finding phase but all patients (those showing a best dose and those failing to demonstrate a best dose) have been entered into the replication phase, the best dose did not necessarily predict response or nonresponse in the replication phase (30).

Because of the potential influence of prior exposure to drug on consolidation processes and the temporally remote effects that prior treatment could have on future test scores, dose-finding paradigms could be particularly susceptible to carryover effects. In the dose-finding phase itself, one could surmise that if the patient were exposed to active drug first, the carryover effect might decrease the likelihood of showing a significant difference from placebo. If this were the case, the proportion of patients demonstrating a best dose should be less in those randomized to active drug first (where there could be a carryover effect), compared with those randomized to placebo first, where one would not expect carryover effects. Rapid 2-week cycles of different doses of active drug and placebo are unlikely to show clear results in terms of efficacy because of the potential for carryover effects.

For example, in the multicenter THA trial, 632 patients received two doses of THA (40 and 80 mg) and placebo in one of three possible titration sequences (40–80–placebo; placebo–40–80; 40–placebo–80). The duration of exposure to each titration sequence was 2 weeks. Interestingly, the best dose rate was 46% when placebo was given first followed by 40 and 80 mg of THA, as opposed to 35% when 40 mg of THA was given first followed by placebo and 80 mg of THA, and 40% when THA 40 and 80 mg was followed by placebo. The different best dose rates for the various titration sequences is suggestive of a carryover effect of prior exposure to active drug. Thus, one potential confounding aspect of the carryover effect is that it may actually decrease the ability of the study to demonstrate a responder, and the "enrichment paradigm,'' in its present form, may actually be having the opposite effect.

Crossover Studies

The two recently completed international studies with THA are also helpful in elaborating on the issue of potential carryover. The Groupe Francais Study (31) administered THA to 60 subjects in a crossover design. One-half of the subjects received 1 month of THA followed by 1 month of placebo, and half received placebo followed by THA. No overall drug effect compared with placebo was reported in the study. However, the two placebo phases differed in that in one placebo phase patients had never been exposed to drug (''true'' placebo), and in the other phase patients had just completed an active drug condition. When the scores for both groups are compared, those who received placebo first followed by active drug showed consistent improvement across all measures compared with those who received active drug followed by placebo, in whom consistent drug effects were not seen, suggesting a potential carryover effect of THA treatment on post-THA placebo scores. To avoid the effect of carryover, a more correct analysis is to compare each group's first treatment phase. When only the parallel data are compared, THA appears to produce consistent improvement in comparison with placebo.

Potential carryover effects are further indicated by the fact that when the two placebo phases are compared (''true'' placebo and placebo following 4 week withdrawal of THA), it is clear that placebo treatment after 4 weeks of THA produced more consistent improvement over baseline than did ''true'' placebo (no prior THA exposure). The end result is that it is difficult to show a significant drug difference over placebo in these studies, possibly because of carryover effects.

Similar conditions may also operate in the interpretation of a recent Canadian study with THA (30,32). In this study, 46 patients were entered into a dose-finding phase of 2 weeks placebo followed by four 2-week treatment epochs of escalating doses of THA, ending with a 4-week washout period. After the dose-finding phase, all patients entered a double-blind crossover treatment of random assignment to 8 weeks of THA or placebo separated by a 4-week washout. Thus, the entire length of this study was 38 weeks.

The 4-week washout period after the dose finding allows some assessment of the duration of THA's effects. After a 4-week washout Mini-Mental State Examination (MMSE) scores had not returned to normal and still exceeded baseline, even when the decay factor had not been taken into consideration. Thus, it would appear that the THA effect persists at 4 weeks after withdrawal of the drug. In the crossover phase, as in the French study, patients with immediate prior exposure to THA had reduced differences between test scores on THA and subsequent placebo, possibly leading to an underestimation of the drug effect seen in patients in the alternate sequence who had received placebo first.

Crossover designs can therefore produce two inherent problems that can influence outcome measures. The first issue is that there is an inadequate washout period, and that the drug is still present during the second phase of the study. This issue can be addressed by lengthening the duration of the washout period to make sure that there is no drug present. The second problem posed by the crossover design is not as easy to remedy. The first treatment period may have produced effects that mean that the subject is no longer in a similar physiologic or psychological state during treatment in the second phase, i.e., the carryover effect (33). The only way to adequately address this issue of design is to avoid the crossover design and opt for the parallel design or, if crossover effects are of concern, to enter enough patients into the study to allow a direct comparison of treatments 1 and 2 using the first phase of the study (in other words, to use a crossover design but utilize only the parallel portion for the analysis).

ASSESSMENT INSTRUMENTS

Many of the assessment tools that are currently being utilized in dose-finding and replication phases of cholinergic trials, such as the Alzheimer Disease Assessment Scale (ADAS) (34) and the MMSE (35), do not have multiple forms, and much of the information on these instruments does not change between administration. With repeated exposure, AD patients could certainly show learning effects from previous and repeated exposure, further adding to any carryover effect.

Thus, there may be two factors operating in these studies where it is difficult to see a difference between drug and placebo conditions: carryover effects from active drug treatment and learning effects following repeated exposure to test material. This learning effect may be less evident in tests with multiple forms or more complex tasks.

CONCLUSIONS

The existence of clinical and neurochemical heterogeneity in AD may mean that drug effects could be hidden by subgroups of responders and nonresponders. One of the real scientific values of the ongoing studies with cholinergic-specific agents is that the results of these studies may support the existence of pharmacological subtypes of AD.

Further consideration must also be given to the issues of potential carryover effects and repeated exposure to cognitive tests in future studies with cholinergic and other agents in Alzheimer's disease. It is unclear whether "enrichment strategies" accomplish their goal or are, in fact, counterproductive. A best dose would be more appropriately defined pharmacokinetically, without earlier exposure in a dose-finding paradigm that clouds the findings in a replication phase.

There appear to be contentious issues with a crossover design, given the ability of cholinergic agents to consolidate information that may not be forgotten for a time period that extends well into the placebo phase. Parallel designs, or a crossover design that enables one to compare a "true" placebo to a post-drug placebo phase, would be more appropriate. Finally, because of potential learning effects by AD subjects on simple tests that do not have multiple forms, further studies need to be conducted to measure the effect of learning by AD patients on these instruments, and how much this "practice" effect could potentially decrease drug–placebo differences during the course of a clinical trial.

REFERENCES

1. Davies P, Maloney AJ. Selective loss of central cholinergic neurons in Alzheimer's disease. *Lancet* 1976;2:1403.
2. Whitehouse PJ, Price DL, Struble RG, Clark AW, Coyle JT, DeLeon MR. Alzheimer's disease and senile dementia: loss of neurons in the basal forebrain. *Science* 1982;215:1237–9.
3. Drachman DA, Leavitt J. Human memory and the cholinergic system. *Arch Neurol* 1974; 30:113–21.
4. Bartus R, Dean R, Beer B, Lapp AS. The cholinergic hypothesis of geriatric memory dysfunction. *Science* 1982;217:400–17.
5. Giacobini E, Becker R. Present progress and future development in the therapy of Alzheimer's disease. *Prog Neuropsychopharmacol Biol Psychiatry* 1989;13:1121–54.
6. David KL, Mohs RC. Enhancement of memory processes in Alzheimer's disease with multiple dose intravenous physostigmine. *Am J Psychiatry* 1982;139:1421–4.
7. Mohs RC, Davis BM, Johns CA, et al. Oral physostigmine treatment of patients with Alzheimer's disease. *Am J Psychiatry* 1985;142:28–33.
8. Sjogren T, Sjogren H, Lindgren AGH. Morbus Alzheimer and morbus Pick. *Acta Psychiatr Scand Suppl* 1952;1–115.
9. Sim M, Sussman I. Alzheimer's disease: its natural history and differential diagnosis. *J Nerv Ment Dis* 1962;135:489–99.
10. Rossor MN, Iversen LL, Reynolds GP, Mountjoy CQ, Roth M. Neurochemical characteristics of early and late onset types of Alzheimer's disease. *BMJ* 1984;288:961–4.
11. Bondareff W, Mountjoy CQ, Roth M. Loss of neurons of origin of the adrenergic projection to cerebral cortex (nucleus locus ceruleus) in senile dementia. *Neurology* 1982;32:164–8.
12. Roth M. Evidence on the possible heterogeneity of Alzheimer's disease and its bearing on future inquiries into etiology and treatment. In: Butler RN, Bearn AG, eds. *The aging process: therapeutic implications.* New York: Raven Press; 1985:251–71.
13. Francis PT, Palmer AM, Sims NR, et al. Neurochemical studies of early-onset Alzheimer's disease: possible influence on treatment. *N Engl J Med* 1985;313:7–11.
14. Haroutunian V, Kanof PD, Tsuboyama G, Davis KL. Restoration of cholinomimetic activity by clonidine in cholinergic plus noradrenergic lesioned rats. *Brain Res* 1990;507:261–6.
15. Berg L, Hughes CP, Coben LA, Danziger WL, Martin RL. Mile senile dementia of Alzheimer type: research diagnostic criteria recruitment, and description of a study population. *J Neurol Neurosurg Psychiatry* 1982;45:962–8.
16. Berg L, Danziger WL, Storandt M, et al. Predictive features in mild senile dementia of the Alzheimer type. *Neurology* 1984;34:563–9.
17. Mayeux R, Stern Y, Spanton S. Heterogeneity in dementia of the Alzheimer type: evidence in subgroups. *Neurology* 1985;35:453–61.

18. Drevets WC, Rubin EH. Psychotic symptoms and the longitudinal course of senile dementia of the Alzheimer type. *Biol Psychiatry* 1989;25:39–48.
19. Pomara N, Deptula D, Singh R. Pretreatment postural drop as a possible predictor of response to the cholinesterase inhibitor velnacrine (HP029) in Alzheimer's disease. *Psychopharmacol Bull* 1991;27:301–7.
20. Sweeney JE, Hohmann CF, Moran TH, Coyle JT. A long-acting cholinesterase inhibitor reverses spatial memory deficits in mice. *Pharmacol Biochem Behav* 1988;31:141–7.
21. Sweeney JE, Puttfarcken PS, Coyle JT. Galanthamine, an acetylcholinesterase inhibitor: a time course of the effects on performance and neurochemical parameters in mice. *Pharmacol Biochem Behav* 1989;34:129–37.
22. Davis KL, Mohs RC, Tinklenberg JR, Pfefferbaum A, Hollister LE, Kopell BS. Physostigmine: improvement of long term memory processes in normal humans. *Science* 1978;201:272–4.
23. Sunderland T, Tariot PN, Cohen RM, Weingartner H, Muekker EA, Murphy DL. Anticholinergic sensitivity in patients with dementia of the Alzheimer's type and age-matched controls. *Arch Gen Psychiatry* 1987;44:418–26.
24. Petersen RC. Scopolamine induced learning failures in man. *Psychopharmacology* 1977; 52:283–9.
25. Kopelman MD. Rates of forgetting in Alzheimer-type dementia and Korsakoff's syndrome. *Neuropsychologia* 1985;23:623–38.
26. Freed DM. Selective attention in Alzheimer's disease: characterizing cognitive subgroups of patients. *Neuropsychologia* 1989;27:325–9.
27. Becker J, Boller F, Saxton J, McGonigle-Gibson KL. Normal rates of forgetting of verbal and non-verbal material in Alzheimer's disease. *Cortex* 1987;23:59–72.
28. Kopelman MD, Corn TH. Cholinergic "blockade" as a model for cholinergic depletion: a comparison of the memory deficits with those of Alzheimer-type, dementia and the alcoholic Korsakoff syndrome. *Brain* 1988;111:1079–1110.
29. Davis KL, Hollister LE, Overall J, Johnson A, Train K. Physostigmine: effects on cognition and affect in normal subjects. *Psychopharmacology* 1976;51:23–7.
30. Gauthier S, Bouchard R, Lamontague A, et al. Tetrahydroaminoacridine—lecithin combination treatment in patients with intermediate stage Alzheimer's disease. *N Engl J Med* 1990;322:1272–6.
31. Chatellier G, Lacomblez L. Tacrine (tetrahydroaminoacridine; THA) and lecithin in senile dementia of the Alzheimer type: a multicenter trial. *BMJ* 1990;300:495–9.
32. Gauthier S, Bouchard R, Bacher Y, et al. Progress report on the Canadian multicenter trial of tetrahydroaminoacridine with lecithin in Alzheimer's disease. *Can J Neurol Sci* 1989; 16:543–6.
33. Hill M, Armitage P. The Two-Period Cross-Over Clinical Trial. *Br J Clin Pharmacol* 1979; 8:7–20.
34. Rosen WG, Mohs RC, Davis KL. A new rating scale for Alzheimer's disease. *Am J Psychiatry* 1984;141:1356–64.
35. Folstein MF, Folstein SE, McHugh PR. "Mini-Mental State": a practical method for grading the cognitive state of patients for the clinician. *J Psychiatr Res* 1975;12:189–98.

Guidelines for Drug Trials in Memory
Disorders, edited by N. Canal, et al.
Raven Press, Ltd., New York © 1993.

30

Functional Metabolic Assessment Using Positron Emission Tomography

J. C. Baron

INSERM U320 and Cyceron, Caen, France

Positron emission tomography (PET) is the only available technique that allows quantitative maps of brain energy metabolism to be obtained in the living human. The technique employs either ^{15}O-labeled molecular oxygen to measure the oxygen consumption rate ($CMRO_2$) or ^{18}F-labeled fluoro-2-deoxy-D-glucose to measure the glucose utilization rate (CMRglu). Because it is known from in vitro and in vivo studies that both parameters reliably reflect the energy expenditure related to local synaptic activity and basic homeostatic mechanisms, their measurement has been widely applied to the study of the cognitive decline related to both normal and abnormal aging. The rationale underlying such investigations is to characterize the nature, extent, and severity of the metabolic/synaptic derangements that presumably form the basis of impairment in selective aspects of cognition and behavior. In a more general sense, the aim of PET studies of brain metabolism is to further our understanding of the pathophysiological mechanisms of brain aging; to improve diagnostic accuracy during the patient's life, and in turn enhance the power of clinical research; and to eventually help design new therapeutic strategies. A final potential use of the PET metabolic paradigm is to evaluate the effects of cognitive enhancers on the brain's metabolic activity, to try and explain their mechanism of action. This chapter concentrates on the latter issue and attempts to define guidelines for the use of PET in drug trials in memory disorders.

RATIONALE

Normal Aging

As shown in Table 1, all studies of $CMRO_2$ (1–5) and six of ten studies of CMRglu (6–15) published to date have reported a decline in metabolic

TABLE 1. *Normal human aging and cortical energy metabolism*

Reference no.	n	Screening[a]	Oxygen consumption	Glucose utilization
1	27	+	↘	
2	27	+	↘	
3	22	+ +	↘	
4	34	+	↘	
5	25	+ + +	↘	
6	40	+		↘
7	37	+ +		→
8	40	+ + +		→
9	53	+ + +		→
10	16	+		↘
11	45	+ +		→
12	44	+		↘
13	42	?		↘
14	36	+ +		↘
15	60	+ + +		↘

[a] Health screening criteria: +, strict; + +, very strict; + + +, extremely strict; →, no decrement with age; ↘, significant decrement with age.

activity of the cerebral cortex in normal aging from the third to the eighth decade of life. The main reason for the lack of total agreement among studies relates to the fact that the metabolic decline is only mild, ranging from 2 to 6% per decade, and hence is subject to statistical uncertainty. Therefore, optimal PET methodology is required to quantitate accurately such small effects (15). Other confounding factors are the lack of consistency in control of the environment during PET scanning (e.g., eyes closed or open) and in the criteria used to define "normal" aging. As shown in Table 1, however, even studies that used extremely strict entry criteria (i.e., lack of any medical or mental illness, biologic abnormality, drug treatment, neuropsychological impairment, or computed tomography scan changes) reported significant effects of aging on cortical metabolism. Studies that compared optimally healthy aging to that occurring in conjunction with minor cardiovascular or metabolic disease suggest that the latter is associated with slightly more conspicuous metabolic decline, particularly affecting the frontal lobe (12). Other brain areas specially affected by the aging process are the perisylvian and parietooccipital areas, whereas the occipital cortex, the basal ganglia, the thalamus, the cerebellum, and the white matter appear to be essentially spared. This preferential functional impairment of the cerebral cortex, and especially of the associative cortex, suggests a role for combined degeneration of several ascending subcortico–cortical systems as well as an impairment in cortico–cortical parallel networks with aging that may underlie the cognitive changes that occur with aging. However, neither Duara et al. (8) nor De Leon et al. (7) found any significant correlation between cognitive and cortical CMRglu changes in their optimally healthy cohorts, but both used only standard, global neuropsychological tests and were unable to observe any metabolic effects of aging. Riege et al. (16) found significant positive correlations between declines in verbal and/or visual memory and metabolic rates in Broca's area and frontal cortex, but also a negative correlation between these memory items and basal ganglia CMRglu. The significance of these findings is uncertain. Haxby et al. (17) reported no significant correlation between resting CMRglu and visual memory across age. The study of aging effects on task-stimulated energy metabolism or blood flow by PET may prove more rewarding in the near future.

Dementia of the Alzheimer Type

The cortical metabolic changes seen in dementia of the Alzheimer type (DAT) with PET have been reviewed in detail recently (18). In patients with NINCDS criteria for probable DAT and moderate to severe dementia, there is an overall reduction in cortical energy metabolism (19). Regionally, there is a consistent predominance of this metabolic depression over the parietooccipital associative cortex. The prefrontal cortex is relatively less affected but the premotor cortex appears to be markedly involved. The primary sensorimotor and visual cortices are essentially spared metabolically. The mediotemporal areas have been difficult to study with PET for reasons of limited spatial resolution, but recent studies using high-resolution machines have reported significant metabolic reductions in these cortical areas, to a lesser extent, however, than corresponding lateral temporal areas. Finally, the metabolic rates of the basal ganglia, thalamus, and cerebellum are relatively preserved until advanced stages of DAT. This pattern of regional metabolic depression was present during life in essentially all cases of autopsy-proven Alzheimer disease (AD). In one patient with pathologically proven AD, however, the prefrontal cortex was the most hypometabolic cortical area (20).

Statistically significant cortical metabolic asymmetries are frequently observed in probable DAT, especially prominent over the posterior associative cortical areas and the prefrontal cortex, with a significantly greater proportion of left-sided hypometabolism.

Cross-sectional studies of probable DAT have shown that the metabolic impairment in the cortex tends to both spread and worsen as a function of dementia severity. In mildly demented patients, the cortical hypometabolism is significant only over the superior parietal cortex, whereas in moderately demented cases, it is also present over the lateral temporal, premotor, and occipital association cortex and in severely demented cases over the prefontal cortex (21). Of interest has been the study of early cases in whom the functional impairment was so mild as to allow only a diagnosis of possible DAT. In these patients, in whom the deficit was mainly confined to memory, a significant parietal cortex hypometabolism was already present and was found to become aggravated as DAT was longitudinally confirmed, suggesting that parietal hypometabolism may represent an early marker for the disease (22). The posterior predominance of cortical hypometabolism typical of early cases tends to disappear in moderately demented patients as premotor–prefrontal metabolism deteriorates. In advanced DAT cases, a pattern of predominantly frontal hypometabolism has been occasionally reported (23).

The posterior associative cortex hypometabolism found in probable DAT is associated with a predominance of the neuropsychological impairment in verbal tasks when it preferentially affects the left hemisphere, and in visuospatial tasks when it preferentially affects the right hemisphere. In patients with predominant memory impairment, the cortical metabolic impairment is essentially symmetrical. In patients with possible DAT and pure memory deficit, a posterior parietal hypometabolism is frequently observed, which lacks a detectable neuropsychological counterpart. At follow-up, however, deficit in visual/verbal tasks develops in these patients, indicating that the initial parietal metabolic impairment preceded the corresponding clinical expression (22,24,25). Initial accounts of mediotemporal cortex metabolism measured by high-resolution PET in DAT indicate less impairment than in the lateral temporal cortex, but reports of the relationships to memory tasks performance are lacking. Metabolic asymmetries in the prefontal cortex correlate with neuropsychological left–right indices in the same way as do those in the parietal cortex. However, posterior–anterior metabolic ratios, (such as parietal/premotor or parietal/prefrontal), have been found to correlate significantly with corresponding neuropsychological indices (such as the verbal–visual over attention–fluency ratio).

The remarkable reproducibility of the metabolic pattern of individual DAT patients over time presumably indicates a permanent impairment of the neuronal circuits involved, which could in turn reflect neuronal death, loss of synaptic contacts, and/or neuronal dysfunction (e.g., "deactivation"). In favor of the neuronal loss hypothesis are three major facts: (i) cortical atrophy, if taken into account in the PET procedure, would account for (part of) the hypometabolic pattern seen; (ii) the distribution of the hypometabolic pattern typical of early DAT is roughly superimposable on that noted post mortem for the neurofibrillary tangles, although metabolic–pathologic discrepancies have been reported (26); and (iii) this pattern is also similar to that of the decrease in cortical somatostatin seen postmortem. Hence, the PET procedure provides a mapping in vivo of the neuronal lesions in the cortex that could be used to assess the long-term effects of therapy.

However, a contribution of neuronal deactivation/disconnection to the cortical metabolic impairment observed by PET should also be considered (18), especially as this would imply that the dysfunctional cortical neurons could still respond to agents that are meant to enhance synaptic processing or adaptation (e.g., transmitter precursors, grafting, growth factors). Putative mechanisms could involve intrinsic or cortico–cortical circuits, cortico–subcortico–cortical loops, or subcortico–cortical projection systems. For example, in patients with DAT the cortical metabolic asymmetries are significantly correlated with corresponding basal ganglia–thalamic and inverse cerebellar metabolic asymmetries (27), according to the concept of diaschisis (28). Transneuronally mediated effects along the cortico–striato–pallido–thalamo–cortical loop may also operate. Hypometabolism of the cerebral cortex associated with behavioral impairment has been clearly demonstrated in patients with uni- or bilateral lesions of the striatum, the pallidum, and the thalamus (29–32). Likewise, lesions of the nucleus basalis of Meynert (nbM), the raphé system, and the locus coeruleus (LC), which are essentially constant in AD, may result in impairment of the cortical neurons. The role of the cholinergic input in the functional activity of the cerebral cortex is well known from electrophysiologic, pharmacologic, and behavioral studies. Cholinergic enhancers (e.g., muscarinic agonists, acetylcholinesterase blockers) increase, and muscarinic antagonists decrease, cortical glucose utilization in animals (33). Unilateral lesions of the nbM or its equivalent in rats and baboons induce a marked ipsilateral depression of cortical glucose use (34–36). These facts tend to favor the use of cholinergic enhancers in DAT. A disturbing factor in this hypothesis comes from the consistent observation made both in rats and in baboons of an effective metabolic recovery despite persisting deficit in cortical ChAT activity (36). It remains possible, however, that such an efficient process of adaptation to cholinergic deafferentation could be impaired in bilaterally lesioned, aged animals, or combined nbM–raphe–LC-lesioned animals, all situations that would more closely mimic the human disease.

In summary, the available data suggest that the reduced cortical metabolic rate in both normal aging and DAT is due to a combination of both direct neuronal lesions and neuronal deafferentation. Therefore, although "restorative" medications would be expected, in the long term, to prevent (or even reverse) the natural decline in CMRglu observed in DAT patients, "cognitive enhancers" may modulate the cortical metabolic activity (e.g., by enhancing cholinergic neurotransmission), in short-term or even acute conditions.

EFFECTS OF PUTATIVE COGNITIVE ENHANCERS ON THE BRAIN'S METABOLIC ACTIVITY

Literature Overview

Table 2 summarizes the available literature data on the effects of putative cognitive enhancers on CMRO$_2$ and/or CMRglu, measured either in healthy animals or in human beings (37–59). Despite a relatively large number of publications on this topic, many are from the 1960s or early 1970s and therefore are often of suboptimal design (e.g., lack of placebo group). In addition,

TABLE 2. *Effects of memory enhancers on brain energy metabolism*

Drug	Reference no.	Species	Mode	Method	Effects
Hydergine	37	Human (CVD)	i.v.	Kety–Schmidt	↗ $CMRO_2$
	38	Human (atheroma)	i.v.	Kety–Schmidt	→ $CMRO_2$
	39	Baboon (anesthetized)	i.v.	Venous outflow	→ $CMRO_2$
	40	Rat (awake)	i.p.	2-DG	↗ CMRglu, ↘ CMRglu specific areas
Piracetam	41	Cat (anesthetized)	i.v.	$AVDO_2$	No clear effect on $CMRO_2$
	42	Human (MID)	oral	Kety–Schmidt	↗ $CMRO_2$, → CMRglu
	43	Human (DAT and MID)	i.v.	PET	↗ CMRglu in DAT
Aniracetam	44	Rat	?	2-DG	→ CMRglu
Pentoxyfilline	45	Dog (anesthetized)	i.v.	Venous outflow	→ $CMRO_2$
	46	Dog (anesthetized)	i.v.	Venous outflow	↗ $CMRO_2$
	42	Human (MID)	oral	Kety–Schmidt	↗ $CMRO_2$, → CMRglu
Vincamine	47	Dog (anesthetized)	i.v.	$AVDO_2$	Biphasic effect on $CMRO_2$
	48	Dog (anesthetized)	i.v.	$AVDO_2$	→ $CMRO_2$
Pyritinol	49	Human (CVD)	oral or i.v.	Kety–Schmidt	↗ CMRglu, → $CMRO_2$
	50	Human (dementia)	oral or i.v.	Kety–Schmidt	→ $CMRO_2$
	42	Human (DAT)	oral	Kety–Schmidt	↗ CMRglu, → $CMRO_2$
THA	51	Rat (awake)	i.v.	2-DG	↗ CMRglu (selective areas)
RS 86	52	Human (DAT)	oral	PET	↘ CMRglu
ACTH 4–9	53	Rat (anesthetized)	i.p.	2-DG	↗ CMRglu in selective areas
	54	Rat (awake)	s.c.	2-DG	→ CMRglu
Naftidrofuryl	55	Rat (awake)	i.p.	2-DG	→ CMRglu
Ginkgo biloba	56	Human (CVD)	oral	$AVDO_2$	↗ $CMRO_2$, ↗
	57	Rat (awake)	?	2-DG	→ CMRglu
Meclofenoxate	37	Human (CVD)	i.v.	Kety–Schmidt	↘ $CMRO_2$
	42	Human (MID)	oral	Kety–Schmidt	→ $CMRO_2$, → CMRglu
Isoxsuprine	37	Human (CVD)	i.v.	Kety–Schmidt	→ $CMRO_2$
Eburnamine	47	Dog (anesthetized)	i.v.	$AVDO_2$	↗ $CMRO_2$
	58	Rat (awake)	i.p.	2-DG	↗ CMRglu (selective areas)
Piribedil	59	Baboon (anesthetized)	i.v.	$AVDO_2$	↗ $CMRO_2$

CVD, cerebrovascular disease; i.v., intravenous; i.p., intraperitoneal; s.c., subcutaneous; MID, multiinfarct dementia; DAT, dementia of Alzheimer type; $AVDO_2$, arteriovenous oxygen difference; 2-DG, [^{14}C]-2-deoxyglucose method; $CMRO_2$, cerebral metabolic rate of glucose; CMRglu, cerebral metabolic rate of glucose; PET, positron emission tomography.

one is struck by the wide diversity in the methods used to measure brain metabolism (i.e., arteriovenous O_2 difference, Kety–Schmidt or PET in humans and venous outflow or [^{14}C]-2-deoxyglucose methods in animals), the clinical status of human subjects (often as vaguely described as "cerebrovascular disease," "multiinfarct dementia," or "atheroma"), the animal species investigated (cat, dog, rat, or baboon), and the arousal status in the latter (awake or anesthetized). Such diversity would make global interpretation of the findings a futile exercise. In addition, the modality employed for drug administration often does not reflect that usually employed in the clinical setting, (i.e., few studies have adhered to the oral route of administration), and only rarely have pharmacokinetic studies and multiple doses been carried out.

With respect to the few agents that have been the matter of at least three studies (i.e., hydergine, piracetam, pentoxyfilline, pyritinol), marked inconsistencies in the findings have been reported. The issue is made even further confusing because studies that have measured either oxygen and glucose consumption for the whole brain, or only CMRglu but in multiple brain areas, have reported either dissociated effects of the drug tested on $CMRO_2$ and CMRglu (42) or regionally selective changes in CMRglu (40,51). Finally, time-dependent changes, such as "biphasic" effects on $CMRO_2$, have also been reported (47).

Positron Emission Tomography

Only two human studies using PET have been published (43,52). The study of Szelies et al. (52) employed [^{18}F]fluoro-2-deoxyglucose to measure CMRglu in several cortical areas and in the cerebellum of eight patients with dementia due to probable AD before and at the completion of 6 weeks of oral treatment with RS 86, a putative central muscarinic receptor agonist. They observed a significant reduction in CMRglu in all association cortex areas, but not in primary sensory cortex or in cerebellum. These effects were similar in all patients regardless of the clinical effects of the drug. However, because there was no placebo group in this study, interpretation of its findings is uncertain. Heiss et al. (43) used the same methodology to evaluate the effects of piracetam (12 g/day i.v. for 2 weeks) on CMRglu in nine patients with probable AD and seven patients with diagnosis of multi-infarct or unclassifiable (presumably mixed) dementia. They reported a small (8–10%), marginally significant increase in CMRglu in the Alzheimer patients in the association cortex areas (except temporal lobe), in the visual, auditory, and cingulate cortex and in the basal ganglia and thalamus, but no effect was seen in the cerebellum. In the demented patients with vascular or undetermined etiology, no significant effects of treatment were observed. As in the study of Szelies et al. (52), however, the lack of placebo group makes such findings of uncertain significance.

Recently, single photon emission computer tomography (SPECT) with [^{99m}Tc]-HMPAO has been used to image brain perfusion patterns before and during central cholinergic stimulation with physostigmine in patients with presumed AD (60) as compared with controls. The authors reported a significant change in the perfusion pattern in AD patients, with lesser reduction in flow in the parietotemporal region relative to other brain areas during treatment, an effect that was not seen in control subjects. Although this effect may well represent increased metabolism in this vulnerable cortical area, the lack of absolute measurement of flow by the SPECT method used prevents such an interpretation. Furthermore, physostigmine may increase flow as a result of a direct vascular effect (i.e., without underlying metabolic change), in a way similar to that reported in a PET study of a cognitive enhancer in multi-infarct dementia (MID) patients (61). Therefore, direct measurement of brain metabolism is necessary to adequately interpret changes in perfusion that may occur as a result of drug treatment.

GUIDELINES

Patient Material

At present, DAT is the only well-defined clinical entity that allows a scientifically sound approach to the study of the effects of memory enhancers. Therefore, clinical diagnoses such as "benign senescent forgetfulness," "frontal-type dementia," "multi-infarct dementia," and "mixed degenerative vascular dementia" all lack a widely accepted as well as a validated criteria checklist that would permit replicability of the paradigm.

In addition to fulfilment of the fundamental inclusion criteria of "dementia" (based on the DSM-III-R criteria) and probable DAT (NINCDS-ADRDA criteria), a number of secondary selection criteria must be considered to improve sample uniformity. These are the following: (a) severity of dementia, which should be mild [Mini-Mental State Examination (MMSE) between 20 and 26) or moderate (MMSE between 10 and 20)], as severely affected patients are presumably beyond therapeutic limits and the effects of drugs on brain metabolism are less to be expected; (b) disease duration, which should be a minimum of 6 months and a maximum of 4–5 years, to exclude both reversible encephalopathies and atypical or advanced AD; (c) age, preferably within the 50–75-year range to avoid inclusion of both atypical dementias of very early onset, and elderly subjects with presumably superimposed cerebrovascular disease; and (d) educational level, as setting a minimal level of schooling (e.g., 6–7 years) facilitates interpretation of the MMSE and makes informed consent to the investigation more reliable.

Exclusion criteria are also of crucial importance. These should preferably include the following. First, significant cerebrovascular disease or risk factors: the modified Hachinski score (62), which includes CT scanning in its criteria and has been validated pathologically, is presently advocated according to a limit score of 2. It should be noted that this limit is practical in that it allows inclusion of patients with uncomplicated arterial hypertension, which is so prevalent in elderly subjects, as well as patients with previous so-called "stroke" (in fact, any type of "spell") as long as no CT scan or focal neurologic signs or symptoms are present. Although "leucoaroiosis," as long as it takes only the form of diffuse white matter hypodensity on CT scan, is not a cause of exclusion using this score (whereas focal or multifocal lesions would be), the status of magnetic resonance imaging (MRI) has not been clarified up to now, especially with respect to "white matter hypersignals" which are often seen in "asymptomatic" elderly people as well as in pathologically proven AD patients. Second, present depression, as assessed by the Hamilton Scale, for example, should be excluded because of risks of both misdiagnosis ("pseudodementia") and interference with brain metabolism. However, a labile affect is widely prevalent in AD, and a relatively high depression score does not necessarily mean "depression" on psychiatric grounds, which require stability of affect. Third, poor cooperation due to mental confusion is an a priori cause of exclusion because PET scanning requires the subject to stand still for a minimum of 10 min twice (or preferably 60 min continuously). Fourth, alcoholism and other addictions, as well as drugs potentially interfering with brain metabolism and/or with the memory enhancer's effects, and, finally, other neurological or systemic disease, should be grounds for exclusion.

Design of the Trial

There are several options in study design, and the choice should be based on both the drug's purported mechanism of action and the constraints of PET methodology.

Timing Options

Three timing options are possible: acute design, short-term design, and long-term design.

In acute design, a single-dose approach is used via an i.v., i.m., or oral route. This design should be considered if the drug to be tested has supposedly immediate biologic and/or cognitive effects (e.g., cholinergic transmission enhancement). In this case, however, careful considerations need be given to the time course of such effects and the pharmacokinetic data in an age-matched population, to determine the most adequate timing between drug administration and PET scanning. In addition, an ideal design would incorporate, in individual subjects, measurement of biologic and/or cognitive effects and assessment of the drug's plasma and/or urine pharmacokinetics.

The short-term design mimics the usual clinical situation in which the cognitive effects of a given orally administered drug reach their optimum after several weeks of regular dosage. In this design, therefore, patients would take the drug for "enough time" before PET scanning is performed; cognitive assessment and plasma drug dosage are also of interest in this design.

Long-term design is a "chronic" paradigm that would apply to putative drugs aimed at preventing (not just compensating for) further deterioration of neuronal function in DAT (e.g., neurotropic agents). Problems in such a design would be variability in natural history (disease progression) among patients and the fact that the pattern of hypometabolism in DAT remains essentially stable in a given individual as disease progresses, making the absolute metabolic rates the main determinant of drug effects.

Structure Options

For obvious reasons, the double-blind versus placebo design is mandatory in the assessment of brain metabolic effects of memory enhancers. Regarding the actual paradigm, the constraints related to PET must be taken into account. In addition to the duration of PET scanning itself, implying the risk of head displacement in poorly cooperative subjects, the two main issues are dosimetry and arterial catheterization (for blood sampling). Dosimetry in PET study is limited to that of the usual nuclear medicine procedures, and is a trade-off of the minimal radioactivity that must be given to obtain statistically meaningful data; most PET investigators set a limit of about two to three studies in a given individual. Arterial (radial) catheterization is mandatory if absolute measurement of CMRglu is considered; although venous "arterialization" by hand heating is possible, it often is not reliable enough for practical purposes. Radial artery catheterization has been shown to be harmless in the PET setting (63); however, to repeat it at regular intervals would cause local discomfort and could be questioned by some Ethical Committees.

These considerations, as well as the actual cost of PET studies, are such that the number of PET sessions in drug trials should be limited as much as possible. Therefore, the ideal paradigm, which would consist of PET studies both before and after treatment in a crossover, placebo versus active agent design, is, practically speaking, unrealistic. There are only two options left: a parallel group design and a crossover design.

The parallel group design (i.e., no crossover) poses a risk of lack of comparability between the two randomized patient groups, in terms of either demographic or cognitive data or metabolic pattern, because the two samples will have to remain small for cost-related reasons.

In the crossover design, each patient is PET scanned only once per arm, i.e., during (but not before) treatment with both active agent and placebo. Although this is the more realistic design, as it avoids the problem of parallel groups and in turn reduces the number of patients to be included, problems with "order" and "carryover" effects must be considered. The former ("order") effect implies that brain metabolism is systematically different at the second PET study, regardless of drug effects. Although such an effect has not been demonstrated with PET in control subjects (64,65), it may still occur in DAT patients. To control for this possible bias, however, the patient sample can be simply balanced into to 1–2 and 2–1 sequence randomized groups. The latter ("carryover") effect should be possible to predict on the basis of prior pharmacodynamic data and drug elimination half-times. Pharmacokinetic assessment before the second study period can assist in evaluating or eliminating this bias.

Potential Pitfalls

Methodological Issues

Accurate head repositioning at repeated PET sessions is mandatory as a good laboratory practice. This can be achieved using either personally molded plastic face masks screwed on a head holder or by x-ray determination of standard bony reference landmarks (e.g., the glabella and the inion).

Reproducibility of measurement of cerebral metabolism is, as for any biologic measurement, subject to some error. In control subjects it has been estimated at about 10% for regional CMRglu (64,65). However, the reproducibility of metabolic patterns (i.e., if absolute rates are normalized for) is much lower (~2%). Because the number of patients to be included in PET trials is necessarily limited by factors such as cost, tight camera schedule, and available computer facilities, reproducibility of measurement must be considered to evaluate the statistical power of any planned trial. Regions of interest (ROIs) are another issue in DAT PET studies. Since it is not always obvious which brain areas should respond most (on a theoretical basis) to the drug, the option is to quantitate the changes in many potentially relevant areas both on the left and on the right hemisphere, thus exposing the study to the risk of spurious findings due to multiple comparisons. This statistical issue requires a fixed schedule well planned in advance, ideally with a limited number of tests based on well-defined anatomic–functional localization hypotheses.

Pharmacologic Issues

In addition to the requirement of obtaining plasma drug pharmacokinetics in each subject, the dose–reponse issue should be addressed. However, it would be unrealistic to submit the same patients to different drug dosages. A parallel group design with two dosages would be possible but would further increase the risk of noncomparability among groups. Otherwise, linearity of the dose–response relationship has to be assumed.

Neurobiologic Issues

Although brain metabolism decreases with dementia severity, it is not known whether it could increase as a result of cognitive enhancement in

DAT. If the metabolic depression of DAT merely reflects loss of synaptic contacts and neurons, one should not expect metabolic changes in response to cognitive improvement (unless the drug is supposed to boost the synaptic plasticity in DAT). If, on the other hand, it represents (at least in part) a "functional" reduction in synaptic activity, then it should react to drugs enhancing synaptic activity. The fact that CMRglu can be modulated by cholinergic agents both in animals and in normal humans obviously speaks in favor of the latter hypothesis (33), but this remains to be demonstrated in AD. At this point, the possibility that metabolic reactivity to memory enhancers might differ according to the clinical stage of the disease must also be considered. Thus, one could speculate that the reduction in CMRglu already seen in moderate dementia represents a complete loss of the "reactive" part of brain energy metabolism. Finally, one could argue that enhancement of brain energy metabolism (if proven to occur) by "cognitive enhancers" might, in the long term, be harmful to the remaining synaptic contacts by inappropriately imposing a burden of energy expenditure. For example, increasing oxidative metabolism could in theory promote oxygen free radical formation or result in accumulation of neurotoxic wastes, and hence exacerbate neuronal death.

Development of in vivo cholinergic markers for PET application may prove useful in the coming years in the evaluation of memory disorders and of the effects of cognitive enhancers. Thus far, succesful developments have been recorded in the study of muscarinic receptors using ^{11}C-labeled methyl-benztropine, [^{11}C]QNB, and [^{11}C]scopolamine (66–68). However, radioligands more selective for the various subtypes of muscarinic receptors will be needed to investigate the pre- and postsynaptic sites of the cholinergic afferents in both the neocortex and the limbic system.

REFERENCES

1. Lenzi GL, Frackowiak RSJ, Jones T, et al. CMRO$_2$ and CBF by oxygen-15 inhalation technique. *Eur J Neurol* 1981;20:285–90.
2. Pantano P, Baron JC, Lebrun–Grandie P, Duquesnoy N, Bousser MG, Comar D. Regional cerebral blood flow and oxygen consumption in human aging. *Stroke* 1984;15:635–41.
3. Yamaguchi T, Kanno I, Uemura K, et al. Reduction in regional cerebral metabolic rate of oxygen during human aging. *Stroke* 1986;17:1220–8.
4. Leenders KL, Perani D, Lammertsma AA, et al. The effects of age on cerebral blood flow, blood volume and oxygen utilization. *Brain* 1990;113:27–47.
5. Marchal G, Rioux P, Petit–Taboue MC, et al. The effects of optimally healthy aging on cerebral oxygen metabolism, blood flow, and blood volume in humans: a PET study. *J Cereb Blood Flow Metab* 1991;11(suppl 2):S785.
6. Kuhl DE, Metter EJ, Riege WH, Phelps ME. Effects of human aging on patterns of local cerebral glucose utilization determined by the ^{18}F fluorodeoxyglucose method. *J Cereb Blood Flow Metab* 1982;2:163–71.
7. De Leon M, George AE, Ferris SH, et al. Positron emission tomography and computed tomography assessment of the aging human brain. *J Comput Assist Tomogr* 1984;8:88–94.
8. Duara R, Grady C, Haxby J, et al. Human brain glucose utilization and cognitive function in relation to age. *Ann Neurol* 1984;16:702–13.

9. De Leon M, George AE, Tomanelli J, et al. Positron emission tomography studies of normal aging: a replication of PET III and ^{18}F FDG using PET VI and 11-CDG. *Neurobiol Aging* 1987;8:319–23.

10. McGeer PL, Kamo H, Harrop R, et al. Positron emission tomography in patients with clinically diagnosed Alzheimer's disease. *Can Med Assoc J* 1986;134:597–607.

11. Junck L, Moen JG, Bluemlein I, et al. Cerebral glucose metabolism in normal aging studied with PET. *J Cereb Blood Flow Metab* 1989;9(suppl 1):S524.

12. Chawluk JB, Alari A, Jamieson DG, et al. Changes in local cerebral glucose utilisation with normal aging. *J Cereb Blood Flow Metab* 1987;7(suppl 1):S411.

13. Pawlik G, Heiss WD, Beil C, Wienhard K, Herholz K, Wagner K. PET demonstrates differential age dependence, asymmetry and response to various stimuli of regional brain glucose metabolism in healthy volunteers. *J Cereb Blood Flow Metab* 1987;7(suppl 1):S376.

14. Hoffmann JM, Guze BH, Baxter L, et al. Familial and sporadic Alzheimer's disease: an FDG-PET study. *J Cereb Blood Flow Metab* 1989;9(suppl):S547.

15. Grady CL, Horwitz B, Schapiro MB, Rapoport SI. Changes in the integrated activity of the brain with healthy aging and dementia of the Alzheimer type. In: Rapoport SI, Petit H, Leys D, Christen Y, (eds) *Aging brain and dementia: new trends in diagnosis and therapy.* New York: Alan R Liss; 1990:355–69.

16. Riege WH, Metter EJ, Kuhl DE, Phelps ME. Brain glucose metabolism and memory functions: age decrease in factor scores. *J Gerontol* 1985;40:459–67.

17. Haxby JV, Grady CL, Duara R, et al. Relations among age, visual memory and resting cerebral metabolism in 40 healthy men. *Brain Cogn* 1986;5:412–27.

18. Baron JC. Cortical functional impairment in dementia of the Alzheimer type (DAT): functional studies in the brain with positron emission tomography. In: Rapoport SI, Petit H, Lays D, Christen Y, eds. *Imaging, cerebral topography and Alzheimer's disease,* Berlin: Springer-Verlag; 1990:129–37.

19. Frackowiak RSJ, Pozzilli C, Du Boulay GH, Marshall J, Lenzi GL, Jones T. Regional cerebral oxygen supply and utilization in dementia: a clinical and physiological study with oxygen-15 and positron tomography. *Brain* 1981;104:753–78.

20. Foster NL, Mann U, Mohr E, Sunderland T, Katz D, Chase TN. Focal cerebral glucose hypometabolism in definite Alzheimer's disease. *Ann Neurol* 1989;26:132–3.

21. Kumar A, Schapiro MB, Grady C, et al. High-resolution PET studies in Alzheimer's disease. *Neuropsychopharmacology* 1991;4:35–46.

22. Haxby JV, Grady CL, Koss E, et al. Longitudinal study of cerebral metabolic asymmetries and associated neuropsychological patterns in early dementia of the Alzheimer type. *Arch Neurol* 1990;47:753–60.

23. Benson DF, Kuhl DE, Hawkins RA, Phelps ME, Cummings JL, Tsai SY. The fluorodeoxyglucose ^{18}F scan in Alzheimer's disease and multi-infarct dementia. *Arch Neurol* 1983;40:711–4.

24. Haxby JV, Grady CL, Duara R, Schlageter N, Berg G, Rapoport SI. Neocortical metabolic abnormalities procede nonmemory cognitive defects in early Alzheimer's type dementia. *Arch Neurol* 1986;43:882–5.

25. Grady CL, Haxby JV, Schageter NL, Berg G, Rapoport SL. Stability of metabolic and neuropsychological asymmetries in dementia of the Alzheimer's type. *Neurology* 1986;36:1390–2.

26. Duara R, Barker WW, Pascal S, Bruce–Gregorios J, Noremberg M, Boothe T. Lack of correlation of regional neuropathology to the regional PET metabolic deficits in Alzheimer's disease (AD). *J Cereb Blood Flow Metab* 1991;11(suppl 2):S19.

27. Akiyama H, Harrop R, McGeer PL, et al. Crossed cerebellar and uncrossed basal ganglia and thalamic diaschisis in Alzheimer's disease. *Neurology* 1989;39:541–8.

28. Baron JC. Subcortical damage and cortical energy metabolism: relevance for dementia. In: Battistin L, Gerstenbrand F, eds. *Aging brain and dementia: new trends in diagnosis and therapy.* New York: Wiley-Liss; 1990:349–54.

29. Metter EJ, Wasterlain CG, Kuhl DE, Hanson WR, Phelps ME. ^{18}FDG positron emission tomography in a study of aphasta. *Ann Neurol* 1981;10:173–83.

30. Laplane D, Levasseur M, Pillon B, et al. Obsessive-compulsive and other behavioral changes with bilateral basal ganglia lesions: a neuropsychological magnetic resonance imaging and positron emission tomography study. *Brain* 1989;112:699–725.

31. Baron JC, D'Antona R, Pantano P, Serdaru M, Samson Y, Bousser MG. Effects of thalamic stroke on energy metabolism of the cerebral cortex, *Brain* 1986;109:1243–59.
32. Levasseur M, Mazoyer R, Sette G, et al. Bilateral paramedian thalamic infarction: a PET study of cortical oxygen consumption. *J Cereb Blood Flow Metab* 1989;9(suppl):S738.
33. Baron JC. Système cholinergique et métabolisme énergétique cérébral. *Cir Métab Cerveau* 1988;5:183–9.
34. London ED, McKinney M, Dam M, Ellis A, Coyle JT. Decreased cortical glucose utilization after ibotenate lesions of the rat ventromedial globus pallidus. *J Cereb Blood Flow Metab* 1984;4:381–90.
35. Orzi F, Diana G, Casamerti F, Palombo E, Fieschi C. Local cerebral glucose utilization following unilateral and bilateral lesions of the nucleus basalis magnocellularis in the rat. *Brain Res* 1988;462:99–103.
36. Kiyosawa M, Baron JC, Hamel E, et al. Time course of effects of unilateral lesions of the nucleus basalis of Meynert on glucose utilization of the cerebral cortex: positron tomography in baboons. *Brain* 1989;112:435–55.
37. Marc–Vergnes JP, Bes A, Charlet JP, Delpla M, Richardot JP, Geraud J. Pharmacodynamie de la circulation cérébrale. *Pathol Biol* 1974;22:815–25.
38. Heyck H. Der Einflurs der Ausganglage auf synpatholytiescher Effect am Kinkreislauf bei zerebrovascularen Erkangurgen. *Arzneimittelforschung* 1961;15:243–51.
39. Szewczykowski J, Meyer JS, Kondo A, Nomura F, Terauza T. Effects of ergot alkaloïds (hydergine) on cerebral hemodynamics and oxygen consumption in monkeys. *J Neurol Sci* 1969;10:25–31.
40. Walovitch RC, Ingram DK, Spangler EL, London ED. Co-dergocrine, cerebral glucose utilization and maze performance in middle-aged rats. *Pharmacol Biochem Behav* 1987;26: 95–101.
41. Vlahov V, Nikolova M, Nikolov P. The effect of piracetam on the local cortical cerebral blood flow in rats. *Arch Int Pharmacodyn* 1980;243:103–10.
42. Hoyer S. Dementia: an incurable mental disability? In: *World Congress of Biological Psychiatry*, 1985.
43. Heiss WD, Hebold I, Klinkhammer P, et al. Effect of piracetam on cerebral glucose metabolism in Alzheimer's disease as measured by positron emission tomography. *J Cereb Blood Flow Metab* 1988;8:613–7.
44. Lorez HP, Martin JR, Keller HH, Cumin R. Effect of aniracetam and the benzodiazepine receptor partial inverse agonist Ro 15-3505 on cerebral glucose utilization, and cognitive function after lesioning of cholinergic forebrain nuclei in the rat. *Drug Dev Res* 1988;14: 359–62.
45. Steen PA, Milde JH, Michenfelder JD. Pentoxyfilline does not change cerebral blood flow or metabolism in the dog. *Acta Anaesthesiol Scand* 1981;25:319–22.
46. Komarek J, Husselrath A, Just M. Die Working von Pentoxyfilin auf die Gelvin durch Blutung und den Gehirn stoff Weechsel beim Hund. *Arzneimittelforschung* 1977;27:1939.
47. Linee PH, Lacroix P, Le Polles JB, et al. Cerebral metabolic, hemodynamic and antithypoxic properties of 1-eburnamonine. *Eur Neurol* 1978;17(suppl 1):113–20.
48. Caravaggi AM, Sardi A, Baldoli E, Francesco GF, Luca C. Hemodynamic profile of a new cerebral vasodilator, vincamine, and one of its derivatives, apovincaminic acid ethyl-ester. *Arch Int Pharmacodyn* 1977;226:139–48.
49. Becker K, Hoyer S. Etudes du métabolisme cérébral lors du traitement par la pirithioxine. *Deut Zeit Nerven* 1966;188:200–9.
50. Hoyer S, Oesterreich K, Stoll KD. Effects of pyritinol-HCl on blood flow and oxidative metabolism of the brain in patients with dementia. *Arzneimittelforschung* 1977;27:671–4.
51. Inglis FM, Dewar D, McCulloch J. Effects on local cerebral glucose utilisation of 9-amino-1,2,3,4-tetrahydroacridine (THA) in the rat brain. *J Cereb Blood Flow Metab* 1989;9(suppl 1):S497.
52. Szelies B, Herholz K, Pawlik G, Beil C, Wienhard K, Heiss WD. Zerebraler Glukosestoffwechsel bei präseniler Demenz vom Alzheimer-Typ. Verlaufskontrolle unter Therape mit muskarinergem Cholinagonisten. *Fortschr Neurol Psychiatr* 1986;54:364–73.
53. McCulloch JM, Kelly PAT, Van Delft AML. Alterations in local cerebral glucose utilization during chronic treatment with an ACTH 4-9 analog. *Eur J Pharmacol* 1982;78:151–8.
54. Dunn AJ, Hund RW. Cerebral 2-deoxyglucose accumulation in mice following chronic treatment with an ACTH 4-9 analog. ORG 2766. *Brain Res Bull* 1984;12:369–71.

55. Orzi F, Schuier F, Fieschi C. Effects of naftidrofuryl on local cerebral glucose utilization in the rat. *J Cereb Blood Flow Metab* 1981;1:137–40.
56. Tea S, Celsis P, Clanet M, Marc–Vergnes JP. Effets cliniques hémodynamiques et métaboliques de l'extrait de Ginkgo biloba en pathologie vasculaire cérébrale. *Gaz Méd France* 1979;86:4149–52.
57. Krieglstein J, Beck T, Seibert A. Influence of an extract of ginkgo biloba on cerebral blood flow and metabolism. *Life Sci* 1986;39:2327–34.
58. Broussolle E, Darriet D, Debilly G, Pujol JF, Bobillier P. RU 24722, a new eburnamine derivative, induces selective alterations in cerebral glucose utilization in freely moving rat. *Eur J Pharmacol* 1989;159:225–31.
59. McCulloch JM, Edvinsson L. The action of piribedil upon the cerebral circulation. *Psychol Med* 1979;11:27–32.
60. Geaney DP, Soper N, Shepstone BJ, Cowen PJ. Effect of central cholinergic stimulation on regional cerebral blood flow in Alzheimer disease. *Lancet* 1990;1:1484–7.
61. Gibbs JM, Frackowiak RSJ. Regional cerebral blood flow and oxygen metabolism in dementia due to vascular disease. *Gerontology* 1986;32(suppl 1):84–8.
62. Loeb C, Gandolfo C. Diagnostic evaluation of degenerative and vascular dementia. *Stroke* 1983;14:399–401.
63. Lockwood AH. Invasiveness in studies of brain function by positron emission tomography (PET). *J Cereb Blood Flow Metab* 1985;5:487–9.
64. Bartlett EJ, Brodie JD, Wolf AP, Christman DR, Laska E, Meissner M. Reproducibility of cerebral glucose metabolic measurements in resting human subjects. *J Cereb Blood Flow Metab* 1988;8:502–12.
65. Tyler JL, Strother SC, Zatorre RJ, et al. Stability of regional cerebral glucose metabolism in the normal brain measured by positron emission tomography. *J Nucl Med* 1988;29:631–42.
66. Dewey SL, MacGregor RR, Brodie JD, et al. Mapping muscarinic receptors in human and baboon brain using [N-^{11}C-methyl]-benztropine. *Synapse* 1990;5:213–23.
67. Frey KA, Koeppe RA, Mulholland GK, et al. Muscarinic receptor imaging in human brain using [C-^{11}] scopolamine and positron emission tomography. *J Nucl Med* 1988;29:808–9.
68. Khalili–Varasteh M, Brouillet E, Chavoix C, et al. Recepteurs cholinergiques muscariniques centraux: étude préliminaire in vivo chez le primate par tomographie par émission de positons (TEP). *Colloq Nat Neurosci* 1989;339.

Guidelines for Drug Trials in Memory
Disorders, edited by N. Canal, et al.
Raven Press, Ltd., New York © 1993.

31

Neurophysiological Assessment of Efficacy in Drug Trials with Memory Disorders

Bernd Saletu

*Department of Psychiatry, School of Medicine, University of Vienna,
A-1090 Vienna, Austria*

Within the rapidly expanding field of neuroimaging methods applied in drug trials concerning memory disorders, quantitative analysis of the electroencephalogram (EEG) and event-related potentials (ERP), supplemented by modern brain mapping techniques have gained increasing interest because they are readily and widely available and are low cost, high-time resolution, and noninvasive methods for objective and quantitative evaluation of the neurophysiologic correlates of memory disorders and their treatment (1–13). Disadvantages of the method include low spatial resolution, two- rather than three-dimensionality, low specificity, and the fact that the P300 paradigm is not often repeatable. A consensus conference on the methodology of clinical trials of nootropics in 1989 came to the conclusion that EEG techniques are sensitive measures of vigilance and may be useful in detecting even small drug-induced changes (14). The relative paucity of behavioral and clinical correlations has been partly offset by recent investigations concerning interrelationships between computed tomography (CT), EEG, clinical and psychometric measures (4,7). This chapter reviews studies that have replicated the above findings, utilizing both confirmatory and descriptive statistics.

METHOD

To replicate previous studies (4,6,7) in 111 demented hospitalized patients on diagnostic aspects of EEG mapping and its relationships to clinical and CT variables, data were obtained as part of a randomized multicenter, parallel-group, double-blind, placebo-controlled comparative trial in mildly to moderately demented patients diagnosed according to the same DSM-III criteria (8). CT, EEG, clinical and psychometric data could be collected in 96 patients in old people's/nursing homes (72 women, 24 men), aged between 61 and 96 years (mean 82 years). The patients had to score on the Shader

Clinical Assessment Geriatric scale (SCAG) between 45 and 90 and on the Mini-Mental State Examination (MMSE) between 10 and 25, and had to be able to complete a labyrinth test. They had to be off pharmaceutical agents for at least 14 days and were subdiagnosed according to the modified Marshall–Hachinski ischemic score [<4, Senile Dementia of the Alzheimer Type (SDAT); >7, multi-infarct dementia (MID)] and CT in 45 SDAT and 51 MID patients. The groups did not differ in regard to sex or age. The study was performed in accordance with the Declaration of Helsinki revised in 1975 (Tokyo) and amended in 1983 (Venice). The approval of an ethical review committee was obtained, as was the patients' informed consent. CT measurements included 10 cerebral spinal fluid space variables as well as 17 cortical density measurements underneath the EEG electrodes (1.7 mm^3 cubes, measured in Hounsfield units). Clinical investigations were carried out by means of SCAG score/factors. Psychometric tests included the digit symbol substitution test (DSST), the trail-making test (TMT), and the digit span (DS) test. Three-minute vigilance-controlled EEGs (V-EEG) were recorded by means of Nihon–Kohden 4317 F and 4321 F polygraphs (time constant 0.3 s; high frequency response 35 Hz; frequency range 0.5–35 Hz; amplification 1-20,000; maximal noise level 2 μ peak to peak). Sixteen leads were digitized on line by a Hewlett–Packard Vectra system with a sampling frequency of 102.4 Hz. The frequency resolution was 0.2 Hz. Topographic brain mapping was carried out based on a method described in detail elsewhere (15–20) by means of Hewlett–Packard Vectra computers. ERPs were recorded utilizing an oddball paradigm.

Pharmaco-EEG trials with the aim of classifying nootropics and to determine their cerebral bioavailability were carried out in double-blind, placebo-controlled trials in groups of 10 to 15 normal healthy volunteers >60 years of age (21–23). They received, randomized in weekly intervals, single oral doses of the experimental compound, placebo, and eventually a reference compound. Evaluations were carried out at 0, 2, 4, 6, and 8 h after oral drug administration. Long-term investigations with nootropics are carried out in patients with adult-onset cognitive disorders (6,21,24,25).

Statistical analysis was based on the concept of descriptive data analysis proposed by Abt (26), including confirmatory statements concerning differences between SDAT, MID, and normals in the absolute δ/θ power as well as regarding the correlations of the latter to a CT variable (greatest distance between lateral ventricles), the SCAG score, and the DSST. α-Adjustment was carried out according to Bonferroni.

EEG Maps of SDAT and MID Patients as Compared with Controls

Previous studies have demonstrated that untreated SDAT patients, as compared with normal aged controls, have increased δ/θ and decreased β activity as well as slowing of the dominant frequency and the centroid of the total activity specifically over the parietal and temporal regions (4,6,7,11,12).

MID patients exhibited these differences from normal controls over all brain regions, which may have been due to the fact that infarcted brain regions and their penumbras produce marked EEG abnormalities and, as they are located in different regions, they might have added up in the mean SPM image of the total patient group. The aforementioned neurophysiological findings in both patient groups indicated a deterioration in vigilance. In recent replicatory studies in patients described in the methodology, confirmatory statistics were carried out regarding differences between SDAT, MID, and normals in absolute δ/θ power. The preselected maximal error probability $\alpha = 0.05$ was corrected for multiple comparisons (2×17 electrode positions) by the procedure of Bonferroni–Holme ($p < 0.05/34 = 0.0015$). The null hypothesis that there is no difference in absolute δ/θ power between controls and SDAT and MID patients, respectively, was rejected. δ/θ Power was increased in SDAT over all brain regions except occipitally, whereas in MID cases this exception was seen left frontally, bioccipitally, and right occipito-temporally (Fig. 1). Descriptive analysis showed no differences in absolute α and β power, whereas relative δ/θ power was enhanced and relative α/β power was reduced in patients compared with controls (Fig. 2). Total power was augmented bitemporally and frontopolarly, and the centroid was slowed over many brain regions. The increase of δ/θ power in SDAT was 3.9 standard deviations of controls and that of MID patients 4.9 in the left temporal region (highest p values) (Table 1). Eighty-six to 88% of the patients showed in the target variable δ and θ power in at least one brain region an increase of over 1 standard deviation from the norm, 67–68% exhibited an increase of at least 2 standard deviations (Fig. 3). These findings obtained in two different studies (6,8) were almost identical. As the maximal difference was taken from any of the 12 electrodes, 14% of normally aged subjects also showed an increase of $\delta/0$ power of at least 2 standard deviations. Improvement of the classification may be obtained by nonlinear statistical approach.

Differences Between SDAT and MID Patients

Between SDAT and MID patients there were few significant differences. The findings were characterized by more slow activity, less β activity, and a slower dominant frequency and centroid of the total activity in MID than in SDAT patients, specifically in the frontal and frontotemporal region (6). The best discrimination between the two subgroups of dementia was obtained utilizing max–min differences of relative power as well as power asymmetry. In our recent investigations, descriptive data analysis of differences in 36 EEG variables demonstrated, again, only few significant findings (β power being lower right parietally and occipitally in MID than SDAT patients, with the former also showing a slower centroid left frontally and centrally and a faster β centroid bifrontally than the latter) (Fig. 4). A better discrimination between the two subtypes of dementia was obtained by means of power asymmetry indices, which revealed more asymmetry in MID than SDAT

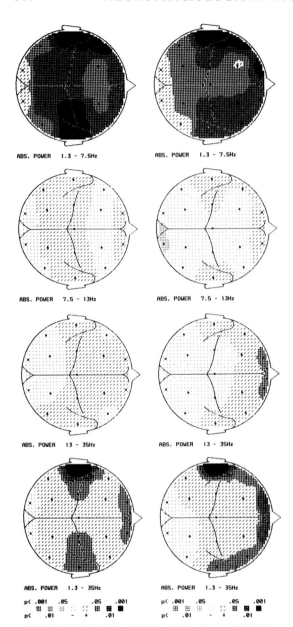

FIG. 1. Differences between SDAT patients and controls (*left side*) and between MID patients and controls (*right side*) in absolute EEG power depicted in brain maps (V-EEG, AV, *n* = 2 × 24). Statistical probability maps (SPM) depicting intergroup differences in absolute power of δ/θ (1.3–7.5 Hz), α (7.5–13 Hz) and β activity (13–35 Hz) and total power (1.3–35 Hz) are shown in the respective four rows. δ/θ Power is increased in SDAT mostly over the left frontotemporal to temporal and right temporal to central regions (*p* < 0.001), and over both parietal, frontopolar, central and right frontotemporal regions (*p* < 0.01), and over both frontal and occipitotemporal regions (*p* < 0.05). MID patients demonstrated the δ/θ augmentation mostly over left temporal to frontotemporal to frontopolar regions (*p* < 0.001), and over both central, the right frontopolar, frontal, frontotemporal and temporal areas (*p* < 0.01), and over the vertex, parietal, and left occipitotemporal regions (*p* < 0.05). The δ/θ augmentation in both subtypes of dementia was significant based on confirmatory statistics. There were generally no differences in absolute α and β power, whereas total power was augmented in SDAT and MID patients over both temporal and frontopolar regions, with an additional augmentation over central regions in SDAT and frontotemporal areas in MID cases.

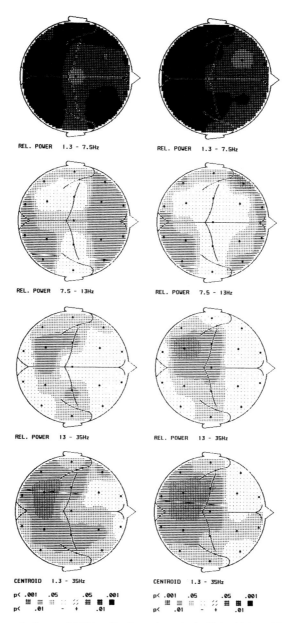

FIG. 2. Differences between SDAT patients and controls (*left side*) and between MID patients and controls (*right side*) in relative power depicted in EEG brain maps (V-EGG, AV, $n = 2 \times 24$). For technical description of maps see legend of Fig. 1. Relative power was augmented ubiquitously in the δ/θ range, relative α and β power was attenuated in both subgroups of dementia over various brain regions. The centroid of the total activity was slowed down in both subgroups of dementia.

TABLE 1. *EEG power spectra data (X, s) in senile dementia of the Alzheimer type and muti-infarct dementia patients and controls II (V-EEG, T_3 = AV)*

Variable	SDAT (n = 24)	MID (n = 24)	Controls (n = 24)
Absolute power (pW)			
Total power (1.3–35 Hz)	71.5 (40.4)***	88.5 (61.1)***	33.6 (23.6)
δ (1.3–3.5 Hz)	14.5 (15.8)**	16.1 (14.5)***	3.9 (2.6)
θ (3.5–7.5 Hz)	19.9 (14.8)***	24.6 (23.8)***	4.9 (4.2)
δ/θ (1.3–7.5 Hz)	34.3 (27.3)***	40.7 (35.1)***	8.8 (6.5)
α (7.5–13 Hz)	21.4 (14.4)	22.6 (16.2)	14.2 (13.1)
β (13–35 Hz)	15.8 (14.2)	25.1 (38.1)	10.7 (7.2)
Relative power (%)			
δ (1.3–3.5 Hz)	19.0 (13.0)*	19.1 (11.8)*	12.3 (4.8)
θ (3.5–7.5 Hz)	25.7 (12.1)***	25.3 (13.4)***	14.0 (6.6)
δ/θ (1.3–7.5 Hz)	44.6 (21.1)***	44.4 (21.5)***	26.3 (10.2)
α (7.5–13 Hz)	30.2 (13.3)*	28.8 (13.7)*	37.8 (9.8)
β (13–35 Hz)	25.1 (17.1)*	26.8 (19.6)	36.0 (14.1)
Centroid total (Hz)	10.2 (3.4)*	10.5 (3.7)*	12.4 (2.5)

* $p < 0.05$, ** $p < 0.01$ (t test), *** $p < 0.001$.

patients concerning δ/θ power frontally, α power parietally, and β power frontopolarly, frontally, and centrally (Fig. 5).

Correlations Between CT, EEG, Clinical, and Psychometric Measurements

Previous investigations utilizing correlation maps regarding the relationship between 11 CT, 9 clinical, and 36 quantitative EEG variables demon-

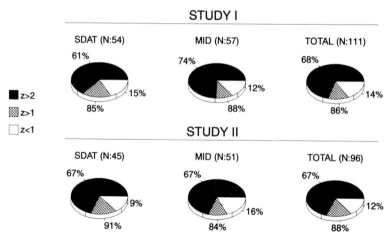

FIG. 3. Percent of patients showing increased slow activity (absolute δ and θ power) in at least one brain region as expressed in z values (number of standard deviations) from the norm. Eighty-six to 88% of demented patients demonstrate in the target variable "δ and θ power" in at least one brain region an increase of over 1 standard deviation from the norm, 67–68% exhibited an increase of at least 2 standard deviations. The results of two different studies are very similar.

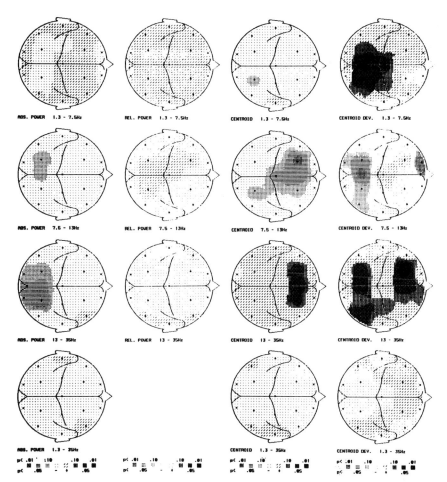

FIG. 4. Topographic EEG differences between MID patients (*n* = 51) and SDAT patients (*n* = 45) as shown in EEG brain maps (V-EEG, AV). Statistical probability maps (SPM) depicting inter-group differences in absolute power (left column), relative power (second column from the left), in centroids (third column from the left), and centroid deviations (right column) in the δ/θ, α, β, and total frequency range (top to bottom rows, respectively) are demonstrated. MID patients show less absolute β activity, no differences in relative power, a slowed α centroid and an accelerated β centroid, as well as an increased centroid deviation in the δ/θ activity, and β frequency range and a decreased centroid deviation in the α range as compared with SDAT patients.

strated that the less the cortical density and the wider the CSF spaces measured in the CT, the higher was the relative power in the δ/θ and the less in the α and β frequency range, and the slower the centroid of the total activity (4,7) (Fig. 6). Furthermore, the more pronounced the slowing of the brain function as determined by quantitative EEG variables, the worse was the psychopathology as evaluated by the clinician, utilizing the SCAG score as

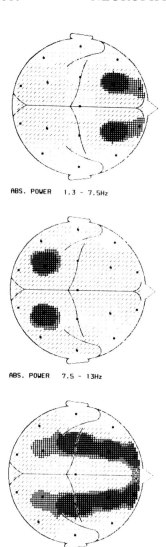

ABS. POWER   1.3 - 7.5Hz

ABS. POWER   7.5 - 13Hz

ABS. POWER   13 - 35Hz

p< .01   .10   .10   .01
p<   .05   -   +   .05

FIG. 5. Differences in power asymmetry indices between MID patients ($n = 51$) and SDAT patients ($n = 45$) shown in statistical probability maps. MID patients, as compared with SDAT patients, revealed an increased power asymmetry in the δ/θ range over the frontal regions (*upper part*), in the α range over the parietal regions (*middle part*), and in the β range frontopolarly to frontally to centrally (*lower part*).

well as SCAG factors. Finally, significant correlations were obtained between EEG mapping and psychometric variables; the slower the brain activity, the worse was the patients' performance in regard to cognition and memory, evaluated by means of the psychometric test battery.

In the recent replication study, confirmatory statistics failed to find significant correlations between the prechosen CT variable (greatest distance be-

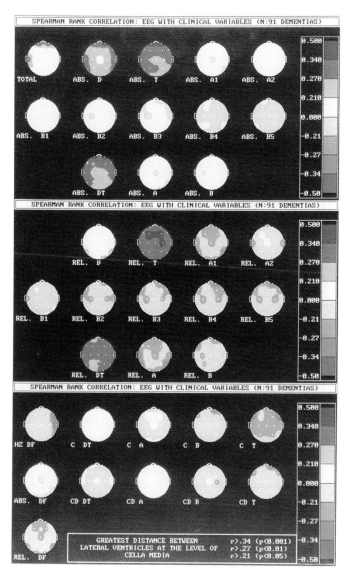

FIG. 6. Brain maps of correlations between a CT measurement (greatest distance between lateral ventricles at the level of cella media) and 36 EEG variables in dementia (*n* = 91). Each of the 36 maps shows the topographic display of correlation coefficients between the CT and a specific EEG variable. The *upper part* of the figure shows 13 correlation maps of absolute power variables, the *middle part* shows 12 relative power variables, and the *lower part* shows 11 centroid and dominant frequency measurements. The eight color key represents positive (hot/red colors) and negative (cold/blue colors) correlation coefficients. Significance levels are shown in the right lower corner. The larger the lateral ventricles (reflecting brain atrophy) in the CT, the more δ/θ activity, the less α (A) and β (B) activity, and the slower the centroid (CT) in the EEG.

tween lateral ventricles) and δ/θ power, whereas significant correlations were found between the latter and the SCAG score and the DSST: the more δ/θ power, the higher was the SCAG score rated by the psychiatrist and the worse was performance in the DSST (Fig. 7).

Descriptive data analysis utilizing Spearman's Rank correlations between 11 CT and 36 EEG variables demonstrated that: the greater the distance between the anterior horns and the candate nuclei and the lower the cortical density, the higher was the δ power. Cortical density was usually negatively correlated with power in all frequency bands. The larger the distance between the chorioid plexus, the less β power and the slower the centroid of the total activity.

More significant and higher correlations were found between EEG measures and clinical variables such as the MMSE (Fig. 8), SCAG, and CGI. The more δ/θ and the less α and β activity, and the slower the centroid of the total activity, the lower was the MMSE (Fig. 8) and the higher was the SCAG and the CGI. Many significant correlations were also found between EEG and psychometric performance measurements: the higher the δ/θ and the less the α and β activity and the slower the centroid of the total activity, the worse was the performance in the DSST, the TMT, and the DS.

Pharmaco-EEG Mapping in the Classification and Determination of Cerebral Bioavailability of Nootropics

Antihypoxidotics/nootropics produce significant changes in the quantitatively analyzed EEGs of normal elderly subjects characterized by a decrease in slow activity and an increase in α and/or β activity (2,3,5,20,23). These changes are opposite to alterations in brain function found during normal and pathologic aging and are indicative of improvement in vigilance. Moreover, the type of change is different from those seen after administration of other psychopharmacologic classes such as neuroleptics, antidepressants, tranquilizers, and psychostimulants (Figs. 9 and 10). Figures 9 and 10 depict pharmaco-EEG maps 1 h after oral administration of 600 mg pyritinol or placebo. Whereas power shows a trend toward a decrease, a significant increase is observed in α and β power. Relative δ/θ power decreases significantly over the vertex region, centrally, left frontotemporally, and parietally, whereas α activity increases. Total power increases, as does the centroid and the absolute power of the dominant frequency. Drugs inducing similar changes include representatives of different drug classes, such as codergocrine mesylate and nicergoline of the ergotalkaloids (2,21,27,28); further vincamine, vinconate, SL76100, and SL76188 of the vincamine alkaloids and analogues (29–31); ifenprodil, tinofedrine, and suloctidile of the phenylethanolamines (32); piracetam, etiracetam, aniracetam and tenilsetam of the pyrrolidine derivatives structurally related to GABA (2,31,33–36); ethophylline of the xanthine derivatives (2); buflomedil (31); ouabaine (g-strophantine) of

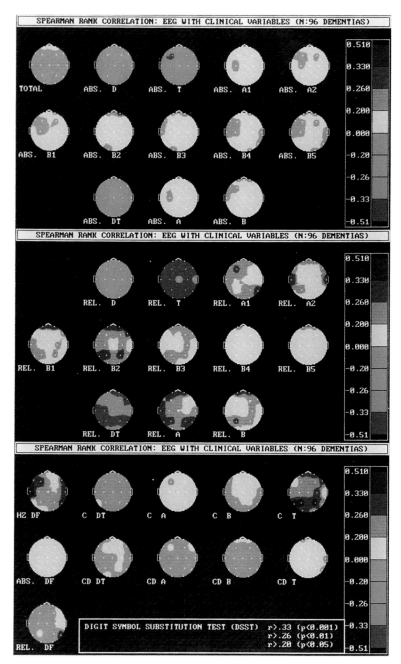

FIG. 7. Brain maps of correlations between psychometric performance (digit symbol substitution test) and 36 EEG variables in dementia (*n* = 96). For technical description of maps and color key, see legend to Fig. 5. The higher the δ/θ activity and the slower the centroid of the total activity, the worse is the performance in the digit symbol substitution test.

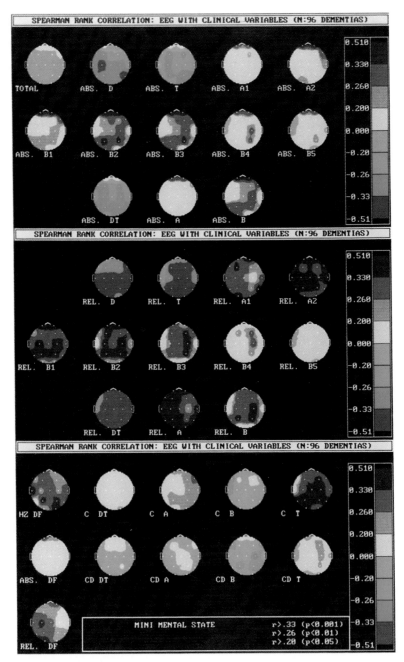

FIG. 8. Brain maps of correlations between cognitive decline evaluated by the Mini-Mental State Examination (MMSE) and 36 EEG variables in dementia (*n* = 96). For technical descriptions of maps and color key, see legend to Fig. 6. The more δ/θ activity, the less α and β activity, and the slower the centroid of the total activity, the lower is the MMS reflecting cognitive decline.

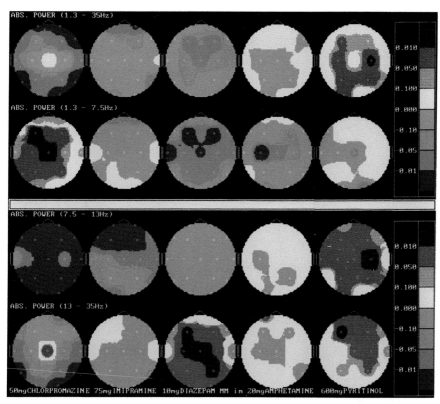

FIG. 9. Topographic pharmaco-EEG changes of absolute power in the 1.3–35 Hz (total power), 1.3–7.5 Hz (δ/θ), 7.5–13 Hz (α), and 13–35 Hz (β) frequency bands (top to bottom row, respectively) after representative drugs of the five main psychopharmacologic classes. Each pharmaco-EEG significance probability image represents the results of a statistical comparison by t test of drug-induced to placebo-induced changes (2 h post-drug, except for pyritinol, 1 h post-drug). The eight-color scale shows differences between drug-induced and placebo-induced changes (based on t values expressed in p = values): dark blue, decrease at $p < 0.01$ level; light blue, decrease at $p < 0.05$; dark green, decrease at $p < 0.10$; light green, trend towards decrease; light yellow, trend toward increase; dark yellow, increase at $p < 0.10$; red, increase at $p < 0.05$; lilac, increase at $p < 0.01$. The neuroleptic chlorpromazine 50 mg decreases total power as well as absolute α and β power (except for the vertex) and increases δ/θ power. The antidepressant imipramine 75 mg attenuates power in the total frequency range as well as in the δ/θ and α bands, mostly over frontal regions. The tranquillizer diazepam 10 mg attenuates total as well as δ/θ power and increases beta power. The psychostimulant amphetamine 20 mg decreases δ/θ power. The nootropic pyritinol 600 mg augments total power as well as α and β power and attenuates δ/θ power only occipitally.

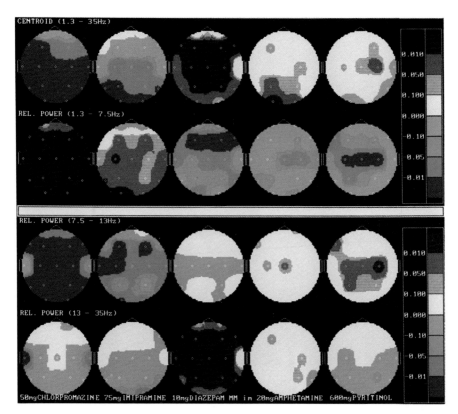

FIG. 10. Topographic pharmaco-EEG changes in the centroid of the total activity (1.3–35 Hz) as well as in relative power of the 1.3–7.5 Hz (δ/θ), 7.5–13 Hz (α), and 13–35 Hz (β) power (top to bottom row, respectively) after representative drugs of the five main psycho-pharmacologic classes. For technical description and color key, see legend in Fig. 8. The neuroleptic chlorpromazine 50 mg slows the centroid, augments δ/θ, and attenuates α and β activity. The antidepressant imipramine 75 mg slows the centroid over posterior parts of the brain, augments moderately δ/θ and attenuates α and occipitally β power. The tranquillizer diazepam 10 mg accelerates the centroid, decreases δ/θ, and increases β activity. The psychostimulant amphetamine 20 mg accelerates occipitally the centroid, decreases centrally δ/θ and increases α activity (vertex). The nootropic pyritinol 600 mg accelerates the centroid centrally, attenuates δ/θ and augments α activity over various brain regions.

the cardiac glycosides; acrihelline of the cardiac steroids; and adrafinil (a benzhydryl-sulfinylacetohydroxamic acid) and its main metabolite modafinil (a benzhydrylsulfinylacetamide) (37). Further drugs inducing such CNS changes were piridoxilate (a glyoxilic acid-substituted pyridoxine), Actovegin (a standardized deproteinized hemoderivative), hexobendine and its combination with ethophylline and ethamivan, Instenon forte, the calcium antagonist cinnarizine, pyritinol and Duxil (an almitrine/raubasin combination) (1,2,20,38–40), and the cholinergic compound linopirdine (DUP 996) (41).

The aforementioned neurophysiologic alterations reflecting an improvement in vigilance were associated with behavior changes such as improvement of complex reaction, psychomotor activity, reaction time, mood, affectivity, attention variability, and tapping, and an increase in critical flicker frequency (CFF) (6). This association was found not only in acute studies but also after chronic administration of antihypoxidotics in the elderly, which supports the idea that improvement of vigilance is linked to improvement in adaptive behavior in humans.

Pharmaco-EEG mapping may also be utilized to explore time–efficacy (Fig. 11) and dose–efficacy relationships (Fig. 12), as well as bioequipotency of different galenic formulations of nootropics (20,22,23).

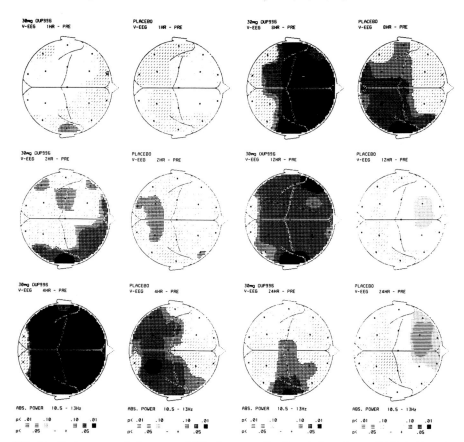

FIG. 11. Brain maps of pharmaco-EEG changes after linopirdine 30 mg (DUP 996) and placebo in absolute power of fast α activity (10.5–13 Hz) at hours 1, 2, 4, 8, 12, and 24 post-oral administration ($n = 13$). Each statistical map represents the result of a statistical comparison by t test of post-drug to baseline power values. DUP 996 30 mg produces, as compared with baseline, a moderate to marked increase of fast α activity from hour 2 through hour 24, whereas after placebo an α augmentation is only seen in hours 4 and 8 to a moderate extent. Conversely, in hours 12 and 24, a decline can be observed.

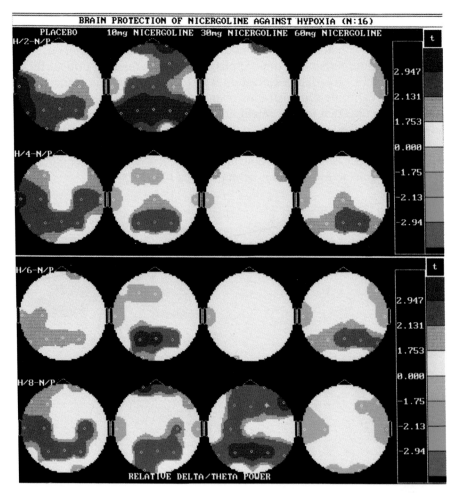

FIG. 12. Brain protection of nicergoline against hypoxia as demonstrated by EEG brain mapping of the relative δ/θ power under hypoxia (H) (9.8% O_2) 2, 4, 6, and 8 h after placebo, 10, 30 and 60 mg nicergoline as compared with normoxia (N) (21% O_2) ($n = 16$). The eight-color scale shows hypoxia-induced changes 2, 4, 6, and 8 h (top to bottom row) after administration of placebo, 10, 30, and 60 mg nicergoline (left to right column) based on t values expressed in p values. For description of the color key, see legend to Fig. 11. Under placebo/hypoxia conditions, δ/θ activity increases specifically over the parietal and temporal and central regions, and is attenuated by 30 and 60 mg nicergoline.

EEG Studies in Experimentally Induced Cognitive Disorders

In the development of new nootropic agents, animal models have been used to produce a state of memory and/or behavior impairment that should be either prevented or reversed by nootropic drugs. Examples are brain lesions, electroconvulsive shock, genetic models, hypoxia, drug-induced deficit models (e.g., scopolamine), and the use of aged animals. In recent years, similar models have been increasingly utilized in human gerontopsychopharmacology as well, specifically the scopolamine and the hypoxia model. In several investigations we could demonstrate that drugs such as co-dergocrine mesylate, nicergoline, aniracetam, tenilsetam, and pyritinol exert brain-protective properties in an experimentally induced hypoxic hypoxidosis (42–47). Hypoxic hypoxidosis was produced by inhalation of a combination of a hypoxic gas mixture (e.g., 9.8% O_2, equivalent to 6,000 m altitude) under normobaric conditions. In the quantitatively analyzed EEG, δ/θ power increased under hypoxia, which was mitigated dose dependently by certain nootropic drugs (Fig. 12).

EEG Mapping in Therapeutic Efficacy Trials in Demented Patients

Topographic mapping of the EEG can be utilized to monitor the therapeutic efficacy of a drug with regard to vigilance improvement both in single patients (Fig. 13) and in large-scale, multicenter therapeutic trials (6,8,48,49). The vigilance-improving property of nootropics, as well as the target area of their action may differ in degenerative and vascular dementia. As can be

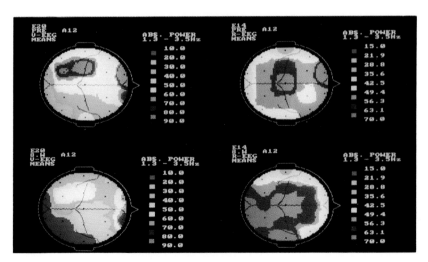

FIG. 13. Topographic brain maps of the absolute power in the δ activity in a therapy-responsive and a therapy-resistant MID patient (left and right row, respectively) before (*upper maps*) and after (*lower maps*) 8 weeks of treatment with nicergoline 20 mg daily. The color key represents absolute δ power in μV^2. Although the therapy-responsive patient shows a decrease of slow activity (vigilance improvement), the therapy-resistant patient shows an increase.

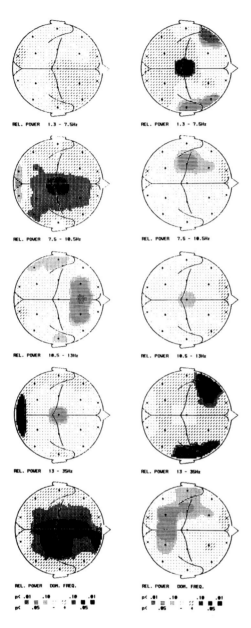

FIG. 14. Pharmaco-EEG maps of differences between xantinolnicotinate- and placebo-treated SDAT patients (*left side*) and MID patients (*right side*). Statistical probability maps concerning relative power of the combined δ/θ, α-1, α-2, and combined β activity as well as the relative power of the dominant frequency, are demonstrated, depicting differences between the drug- and placebo-induced changes in terms of *p* values. In SDAT patients, 8 weeks of treatment with 3 g xantinolnicotinate per day (*n* = 19) results (as compared with placebo) (*n* = 21) in an increase of slow α, a decrease of fast α, an increase of occipital, and a decrease of vertex β activity as well as an augmentation of relative power of the dominant frequency over various brain regions. In MID patients, 8 weeks of therapy with 3 g xantinolnicotinate (*n* = 26) induces (as compared with placebo) (*n* = 23) an attenuation of δ/θ activity and an augmentation of β activity over the FT-T regions as well as a decrease of relative power of the dominant frequency and slow α activities over the left C and P regions.

seen in Fig. 14, the most prominent change exhibited by SDAT patients is increase of relative α-1 power, mostly over the vertex region, after 8 weeks of treatment with 3 g xantinolnicotinate daily, whereas vascular dementia patients exhibit as the most prominent change a decrease of δ/θ activity and an increase of β activity. This is of interest because CGI, SCAG, DSST,

TMT, and DS test performance improved in both subgroups of dementia to a similar extent as compared with placebo (Table 2). However, if one analyzes EEG drug effects by MANOVA considering time (week 0, 8), groups (drug, placebo), and relative power variables (δ/θ, α-1 and -2, and β), the action of the drugs in SDAT patients is seen mostly over the frontal region, whereas in MID patients the action is seen mostly over both FT regions (significant Hotelling's T^2 values >2.57, $p < 0.05$).

Event-Related Potentials in Gerontopsychopharmacology

ERPs and specifically the P300 cognitive potential, have been increasingly utilized in gerontopsychopharmacology for several reasons. First, there is a strong relationship to cognitive aspects of controlled information processing (see refs. 50–52 for review). In signal detection paradigms, latencies of the P300 complex, specifically the so-called P3b first described by Squires et al. (18) appear to reflect stimulus evaluation time but not response selection time. Amplitudes of these components have been shown to be related to processing resources that are requested when a perceptual set has to be changed according to the environmental demands. Second, age-related changes in a variety of cognitive functions are correlated with changes in ERP components evaluated by means of different experimental approaches in the auditory, visual, and somatosensory modality and by different recording and analysis techniques. Many studies have demonstrated that the latency of P300 increases with increasing age (53). There is also strong evidence that P300 amplitude decreases over central and parietal regions and that the scalp distribution changes to a more frontal orientation (54). Third, in various neurologic disorders P300 seems to be abnormal, e.g., in dementia of the Alzheimer type, amplitude was reduced and latency was lengthened (55,56), and in multiple sclerosis latency was prolonged (57). Goodin and Aminoff (58,59) suggested that ERPs may be helpful in elucidating the underlying pathogenesis of different dementia syndromes, such as dementia associated with Alzheimer disease (AD), Parkinson disease, and Huntington's disease. Abnormal ERPs are interpreted in dementia and for pharmacologic effects on ERPs, it is important to consider the cortex as a major current source of the P300, although various subcortical generators, such as the hippocampus and amygdala, have also been proposed (60). Finally, different drugs have been reported to affect P300 ERPs, e.g., the catecholaminergic psychostimulant methylphenidate enhanced P300 amplitude depending on the subject's state and task demands (61), the anticholineric drug scopolamine slowed P300 in young women (62), and the neuroleptic flupentixol suppressed P300 amplitude, indicating an impairing effect on human information-processing resources (63). A cholinergic nootropic (WEB 1881 FU) significantly influenced the overall amplitude of cognitive ERP components in incidental and

TABLE 2. Clinical changes of SDAT and MID patients after 8 weeks of therapy with 3 g xantinolnicotinate and placebo[a]

| | | SDAT (n = 52) | | | | | MID (n = 56) | | | | | |
| | | Xantinolnicotinate (n = 26) | | Placebo (n = 26) | | Diff. SX-SP U test | Xantinolnicotinate (n = 28) | | Placebo (n = 28) | | Diff. MX-MP U test | Other Diff. U test |
Test		Pre	8 wk	Pre	8 wk		Pre	8 wk	Pre	8 wk		
CGI	MD	6.00	4.00**	6.00	6.00	++	6.00	4.00**	6.00	6.00	++	SP vs MX++
	X̄	5.38	4.23	5.46	5.38		5.43	4.39	5.39	5.50		SX vs MP++
	SD	0.75	1.27	0.81	0.85		1.03	1.26	1.10	1.35		
SCAG	MD	69.0	63.5**	71.5	71.0	++	70.5	63.0**	71.0	70.0	++	SP vs MX++
	X̄	69.7	64.5	70.7	69.5		69.6	64.1	69.5	69.1		SX vs MP++
	SD	5.5	6.5	6.3	6.8		7.4	8.3	7.9	8.8		
Digit symbol substitution test (DSST)	MD	11.5	16.5**	9.5	12.0**	++	11.5	17.0**	11.0	13.0**	++	SP vs MX++
	X̄	12.2	16.9	10.8	12.9		11.3	17.3	11.9	13.6		SX vs MP++
	SD	4.6	5.8	4.7	6.7		3.8	5.4	6.3	6.8		
Trail-making test (TMT)	MD	91.5	82.8**	117.8	108.3**	n.s.	102.3	93.3**	98.0	93.3**	++	n.s
	X̄	99.8	93.4	117.1	111.4		110.9	104.3	113.9	106.9		
	SD	47.6	47.0	33.3	35.2		42.8	43.4	51.1	39.5		
Digit (DS)	MD	7.0	8.0**	6.0	6.5	++	7.0	8.0**	7.0	6.0	++	SP vs MX++
	X̄	6.8	7.7	6.7	6.7		6.9	7.6	6.8	6.6		SX vs MP++
	SD	1.0	1.2	1.2	1.3		1.4	1.1	1.6	1.5		

[a] ** $p < 0.01$ (Wilcoxon); ++ $p < 0.01$ (Mann–Whitney U test).

intentional memory tasks in young, healthy subjects, suggesting effects on the cognitive processes (64). On the other hand, there was no effect on ERP correlated with visuospatial attention, suggesting that early perceptual processes are not influenced by this cholinergic nootropic drug (65). In our own psychophysiological study using of the Viennese Psychophysiological Test System (VPTS) described by Semlitsch et al. (19), the antihypoxidotic/nootropic drugs tenilsetam and co-dergocrine mesylate increased P300 amplitudes as compared with placebo, which suggests an improving effect on information processing resources (66) (Fig. 15). P300 latencies were unchanged, which indicated no effect on stimulus evaluation time. In addition, tenilsetam also affects early stages of information processing (66).

With the advent of mini- and microcomputers, topographic distributions of event-related potentials came into the center of research. Topographic variations indicate that P300 (P3b) is not a unitary phenomenon but rather is a composite of activities arising from multiple intercranial sources of bioelectric generators (67), suggesting multiple contributions to scalp-recorded P300 (68). In a double-blind, placebo-controlled study, the effects of the hemoderivative Actovegin on cognitive event-related potentials were studied in 18 age-associated memory impairment (AAMI) patients. P300 latencies are delayed in AAMI (393.8 ms) as compared with young subjects (349.0 ms). Moreover, P300 amplitude was reduced in central and parietal leads (e.g., at Cz 12.7 vs. 13.7 μV and at Pz 14.5 vs. 16.9 μV for AAMI and young subjects, respectively) and augmented in frontal leads (e.g., at Fz 11.9 vs. 7.3 μV for AAMI and young subjects, respectively). These findings are in accordance with the reported change in the scalp distribution of P300 amplitude in the elderly to a more frontal orientation (54). P300 amplitude increased after acute, subacute, and superimposed infusion of 250 ml 20% Actovegin as compared with placebo, confirming the hypothesis that nootropic drugs influence the P300 amplitude in the sense of an improved availability of cognitive processing resources (Fig. 16). This increase of P300 amplitude (up to 4.8 μV), seen specifically in central and parietal regionss, proved to be significant in a confirmatory test (69). There was no effect on earlier stages of information processing measured by N1 and P2 components of nontarget ERP or on ERP latencies. Our P300 findings were therefore of interest, as in psychometric tests Actovegin mostly improved the noopsyche with regard to attention, memory, and rigidity/perseveration measurements (70). With regard to the thymopsyche, an improvement was noted in mood, affect, wellbeing, and sedation. Last but not least, we found an improvement in vigilance, as reflected in the EEG mapping (70).

Studying the acute effects of amantadine infusions on ERP in 20 mildly demented patients diagnosed according to DSM-III-R criteria, we found no amantadine effect on ERP latencies (71). N1 of the nontarget showed a trend toward amplitude augmentation; P2 amplitude was reduced. As compared with placebo, P300 amplitude of targets was significantly augmented by 3.1

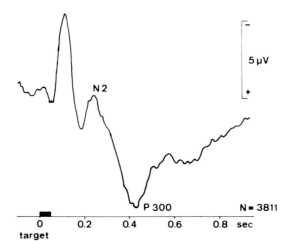

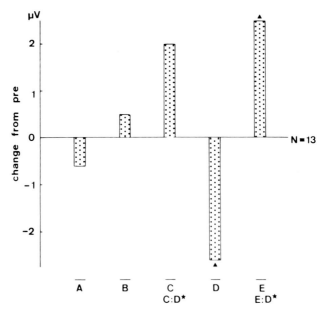

FIG. 15. Grand average and drug-induced changes of the event-related potential (ERP, P300) obtained in elderly patients in the signal detection test (SIG-DET) 2 h after tenilsetam (TEN), co-dergocrine mesylate (CDM), and placebo (*n* = 13). *Upper,* grand average. The grand average ERP evoked by the targets in the SIG-DET test is shown. The latency of N2 is 247.5 ms, the amplitude is 0.2 μV. The latency of P300 is 427.7 ms, the amplitude is 7.6 μV. *Lower,* Drug effect. Changes of N2-P300 amplitudes are demonstrated as obtained 2 h after 150 mg TEN (*A*), 300 mg TEN (*B*), 900 mg TEN (*C*), placebo (*D*), and 5 mg CDM (*E*). A significant *p* value of the paired sampled *t* test (post- and pretreatment) is marked by a triangle (*p* < 0.05). Significant differences between the drugs and placebo are marked by an asterisk (*p* < 0.05 for the Newman–Keuls test). A dose-dependent increase of the N2-P300 amplitude can be seen after TEN and CDM as compared with placebo.

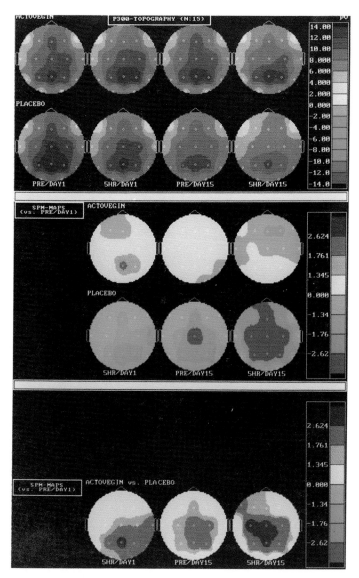

FIG. 16. Changes in P300 topography during acute, subacute and super-imposed infusion therapy of AAMI patients with Actovegin and placebo. *Upper:* topographic distribution of P300 amplitudes at peak latency of spatial average before (pre/day 1) as well as after acute (5 h/day 1), subacute (pre/day 15), and superimposed (5 h/day 15) infusion of Actovegin (250 ml 20% Actovegin) and placebo (n = 15). To allow comparison the scale is set to −14 μV. Middle part: descriptive significance probability maps (SPM) based on t values as compared to pre/day 1. *Lower:* placebo-corrected descriptive significance probability maps (SPM) based on *t* values as compared to pre/day 1. Hot colors represent an increase, cold colors a decrease (*t* > 1.34; *p* < 0.10; *t* > 1.76, *p* < 0.05; *t* > 2.62, *p* < 0.01). Actovegin significantly augments P300 amplitude in the sense of an improved availability of cognitive processing resources.

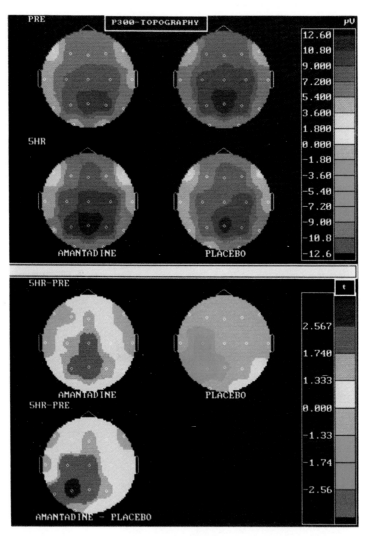

FIG. 17. P300 topography. *Upper part:* topographic distribution of P300 amplitudes at peak latency of spatial average before (PRE) as well as after infusion (5 h) of amantadine (0.2 g) and placebo in mildly demented patients ($n = 15$). To allow comparison, the scale is set to -12.6 μV to $+12.6$ μV. *Lower part:* descriptive significance probability maps (SPM) based on t values as compared with PRE (upper row) and placebo-corrected descriptive significance probability map (SPM) based on t values as compared with PRE (lower row). Hot colors represent an increase, cold colors a decrease ($t > 1.333$: $p < 0.10$; $t > 1.740$: $p < 0.05$; $t > 2.567$: $p < 0.01$). For the judgment of the hypothesis of increased P300 amplitude after infusion of amantadine as compared with placebo, descriptive p values for one-tailed test ($p < 0.05$) were chosen.

μV (30% of pretreatment value), confirming the hypothesis that amantadine (0.2 g) may influence the P300 amplitude in the sense of an improved availability of cognitive processing resources (Fig. 17).

SUMMARY

EEG/EP mapping is a readily available, noninvasive, high-time resolution method for objective and quantitative evaluation of the neurophysiologic basis of cognitive disorders.

On EEG maps the demented patients showed more slow activity and less α and β activity, as well as a slowing of the dominant frequency and the centroid. Changes were most prominent in parietal and temporal regions. MID patients exhibited markedly augmented δ/θ activity and attenuated α and β activity, with ubiquitous slowing of the dominant frequency and centroid. These neurophysiologic findings suggest a deterioration of vigilance. Differences between AD and MID patients were found primarily in differences between maximal and minimal power and right–left differences.

Correlation coefficients between CT and EEG variables demonstrated that the greater the anterior horn distance, lateral ventricle distance, and Evans' index, and the less the cortical density, the more the δ/θ activity and less the α and β activity. Moreover, higher δ/θ activity and lower α and β activity correlated with higher SCAG scores and worse psychometric performance. In human psychopharmacology, pharmaco-EEG/EP analysis and subsequent mapping can be utilized for classification and determination of cerebral bioavailability of nootropics. With regard to experimentally induced cognitive disorders, the hypoxia model seems to be a valuable specific method, as brain function slows under hypoxia, which is mitigated dose dependently by certain nootropic drugs.

Topographic mapping of the EEG can also be utilized to monitor the therapeutic efficacy of a drug with regard to vigilance improvement both in single patients and in large-scale multicenter therapeutic trials. Brain region differences in drug action can be demonstrated in SDAT and MID patients.

Finally, mapping of ERPs and specifically of P300 cognitive potentials, has been increasingly utilized in gerontopsychopharmacology to demonstrate improved availability of cognitive processing resources. Examples of drug-induced EP changes are shown in normally aged subjects, in AAMI as in mildly demented patients.

REFERENCES

1. Saletu B. *Psychopharmaka, Gehirntätigkeit und Schlaf*. Basel: Karger; 1976.
2. Saletu B. Application of quantitative EEG in measuring encephalotropic and pharmacodynamic properties of antihypoxidotic/nootropic drugs. In: Scientific International Research,

ed. *Drugs and methods in C.V.D. Proc. Int. Cerebrovascular Diseases*, France. New York: Pergamon Press; 1981:79–115.

3. Saletu B. The use of pharmaco-EEG in drug profiling. In: Hindmarch I, Stonier PD, eds. *Human psychopharmacology, measures and methods*, Vol 1. Chichester: John Wiley & Sons; 1987:173–200.

4. Saletu B. EEG brain mapping in dementia and gerontopsychopharmacology. In: Hindmarch I, Hippius H, Wilcock GK, eds. *Dementia: molecules, methods and measures*. Chichester: John Wiley & Sons Ltd; 1991:151–60.

5. Saletu B, Grünberger J. Memory dysfunction and vigilance: neurophysiological and psychopharmacological aspects. *Ann NY Acad Sci* 1985;444:406–27.

6. Saletu B, Anderer P, Paulus E, et al. EEG brain mapping in SDAT and MID patients before and during placebo and xantinolnicotinate therapy: reference considerations. In: Samson–Dollfus D, Guieu JD, Gotman J, Etevenon P, eds. *Statistics and topography in quantitative EEG*. Paris: Elsevier; 1988:251–75.

7. Saletu B, Anderer P, Paulus E, et al. EEG brain mapping in diagnostic and therapeutic assessment of dementia. *Alzheimer Dis Assoc Disord* 1991;5:57–75.

8. Saletu B, Anderer P, Fischhof PK, Lorenz H, Barousch R, Böhmer F, Paroubek J. EEG mapping and psychopharmacological studies with denbufylline in SDAT and MID. *Biol Psychiatry* 1992;32:668–81.

9. Itil TM, Shapiro DM, Eralp E, Akmann A, Itil KZ, Garbizu C. A new brain function diagnostic unit, including the dynamic brain mapping of computer analyzed EEG, evoked potentials and sleep (a new hardware/software system and its application in psychiatry and psychopharmacology). *New Trends Exp Clin Psychiatry* 1985;1:107–77.

10. Herrmann WM, Schärer E. Das Pharmako-EEG und seine Bedeutung für die klinische Pharmakologie. In: Kuemmerle HP, Hitzenberger G, Spitzy KH, eds. *Klinische Pharmakologie*, 4th ed. München: Landsberg; 1986:1–71.

11. Duffy FH, Albert MS, McAnulty G. Brain electrical activity in patients with presenile and senile dementia of the Alzheimer type. *Ann Neurol* 1984;16:439–48.

12. John ER, Prichep LS, Fridman J, Easton P. Neurometrics: computer assisted differential diagnosis of brain dysfunctions. *Science* 1988;239:162–9.

13. Maurer K. *Topographic brain mapping of EEG and evoked potentials*. Berlin: Springer Verlag; 1989.

14. Amaducci L, Angst J, Bech P, et al. Consensus conference on the methodology of clinical trials of "nootropics," Munich, June 1989. *Pharmacopsychiatry* 1990;23:171–5.

15. Bartels PH, Subach JA. Automated interpretation of complex scenes. In: Preston E, Onoe M, eds. *Digital processing of biomedical imagery*. New York: Academic Press; 1976: 101–14.

16. Duffy FH, Bartels PH, Burchfield JL. Significance probability mapping: an aid in the topographic analysis of brain electrical activity. *Electroencephalogr Clin Neurophysiol* 1981; 51:455–62.

17. Anderer P, Saletu B, Kinsperger K, Semlitsch H. Topographic brain mapping of EEG in neuropsychopharmacology—part I. Methodological aspects. *Methods Find Exp Clin Pharmacol* 1987;9:371–84.

18. Squires NK, Squires KC, Hillyard SA. Two varieties of long-latency positive waves evoked by unpredictable auditory stimuli in man. *Electroencephalogr Clin Neurophysiol* 1975;38: 387–401.

19. Semlitsch H, Anderer P, Saletu B, Resch F, Presslich O, Schuster P. Psychophysiological research in psychiatry and neuropharmacology. I. Methodological aspects of the Viennese Psychophysiological Test-System (VPTS). *Methods Find Exp Clin Pharmacol* 1989;11: 25–41.

20. Saletu B, Anderer P, Kinsperger K, Grünberger J. Topographic brain mapping of EEG in neuropsychopharmacology—part II. Clinical applications (pharmaco EEG imaging). *Methods Find Exp Clin Pharmacol* 1987;9:385–408.

21. Saletu B, Grünberger J, Anderer P. Proof of antihypoxidotic properties of tenilsetam in man by EEG and psychometric analyses under an experimental hypoxic hypoxidosis. *Drug Dev Res* 1987;10:135–55.

22. Saletu B, Anderer P, Grünberger J. EEG brain mapping in gerontopsychopharmacology: on protective properties of pyritinol against hypoxic hypoxidosis. *Psychiatry Res* 1989;29: 387–90.

23. Saletu B, Anderer P, Grünberger J. Topographic brain mapping of EEG after acute application of ergotalkaloids in the elderly. *Arch Gerontol Geriatr* 1990;11:1–22.
24. Saletu B, Saletu M, Grünberger J, Mader R. Spontaneous and drug-induced remission of alcoholic organic brain syndrome. *Psychiatry Res* 1983;10:59–75.
25. Saletu B, Linzmayer L, Grünberger J, Pietschmann H. Double-blind, placebo-controlled, clinical, psychometric and neurophysiological investigations with oxiracetam in the organic brain syndrome of late life. *Neuropsychobiology* 1985;13:44–52.
26. Abt K. Descriptive data analysis (DDA) in quantitative EEG studies. In: Samson-Dollfus D, Guieu JD, Gotman J, Etevenon P, eds. *Statistics and topography in quantitative EEG,* Amsterdam: Elsevier; 1988:150–60.
27. Saletu B, Grünberger J, Linzmayer L. Bestimmung der encephalotropen, psychotropen und pharmakodynamischen Eigenschaften von Nicergolin mittels quantitativer Pharmakoelektroenzephalographie und psychometrischer Analysen. *Arzneimittelforschung* 1979; 29:1251–61.
28. Saletu B, Grünberger J, Linzmayer L, Anderer P. Proof of CNS efficacy and pharmacodynamics of nicergoline in the elderly by acute and chronic quantitative pharmaco-EEG and psychometric studies. In: Tognoni G, Garattini S, eds. *Drug treatment in chronic cerebrovascular disorders.* Amsterdam: Elsevier/North Holland Biomedical Press; 1979:245–72.
29. Saletu B, Grünberger J. Zur Pharmakodynamik von Vincamin: Pharmako-EEG und psychometrische Studien bei Alternden. In: Lechner H, ed. *Fortschritte in Pathophysiologie, Diagnostik und Therapie cerebraler Gefβkrankheiten,* Amsterdam: Excerpta Medica; 1982: 154–177.
30. Grünberger J, Saletu B, Linzmayer L, Stöhr H. Objective measures in determining the central effectiveness of a new antihypoxidotic SL-76188: pharmaco-EEG, psychometric and pharmacokinetic analyses in the elderly. *Arch Gerontol Geriatr* 1982;1:261–85.
31. Saletu B, Grünberger J, Linzmayer L, Wittek R. Classification and determination of pharmacodynamics of a new antihypoxidotic drug, vinconate, by pharmaco-EEG and psychometry. *Arch Gerontol Geriatr* 1984;3:127–46.
32. Saletu B, Anderer P. Double-blind placebo-controlled quantitative pharmaco-EEG investigations after tinofedrine i.v. in geriatric patients. *Curr Ther Res* 1980;28:1–15.
33. Saletu B, Grünberger J. Antihypoxidotic and nootropic drugs: proof of their encephalotropic and pharmacodynamic properties by quantitative EEG investigations. *Prog Neuro-Psychopharmacol* 1980;4:469–89.
34. Saletu B, Grünberger J, Linzmayer L. Quantitative EEG and psychometric analyses in assessing CNS-activity of RO 13-5057—a cerebral insufficiency improver. *Methods Find Exp Clin Pharmacol* 1980;2:269–85.
35. Saletu B, Grünberger J, Cepko H. Pharmacokinetic and -dynamic studies in elderlies with a potential antihypoxidotic/nootropic drug tenilsetam utilizing pharmaco-EEG and psychometry. *Drug Dev Res* 1986;9:95–113.
36. Bente D. Vigilanz: psychophysiologische Aspekte. *Verh Dtsch Ges Inn Med* 1977;83: 945–52.
37. Saletu B, Grünberger J, Linzmayer L, Stöhr H. Pharmaco-EEG, psychometric and plasma level studies with two novel alpha-adrenergic stimulants CRL 40476 and 40028 (Adrafinil) in elderlies. *New Trends Exp Clin Psychiatry* 1986;2:5–31.
38. Saletu B, Grünberger J, Rajna P, Stöhr H. Vigilanzverbesserung bei alternden Menschen: Doppelblinde, placebokontrollierte neurophysiologische und psychometrische Studien mit Pridoxilat. *Therapiewoche* 1982;32:5590–603.
39. Saletu B, Grünberger J, Linzmayer L, Stöhr H. Zur Funktionsbesserung des alternden Gehirns: Placebokontrollierte Pharmako-EEG und psychometrische Studien mit einem stoffwechselaktiven Hämoderivat (Actovegin). *Z Gerontol* 1984;17:271–9.
40. Saletu B, Grünberger J, Linzmayer L, Anderer P. Einfluβ eines eiweiβfreien Organextraktes auf die Vigilanz alternder Menschen. Doppelblinde, placebokontrollierte Pharmako-EEG-Untersuchungen mit zwei verschiedenen galenischen Formulierungen. *Therapiewoche* 1986;36:4131–48.
41. Saletu B, Darragh A, Salmon P, Coen R. EEG brain mapping in evaluating the time-course of the central action of DUP 996—a new acetylcholine releasing drug. *Br J Clin Pharmacol* 1989;28:1–16.
42. Saletu B, Grünberger J. Cerebral hypoxic hypoxidosis: neurophysiological, psychometric and pharmacotherapeutic aspects. *Adv Biol Psychiatry* 1983:146–64.

43. Saletu B, Grünberger J. The hypoxia model in human psychopharmacology: neurophysiological and psychometric studies with aniracetam i.v. *Hum Neurobiol* 1984;3:171–81.
44. Saletu B, Grünberger J, Anderer P. Proof of antihypoxidotic properties of tenilsetam in man by EEG and psychometric analyses under an experimental hypoxic hypoxidosis. *Drug Dev Res* 1987;10:135–55.
45. Saletu B, Anderer P, Grünberger J. EEG brain mapping in gerontopsychopharmacology: on protective properties of pyritinol against hypoxic hypoxidosis. *Psychiatry Res* 1989;29: 387–90.
46. Saletu B, Grünberger J, Anderer P. On brain protection of co-dergocrine mesylate (Hydergine[R]) against hypoxic hypoxidosis of different severity: double-blind placebo-controlled quantitative EEG and psychometric studies. *Internation* 1990;28:510–24.
47. Saletu B, Grünberger J, Linzmayer L, Anderer P. Brain protection of nicergoline against hypoxia: EEG brain mapping and psychometry. *J Neural Transm Park Dis Dement Sect* 1990;2:305–25.
48. Saletu B, Hochmayer I, Grünberger J, et al. Zur Therapie der Multiinfarktdemenz mit Nicergolin: doppelblinde, klinische, psychometrische und EEG-Imaginguntersuchungen mit 2 Dosierungsschemata. *Wien Med Wochenschr* 1987;137:513–24.
49. Fischhof PK, Saletu B, Rüther E, Litschauer G, Möslinger-Gehmayr R, Herrmann WM. Therapeutic efficacy of pyritinol in patients with senile dementia of the Alzheimer type (SDAT) and multi-infarct dementia (MID). *Neuropsychobiology* 1992;26:65–70.
50. Johnson R Jr. A triachic model of P300 amplitude. *Psychophysiology* 1986;23:367–84.
51. McCarty G, Donchin E. Chronometric analysis of human information processing. In: Gaillard, Ritter, eds. *Tutorials in ERP research: endogenous components*. Amsterdam: Elsevier; 1983:251–68.
52. Rösler F, Sutton S, Johnson R, et al. Endogenous ERP components and cognitive constructs. A review. *Electroenceph Clin Neurophysiol* 1986;38:51–92.
53. Pfefferbaum A, Ford JM, Wenegrat BB, Roth WT, Kopell BS. Clinical application of the P3 component of event-related potential. I. Normal aging. *Electroenceph Clin Neurophysiol* 1984;59:85–103.
54. Friedman D, Hamberger M, Putnam L. The frontal lobe dysfunction hypothesis in the elderly: evidence from event-related potentials [Abstract]. 9th International Conference. Event-related potential of the brain. Noordwijk; 1985.
55. Ito J, Yamao S, Fukuda H, Mimori Y, Nakamura S. The P300 event-related potential in dementia of Alzheimer type. Correlation between P300 and monamine metabolites. *Electroenceph Clin Neurophysiol* 1990;77:174–8.
56. Polich J, Ladisch C, Bloom RE. P300 assessment of early Alzheimer's disease. *Electroenceph Clin Neurophysiol* 1990;77:179–89.
57. Newton MR, Barret G, Callanan MM, Towell AD. Cognitive event-related potentials in multiple sclerosis. *Brain* 1990;112:1637–60.
58. Goodin DS, Aminoff MJ. Electrophysiological differences between subtypes of dementia. *Brain* 1986;109:1103–13.
59. Goodin DS, Aminoff MJ. Electrophysiological differences between demented and nondemented patients with Parkinson's disease. *Ann Neurol* 1987;21:90–4.
60. Rockstroh B, Elbert T, Canavan A, Lutzenberger W, Birbaumer N. *Slow cortical potentials and behavior*. Baltimore: Urban & Schwarzenberg; 1989.
61. Klorman R, Brumghim JT, Salzman LF, et al. Effects of methylphenidate on stimulus evaluation and response processes: evidence from performance and event-related potentials. *Psychophysiology* 1988;25:292–304.
62. Callaway E. Human information processing: some effects on methylphenidate age and scopolamine. *Biol Psychiatry* 1984;19:649–62.
63. Rösler F, Manzey D, Sojka B, Stieglitz RD. Delineation of pharmacopsychological effects by means of endogenous event-related potentials: an exemplification with flupentixol. *Neuropsychobiology* 1985;13:81–92.
64. Münte TF, Heinze HJ, Scholz M, Künkel H. Effects of a cholinergic nootropic (WEB 1881 FU) on event-related potentials recorded in incidental and intentional memory tasks. *Neuropsychobiology* 1988;19:158–68.
65. Münte TF, Heinze HJ, Scholz Mb, Bartusch SM, Dietrich DE. Event-related potentials and visual spatial attention: influence of a cholinergic drug. *Neuropsychobiology* 1989;21: 94–9.

66. Saletu B, Semlitsch H, Anderer P, Resch F, Presslich O, Schuster P. Psychophysiological research in psychiatry and neuropsychopharmacology. II. The investigation of antihypoxidotic/nootropic drugs (tenilsetam and co-dergocrine-mesylate) in elderlies with the Viennese Psychophysiological Test-System) (VPTS). *Methods Find Exp Clin Pharmacol* 1989;11: 43–55.
67. Ruchkin DS, Johnson RJ, Canoune HL, Ritter W, Hammer M. Multiple sources of P3b associated with different types of information. *Psychophysiology* 1990;27:157–76.
68. McCarthy G, Wood CC. Intracranial recordings of endogenous ERPs in humans. *Electroencephalogr Clin Neurophysiol* 1987;39:331–7.
69. Semlitsch HV, Anderer P, Saletu B, Hochmayer I. Topographic mapping of cognitive event-related potentials in a double-blind placebo-controlled study with the hemoderivative actovegin in age-associated memory impairment. *Neuropsychobiology* 1991;24:49–56.
70. Saletu B, Grünberger J, Linzmayer L, Anderer P. EEG brain mapping and psychometry in age associated memory impairment after acute and two weeks infusions with the hemoderivative Actovegin: double-blind, placebo-controlled trials. *Neuropsychobiology* 1990–91; 24:135–48.
71. Semlitsch HV, Anderer P, Saletu B. Topographic mapping of long latency 'cognitive' event-related potentials (P300): a double-blind, placebo-controlled study with amantadine in mild dementia. *J Neural Transm Park Dis Dement Sect* 1992;4:319–36.

Guidelines for Drug Trials in Memory Disorders, edited by N. Canal, et al.
Raven Press, Ltd., New York © 1993.

32

Noncognitive Symptoms in Dementia

Peter J. Whitehouse

Alzheimer Center, University Hospitals of Cleveland, Cleveland, Ohio 44106

The noncognitive symptoms present in many dementias represent a vital opportunity to understanding the biologic basis of such psychiatric symptoms and to develop therapies that could have major impact on improving the quality of life for patients with dementia and their families. The primary scientific focus in dementia has been on the cognitive symptoms such as memory, language, praxis, and perception, and on their biologic substrate(s). For example, in Alzheimer disease (AD) and several other dementias, dysfunction in cholinergic basal forebrain neurons correlates with the severity of cognitive impairment and has led to the development of major programs around the world to develop drugs that enhance activity in the system.

The so-called noncognitive symptoms are more difficult to characterize. Whether it is best to refer to these symptoms as a psychological, psychiatric, or behavioral phenomenon is unclear. Frequently they are defined by the word "noncognitive" to include all clinical manifestations other than the disturbance in intellectual activities. Some of these behavioral symptoms can be labeled with terms that have been well defined in traditional psychiatric literature, including anxiety, depression, psychosis, hallucinations, and delusions. Others, such as screaming, wandering, and agitation, are less well defined and are not included in formal psychiatric nosologies.

This chapter reviews the impact of these symptoms on lay and professional caregivers, considers the possible biologic substrate(s) for these symptoms, and reviews what is known about their clinical characteristics. Finally, it will review the biologic treatment of these conditions, followed by consideration of the need for integrated behavior management. A consistent theme will be that the importance of these symptoms is out of proportion to the attention they have received from the scientific community. For the most part, this chapter will focus on AD, the most common cause of dementia in most countries. Behavioral symptoms are even more common in other dementias, which will be mentioned briefly. Data from our NIMH- and NIA-supported Alzheimer Center in Cleveland will be emphasized.

IMPACT OF NONCOGNITIVE SYMPTOMS

Although the cognitive symptoms in AD are considered the so-called core symptoms, it is the noncognitive symptoms that wreak havoc with family and professional caregivers in a variety of settings. Early changes in personality and depression are common causes of stress in patients and families, and these may occur before frank cognitive impairment allows a diagnosis of dementia. Later in the illness psychotic manifestations, including hallucinations and delusions, may be more common and more disabling.

A number of studies (1,2) have convincingly documented that the psychopathology is a major source of caregiver stress and a frequent reason for institutionalization. Caregivers report considerable stress due to these behavioral symptoms at home. Deimling and Bass (3) measured different aspects of older persons' abilities, including social skills, performance of activities of daily living, cognition, and disruptive behaviors. In a statistical path analysis, the behavior disturbances were the major determinant of caregiver stress. Moreover, in day-care programs and in nursing homes these behavior problems often lead to exclusion of patients from participation in programs and result in transition to the next level of care (e.g., from day care to nursing home).

BIOLOGY

A vast literature exists in biologic psychiatry and neuropsychiatry concerning the search for the biologic basis of affective and psychotic disorders (4). Many different theories relate psychiatric symptoms to the cerebral hemispheres, the limbic system, the basal ganglia, the diencephalon, and to brainstem function. Clearly, a major clue to the biologic substrate of some of these behaviors and states lies in understanding the mechanism of actions of drugs that have proven to be effective in treating these conditions. For example, antidepressants are believed to act by altering bioaminergic mechanisms. Moreover, psychosis can be produced by drugs that interact with noradrenergic and serotoninergic systems, such as amphetamine and LSD. Attempts to find biologic markers for psychiatric diseases in autopsy studies and in in vivo studies, such as positron emission tomography (PET) scanning, have been only partially successful, although progress is being made. In many degenerative diseases, frank pathology, including neuron loss, occurs in some of these systems and is thought to underlie psychiatric symptoms. For example, in AD the loss of neurons in the locus coeruleus and the raphe nuclei has been related to the presence of affective symptoms (5–7). Although these studies should be considered preliminary because they are based on a small number of cases in which many variables were measured, they are intriguing and are consistent with the neuropsychiatric literature suggesting that dysfunction in these brain regions may cause psychiatric symptoms. Other brain areas are affected in AD, and these may also be biologic substrates for some of these psychiatric symptoms. They include the hippocampus, amygdala, hypothalamus, and basal ganglia. Psychiatric symptoms are also common in other neurodegenerative diseases, some of which may mimic AD. Huntington's disease is frequently associated with manic depressive illness and, more rarely, with schizophrenia. Changes in personality may precede frank dementia and chorea by many years. Pick's disease and progressive subcortical gliosis are additional examples of disorders that can mimic AD. However, Pick's disease can often be differentiated from AD because of the early psychiatric manifestations, including disinhibition, which are characteristic of the predominantly frontal lobe pathology.

CLINICAL PHENOMENOLOGY

Premorbid clinical factors may contribute to the clinical course in AD and related disorders. We have reported (8,9) that there is some evidence that exaggerations in premorbid personality occur in AD. For example, patients who were suspicious for most of their lives tend to become more paranoid when they become demented. Most AD patients show characteristic changes in personality when the disease progresses, including, for example, increased passivity. Retrospective studies of the effect of premorbid personality on the disease are difficult. Further studies will be required to understand the complex interactions between the premorbid personality and the psychopathology that develops when the illness occurs.

In the literature, studies report wide ranges in the frequency of psychiatric symptoms (1,10–12). This variability is probably due to differences in referral populations associated with the different centers that report their results and with different methods of assessment. Psychiatric clinics, for example, probably have a higher percentage of patients who show severe psychopathology. Moreover, unlike the tests for assessment of cognitive symptoms in AD, instruments to quantitate the noncognitive symptoms are less well developed. Attempts have been made to use instruments that have been standardized in nondemented populations, such as the Brief Psychiatric Rating Scale (BPRS), and to develop new instruments such as the Behave-AD (13), and the Cornell Scale for Depression in Dementia (11) to assess the presence of these symptoms in dementia. These latter instruments are likely to be more helpful than instruments developed for use in cognitively intact patients, in part because of the overlap in symptoms that may occur between dementia and these other psychiatric conditions. For example, the problems of differentiating the symptoms of depression, such as apathy and cognitive retardation, from dementia are well known. Tests such as the BPRS may be useful, but the clinician must be aware of the potential dangers in using these in a population for which the test was not designed. Recently, we have shown (Ownby, et al., unpublished observations) that the factor structure of the BPRS in dementia overlaps with that found in normal elderly subjects, although a completely new factor emerged, probably related in part to the cognitive difficulties.

Because of the difficulties in using currently available instruments, efforts to develop an instrument that will be more widely accepted for the assessment of noncognitive symptoms are being made. One major effort is being coordinated through the Consortium to Establish a Registry for Alzheimer's Disease (CERAD). Several hundred patients have been tested with an item pool that represents the collaborative efforts of major workers who have agreed to work to combine the best of different scales in the field (Tariot, Patterson, and Mack, unpublished observations). We have also been using this item pool in collaboration with CERAD to assess differences between Japan and the United States in the assessment and frequency of these symptoms (Whitehouse and Homma, unpublished observations).

One problem with using these newly developed screening instruments is one of validation. We (Strauss, Kennedy, Friedman, and Whitehouse, unpublished observations) have developed a semistructured psychiatric interview with adequate reliability which can be used to validate these instruments. By use of our semistructured interview, the DSM-III-R diagnoses can be made, in addition to assessments of behavioral symptoms. By comparing the results of our assessment instrument, which can be administered by a variety of clinicians, to this more intensive formal psychiatric evaluation, we can better understand the strengths and weaknesses of our screening approaches.

Although general-purpose screening instruments are useful for assessing the effects of interventions and for study of the natural history of the disease, more focused assessments of specific behaviors are likely to be important for interventional studies as well. For example, a scale such as the Cornell Scale for Depression in Dementia would be more appropriate than a general screening instrument to measure the effects of antidepressants (11). Moreover, Cohen–Mansfield and Billig (14) have developed a specific instrument that may be better for quantifying agitation. Direct observation of behavior may also be important. For example, monitoring devices, either worn by the patient or located in the environment, can be used to measure the amount of wandering in individual patients.

In summary, our understanding of the natural history of the behavioral symptoms in AD and related disorders, as well as the relationships among these behaviors, cognitive symptoms, and caregiver stress, will depend on the development of more reliable and valid assessment tools. In addition, these tools can be used to assess interventions, to be discussed below.

MANAGEMENT OF NONCOGNITIVE SYMPTOMS

In the practical world of the care of patients with dementia, clinicians spend an inordinate amount of time using both biologic and behavioral interventions to manage the noncognitive symptoms. Unfortunately, much of this is done without the guidance of empirical studies. The usual approach is to start with behavioral interventions rather than drugs and then, when necessary, to add drugs at the lowest possible dosage and to change the dosage slowly, while carefully monitoring well-defined target behaviors for positive action as well as for harmful side effects.

When a noncognitive symptom is to be analyzed, defining the target behavior as precisely as possible is essential. Caregivers' descriptions should not be accepted at face value, as they will use terms such as "depression" or "agitation" differently. It is best to elicit an actual physical description of the behaviors that stress the caregiver. Once the target behavior is defined, it is important to have an accurate assessment of its frequency. Use of a diary by the caregiver often helps in this process. The diary will also contribute to assessment of factors that appear to precipitate or prevent the behavioral symptom. Changes in routine frequently contribute to the appearance of noncognitive symptoms. During this evaluation process, it is important to try, as much as possible, to put oneself in the place of a cognitively impaired patient and to interpret the environment as the patient might perceive it.

Well-defined target symptoms may respond to behavior modification approaches. A variety of behavior therapy techniques can be used in which social or other reinforcements are appropriately linked to behavioral change. In patients with mild dementia, various forms of psychotherapy may assist the patient's response to anxiety in ways that are more adaptive than agitation or verbal aggression. Confrontation of the patient usually is not helpful, whereas redirection of the patient away from the situation that creates the behavioral problem may work effectively. Family therapy can be helpful in aiding family members to interpret and respond to the noncognitive symptoms in more constructive ways.

Certain other interventions, such as art therapy, music therapy, and recreation therapy, although not directly targeted at the behavioral symptoms may, in fact, contribute to their prevention. Wandering, for example, can be managed in part by presenting other opportunities for activity through recreation and exercise programs.

In institutional long-term care, new attention is being given to behavioral symptoms and management. Physical restraints are being recognized as potential causes rather than treatments of behavior disturbances, and major efforts are under way to reevaluate the use of these devices. The use of psychoactive medications to control behavioral symptoms is being examined carefully. The words "chemical straitjacket" raise the specter of concern for medication misuse. Nevertheless, the appropriate use of psychoactive medications may be very helpful in improving the quality of life for both the patient and the staff.

Empirical studies of drugs to improve noncognitive symptoms are rare in nursing homes or, in fact, in any setting. Some clinicians use major tranquilizers, others minor tranquilizers. New-generation antidepressants, such as serotoninergic uptake blockers, may have broad positive effects on behavior. More systematic studies of other classes of drugs (e.g., β-blockers and anticonvulsants) are also needed. Over the long term, therapies are required that can provide more than merely relief of symptoms. For example, growth factors may enhance neuron viability and slow progression of disease. Much attention has focused on the positive effects of nerve growth factor and related members of the same family on cholinergic basal forebrain neurons. However, other factors may enhance neuronal viability in other brain regions. Recently, for example, members of our group (15) demonstrated that fibroblast growth factor may be trophic to the locus coeruleus.

CONCLUSION

In summary, the noncognitive symptoms of dementia are common and represent a major cause of stress on the health-care system. Whether these symptoms are core symptoms of dementia or not is an interesting conceptual question that may be moot from the point of view of the practitioner, to whom it is clear that these symptoms have not received adequate attention from researchers. This lack of attention is particularly surprising because these diseases offer an opportunity to understand fundamental aspects of the biologic bases of emotions.

REFERENCES

1. Ryden MB. Aggressive behavior in persons with dementia who live in the community. *Alzheimer Dis Assoc Disord* 1988;2:342–55.
2. Kumar A, Koss E, Metzler D, Moore A, Friedland RP. Behavioral symptomatology in dementia of the Alzheimer type. *Alzheimer Dis Assoc Disord* 1988;2:363–5.
3. Deimling GT, Bass DM. Symptoms of mental impairment among elderly adults and their effects on family caregivers. *J Gerontol* 1986;41:778–84.
4. Meltzer HY, ed. *Psychopharmacology: the third generation of progress.* New York: Raven Press; 1987.
5. Zweig RM, Ross CA, Hedreen JC, et al. The neuropathology of aminergic nuclei in Alzheimer's disease. *Ann Neurol* 1988;24:233–42.
6. Zubenko GS, Moossy J, Kopp U. Neurochemical correlates of major depression in primary dementia. *Arch Neurol* 1990;47:209–14.
7. Zubenko GS, Moossy J, Martinez AJ, et al. Neuropathologic and neurochemical correlates of psychosis in primary dementia. *Arch Neurol* 1991;48:619–24.
8. Petry S, Cummings JL, Hill MA, Shapira RN. Personality alterations in dementia of the Alzheimer type. *Arch Neurol* 1988;45:1187–90.

9. Chatterjee A, Strauss M, Smyth K, Whitehouse PJ. Personality changes in Alzheimer's Disease. *Arch Neurol* 1992;49:486–91.
10. Rubin EH, Kinscherf DA. Psychopathology of very mild dementia of the Alzheimer type. *Am J Psychiatry* 1989;146:1017–21.
11. Alexopoulos GS, Abrams RC, Young RC, Shamoian CA, Berrios GD, Brook P. Delusions and psychopathology of the elderly with dementia. *Acta Psychiatry Scand* 1985;72:296–301.
12. Mendez MF, Martin RJ, Smyth KA, Whitehouse PJ. Psychiatric symptoms associated with Alzheimer's disease. *J Neuropsychiatry* 1990;2:28–33.
13. Reisberg B, Borenstein J, Salob SP, et al. Behavioral symptoms in Alzheimer's disease: phenomenology and treatment. *J Clin Psychiatry* 1987;48(suppl):9–15.
14. Cohen–Mansfield J, Billig N. Agitated behaviors in the elderly. *J Am Geriatr Soc* 1986;34: 711–21.
15. Wilcox BJ, Unnerstall JR. Identification of a subpopulation of neuropeptide Y-containing locus coeruleus neurons that project to the entorhinal cortex. *Synapse* 1990;6:284–91.

Guidelines for Drug Trials in Memory
Disorders, edited by N. Canal, et al.
Raven Press, Ltd., New York © 1993.

33

Discussion

Dr. Thal: Dr. Sano, you said that the groups you examined started out at the same degree of dementia. However, according to your Mini-Mental scores for the three groups, it looked like there was almost a twofold difference in the starting scores of psychotic patients without, as opposed to those with, extrapyramidal signs.

Dr. Sano: That's correct. There's also a difference in the duration of illness. When the Mini-Mental scores are used across duration of illness, and then you change the level—shifting it, choosing people selectively who had the same duration and who are similar otherwise (the same age of onset, for example)—then the Mini-Mental score is equivalent. But because we're looking at retrospective data, the difference at the time of initial visit was different.

Dr. Thal: What happens when you match the patients for severity of disease? What if you take a group of patients with and without extrapyramidal features and match them so that they all have the same average Mini-Mental score, and then do a survival analysis?

Dr. Sano: We match patients on duration of illness, and we find that the survival analysis demonstrates that myoclonus predicts death quite significantly.

Dr. Thal: I don't think that's the right match.

Dr. Sano: If we match then on Mini-Mental scores, would it be to predict death or to predict functional outcome?

Dr. Thal: Functional outcome.

Dr. Sano: If we match them on Mini-Mental for extrapyramidal signs we can more predict more rapid functional decline. We haven't been able to do that with myoclonus because we don't have a large enough cohort.

Dr. B. Reisberg: What do you mean by extrapyramidal symptoms? Do you mean rigidity?

Dr. Sano: We definitely mean rigidity; and we actually find that it occurs a bit earlier than generally reported. We agree that you see it at a very high incidence in people who are in stage 7 or in very late stages, but it starts to occur much earlier. The problem is that you don't readily see rigidity, and unless you specifically examine the patient with this in mind, it may go unnoticed. Just as in psychosis, it's primarily delusions that we're talking about.

Dr. Reisberg: We reported that 50% of Alzheimer patients at stage 6 manifested paratonic rigidity to a moderate to severe degree, but you can sometimes pick it up earlier.

Dr. Roth: Did the personality factor predict anything with respect to functional outcome or death?

Dr. Sano: Actually, we haven't examined it as a predictor. What we did find is that it didn't systematically decrease. In this case the scores go up over time.

Dr. Korczyn: Did I understand you correctly, that myoclonus was as frequent as rigidity in these patients?

Dr. Sano: If you look at the number of years' duration (those people who reach a certain level of duration), what you find is that myoclonus occurs as frequently as extrapyramidal signs and psychosis. Myoclonus occurs later but as frequently. The dilemma is that it also seems to occur in younger patients, equal duration but younger patients, which suggests that perhaps there is another domain here.

Dr. Korczyn: Therefore, these are cumulative curves? What was the frequency that it reached?

Dr. Sano: Yes, these are cumulative curves. I believe the frequency in the 10-year period was 75%. Obviously, you don't have as big a cohort out of the 10-year period.

Dr. Korczyn: Was the existence of rigidity a predictor for myoclonus?

Dr. Sano: The details of separating out extrapyramidal signs in myoclonus in predicting death, is that most of those patients who have extrapramidal signs eventually develop myoclonus. Therefore, independently, extrapyramidal signs—if a person survives to myoclonus—do not predict death. If a person doesn't survive that long, then the extrapyramidal signs predict death at a statistically significant level. Clearly, they are an earlier milestone and they do seem to be associated with later development of myoclonus.

Dr. Korczyn: Do you know about how many of those patients with or without rigidity or myoclonus have diffuse Lewy body disease?

Dr. Sano: In our experience, those patients did not have Lewy body disease. In this particular cohort, those who have come to autopsy, Lewy body disease was not a complicating factor.

Dr. Korczyn: With ubiquitin stains?

Dr. Sano: Absolutely.

Dr. Salazar: Are you suggesting that the patients who have rigidity or delusions should be separated or should be stratified in drug trials?

Dr. Sano: On the contrary, I have two suggestions: One is that rigidity and myoclonus can be used as outcome measures because they would predict a decline that we don't have time to look for in a trial. Second, the high frequency of both rigidity and myoclonus suggests that they are, in fact, showing us milestones rather than subclasses. Our initial idea was that they identify subgroups, but the later inception studies make us believe that perhaps they exist for all patients.

Dr. Salazar: Dr. Lawlor, I was intrigued by your discussion of the problem of carryover effects. In looking at our own heterogeneous data, perhaps indicating a therapeutic opportunity is not as much of a problem as it might be. In the studies of Feeney et al., after cortical ablation experiments in rats, he was able to demonstrate a beneficial synergistic effect of amphetamines plus physical therapy. Amphetamines by themselves or the physical therapy task by itself did not produce that benefit. What you seem to be showing is that giving drugs to animals or to people and then administering a test, which in essence is a training session, appears to improve performance. Perhaps we could use that type of strategy to improve the results in clinical trials—combining specific training with drugs.

Dr. Lawlor: This is a very interesting idea. However, the thrust of my article was to highlight the problems caused by carryover and practice effects on the results of clinical trials in Alzheimer disease.

Dr. Thal: I've looked at the same data and have come to some slightly different conclusions. First, I think the issue about heterogeneity is quite interesting and very relevant, and it may help to explain some of the differences in response to drugs. The problem is, how do we identify the so-called subgroups? If patients have different biochemical lesions, we do not have the means of clinically identifying them. Another issue is that although it is interesting to model this after animals, when you have an nbM lesion or an nbM plus a dorsonoradrenergic bundle lesion, you have disturbed neurotransmitters, but how many neurotransmitters are disturbed in the Alzheimer brain? As the neurochemical evidence has evolved, it's clear that there are at least six neurotransmitters that are probably involved in most Alzheimer brains. Therefore, the issue becomes much more complex and we don't have ways of identifying the patients.

My second point deals with rates of forgetting. There is extremely compelling evidence that has recently been published indicating that patients with Alzheimer disease have dramatically more rapid rates of forgetting than patients without Alzheimer disease. In looking over the literature very carefully, it seems that the only area in which Alzheimer patients do not have rapid rates of forgetting is for a picture recognition task. But if you look at any other paradigm, any other type of memory task, these individuals do have rapid rates of forgetting and, indeed, that is probably one of the hallmarks of the disease.

The third point deals with the issue of carryover effects. You brought up some very good points, one of which is that animals and humans, when they have learned certain information, will never forget it. This is a permanent carryover in a sense. This may be relevant to drug trials, as we are looking for very small differences using cholinesterase inhibitors and these permanent carryover effects may make it difficult to identify such effects.

Dr. Lawlor: This issue of identifying subgroups of responders to cholinomimetic therapy is important. In vivo imaging with SPECT, direct imaging of cholinergic and other receptors with PET, or the short-term cognitive effect of a test dose of a rapidly acting cholinesterase inhibitor might allow us to predict who is likely to show positive effects following cholinesterase inhibitor therapy.

Dr. Gottfries: We investigated both CAT activity and that of monoamines in Alzheimer brains and found that there was variation in these different markers that overlapped with control series. In some brains we noticed that there were rather slight disturbances or reduced activity of CAT, although the patient was demented. We found that the dementia was related to the summarized lesions in these brains and not necessarily to the CAT activity. Memory is a complex process and should be related not only to the disturbance in the CAT activity or the cholinergic system, but possibly to the summarized lesions of these transmitters.

Dr. Lawlor: I agree with you. Although I focused primarily on memory and the cholinergic system, it would be important to try to understand the clinical correlates of the other neurotransmitter deficits in Alzheimer disease. For example, it would be interesting to examine serotoninergic and noradrenergic dysfunction in relation to behavioral abnormalities as well as cognitive abnormalities. I believe that a number of groups are actually addressing these issues now.

Dr. Roth: It's true that there aren't any clear clinical correlates of type 1 and type 2, and we did not anticipate these neurochemical changes you described in the original studies. We need to return to the original cases to separate them on the basis of all the data we have neurobiologically. Familial cases in our experience, whether old or young, tend to be extensively lesioned with respect to neurochemical abnormalities. Also, I'm surprised that the GABA lesion received so little attention. GABA mediates far more synapses than any other neurotransmitter and I don't know what the GABAergic lesion means, but it should to be receiving more attention.

Dr. Lawlor: I believe there are a number of laboratories beginning to investigate GABA and glutamate, and it's a question of having the pharmacological probes to look at those neurotransmitter systems.

Dr. Lader: I'm a little disconcerted by some of your designs, which were notable for their symmetry. If you got these carryover effects in an asymmetrical design, is it not a danger that you might be magnifying or diminishing real placebo–drug differences according to which elements of the design you incorporate?

Dr. Lawlor: The point I was making is that it will be difficult to show drug–placebo differences with these types of study design.

Dr. Lader: Essentially, what you are doing initially is a sophisticated, flexible dose approach. You actually have three doses of the placebo. We have a very similar situation when we are dealing with all sorts of conditions where the usual procedure is either to do very large, very expensive, fixed-dose multi-arm studies of placebo at three doses, or a flexible dose study with unsatisfactory criteria for manipulating the dose. What we've got here is a rather curious case where you're going in and you're putting people onto these doses in succession, but not in a flexible, increasing dose. Also, the design is not fully balanced, so you don't get people starting on a highest dose. I would question whether there is a danger of actually biasing the results, one way or the other, depending on which of those dosage patterns you choose initially.

Dr. Lawlor: Just to clarify, those were two dose-finding paradigms. In one, there was a random allocation of different doses and placebo, but in the Canadian study there was a fixed-dose escalation during dose finding.

Dr. Whitehouse: Dr. Baron, you mentioned cognitive activation, a new technique using MRI to measure volume and blood flow. This new technique offers the promise of measuring functional aspects of brain activity with much higher resolution. Do you envision that we're going to be able to use MRI and in some sense obtain the same kinds of results with a higher resolution?

Dr. Baron: Yes, I think that if PET studies had not existed before, and before PET if xenon studies had not existed, they would not be conducting those studies with MRI. I believe it's just the natural evolution of techniques. However, what's important is not the technique, it's the ideas that provide the foundation for the technique. If you have a technique that is sensitive to cognitive activation, which I think has not been shown so far, and which is less invasive, it should be used. It's important to understand that for these activation studies using PET you don't necessarily need to do arterial puncture. You can do imaging alone, so the only invasive part that remains is the dose of radiation.

Dr. T. Erkinjuntti: Dr. Saletu, using the McKhann criteria for probable Alzheimer disease, you said that in about 20 to 30% of the cases you did not see the reduction of occipital α-frequency during disease progression. What could this mean? Also, if the accuracy of the antemortem diagnosis using these criteria is nearly 90% and if the power of the occipital EEG for differentiation is 66%, how can you use it in clinical everyday practice?

Dr. Saletu: Concerning the α-activity, there was little difference as compared with normal aging people. In both studies the difference was actually the δ/θ range. With regard to differential diagnosis, I didn't say that we could demonstrate 90% classification, although I must say it retrospectively now, if I look at the data utilizing a set score as compared with normal controls. I remember that almost all patients showed this increase of slow activity. That was the outcome and I don't know whether we can improve on that or not. I believe that data opposite to that was given during the meeting. We had, for instance, tremendous problems when we correlated CT data to the Hachinski score; there was not good agreement between radiologic and clinical diagnosis.

Dr. Gottfries: Dr. Whitehouse, in brains of patients with Alzheimer disease, there is a decrease of the amount of neurons in the locus coeruleus, but in one investigation we made a couple of years ago, we found that the metabolite HMPG was significantly increased. Although that finding has been confirmed by one group, I believe additional confirmation is needed from more groups. The only way we could interpret that finding was that there was an increased speed in turnover in the locus coeruleus in brains of patients with Alzheimer-type dementia. Have you done any studies of the metabolite HMPG in your investigation and have you any comments on the high activity of this system?

Dr. Whitehouse: No, we've never measured the metabolite HMPG. We've measured norepinephrine levels, and in some cases it's down and in others it's not. I would interpret your result as you did, that the remaining neurons are turning over faster and that is why you have more metabolites.

Dr. Gottfries: I don't believe that they compensate the loss, because at least our increase was up to 200%. You should assume an increase to the same level as the normal, but a high activity was indicating, for example, a running of this nucleus to a higher speed than usual.

Dr. Whitehouse: Another explanation could be that there may be changes in noradrenergic regulation of blood vessels in Alzheimer disease. We found increases in β-receptors in blood vessels, so possibly some of the sources are coming from there. Also, according to Crutcher's work and others, when you lesion the cholinergic base of the forebrain, you got sympathetic ingrowth. Therefore, there may be a sprouting of sympathetic fibers, either in blood vessels or from other noradrenergic sources. Perhaps that is more comparable with your large increase.

Dr. Hachinski: Dr. Whitehouse, please provide more details on the innervation that arises from the locus coeruleus that has to do with the blood–brain barrier and the blood vessels. How would this affect the blood–brain barrier and the regulation of the caliber of the vessels?

Dr. Whitehouse: We have been taking cerebral cortex and isolating microvessels, so it's a purely chemical approach, and we demonstrated that there are neurochemical alterations in the blood vessels. There are reductions in the glucose transporter and there are increases in β-receptors, just as there are in the cortical specimens that represent neuronal tissue after the microvessels have been removed. The consequences of these neurochemical changes for alterations in the blood–brain barrier are not so clear. Obviously, the enervation of the blood vessels would affect caliber, but the full range of effects is another matter.

Dr. T. Crook: With regard to noradrenergic involvement, we looked at the α_2-agonist guanfacine in both Alzheimer disease and AAMI patients. We were looking at mildly impaired, relatively young Alzheimer disease patients. In AAMI we found nothing. In Alzheimer disease the finding was interesting; family members reported that patients were improved, particularly with regard to agitation, but also improved with regard to memory and other cognitive symptoms. Because we believed that we had a real drug effect, we kept the patients on the drug for about a year after the double-blind phase of the study. We found that, in fact, family members were distinguishing the drug from placebo. However, on psychometric testing the drug-treated patients were substantially worse, particularly with regard to reaction time. Therefore, whether we were simply sedating the patients so that the pathology was less apparent, or whether we were doing something more profound neurochemically, is open to question.

Dr. Whitehouse: Professor Goldman has been studying clonidine in animal models, and John Growdon and others have tried clonidine in humans, and I don't believe that anybody has convincingly demonstrated a positive cognitive effect. Clearly, drugs that act on adrenergic mechanisms, like stimulants, can be powerful in their effect on behavioral tests.

Dr. Crook: I think that in this session we have seen that some real advances have been made with regard to measurements for assessing clinical efficacy and also some clear needs pointed out for other measurements. Some of the most interesting findings may relate not so much to establishing efficacy, which ultimately, of course, is a matter of clinical measurements, but to the electrophysiologic measurements and the neuradiologic measurements. I believe that these are now proving very useful in terms of identifying drugs that operate at sites of interest and identifying appropriate dosage levels, and will provide the basis for a trial.

Guidelines for Drug Trials in Memory Disorders, edited by N. Canal, et al. Raven Press, Ltd., New York © 1993.

34

Concluding Remarks

Robert J. Joynt

Department of Neurology, University of Rochester, Rochester, New York 14642

The goal of the conference was guidelines for development and evaluation of clinical trials and disorders in memory. We looked first at the ethical problems involved in using patients—largely incompetent—and obtaining the proper approval to proceed with some of the trials that are so necessary. We have to use the affected population as good therapies are not available. Dr. McKhann identified several major problems: the diagnostic groups, the heterogeneous population, the identification, getting meaningful end points, drug selection, duration of trials, the types of trials, and the assessment. These diagnostic groups and the problems with Alzheimer disease have been emphasized here. In addition to the clinical heterogeneity that we know about—some more right hemisphere, some more left hemisphere, some with extrapyramidal signs, some with none—now there has come to light a genetic heterogeneity—problems with chromosomes 21 and 19, problems with probably neither 19 or 21, and some mutations in a few cases. So there are great problems from the standpoint of identifying these. Are we dealing with one disease? Are we dealing with several? As Dr. Drachman pointed out, could Lewy body disease merely be clumped up ubiquitin, or is it a separate disease?

With regard to vascular disease, Dr. Hachinski emphasized that vascular dementia is not an entity unto itself, but when you're talking about degenerative dementia you have to be careful to look at the mechanism for pointing out that vascular dementia can coexist with, contribute to, or cause dementia. The approach should be undertaken early on the brain at risk, the predemented stage and the demented stage, and the issue of the white matter changes. However, there is a great deal of controversy about this. Head injury is considered an excellent model to look at as there are a variety of pathologies in this type of injury and various opportunities for treatment.

How to handle the heterogeneous populations is obviously a difficult problem. We have to select the best groups, but how this can be done is not clear. We may have to use the best selection criteria and separate as we go along. With regard to identification and mid points or end points, there are many of these that can be followed. One of the problems, of course, is with early diagnosis. For instance, with regard to norms, what is normal behavior? It is very difficult to identify what is normal at the age of 85 years: Should we look mainly at cognitive functions, or should we look at functional scales? Quality of life both for the patients and the caregivers is important.

With regard to drug selection, again, there are a number of different modes: intervention, substitution, facilitation, or serendipity. The approaches are several. And many of you talked about the different neuropharmacological problems were addressed, noting that most of the research is on neurotransmitter systems. What was not fully addressed was the neurotropic factors or how to manipulate the APP gene, which may in fact turn out to be one of the more important ways to attack this particular disease.

Many important topics with regard to duration and type of trials were addressed: time to reach the end point and what the end points are that you want to reach along the way, what the stratification is and whether you should start by stratifying by severity in doing the actual assessment, how long the tests are clinically relevant to the problem, and the problem of learning with repeated trials. In addition to the cognitive functions, we learned a great deal about some of the functional tests that might be used, i.e., PET scanning and brain mapping, that are important not only in diagnosis but also in assessing treatment trials.

Vascular dementia and Alzheimer disease remain difficult problems for therapeutic intervention, vascular dementia because of the difficulty with diagnosis and Alzheimer disease because of the uncertainty of the mechanism or the various mechanisms that may be present. Therapies need to be based on understanding basic mechanisms. Take, for instance Parkinson's disease: we had a clue and went ahead. However, we can't stand by and wait for all the explanations for these memory disorders before we try out possible therapies. Drug selection is a limiting factor. Pharmaceutical strategies should not be discouraged by the complexity of the problem. I think we can be assured that they will not. Finally, single therapeutic strategies, such as the idea of a central cholinergic deficit, may not work; consider the cancer model and our Parkinson disease model as we move forward.

In conclusion, I thank Professor Canal and his staff for this wonderful and informative conference.

Subject Index